Think Like a Dietitian

While courses in nutrition counseling teach providers to listen to their patients, this book gives registered dietitian nutritionists (RDNs) a heads-up on what to listen *for*, with educational materials that address the everyday challenges many people, hence many RDNs, face.

Split into four distinct sections, this book equips readers to provide comprehensive education and counseling for the most common nutrition referrals.

Topics include:

- How to structure a nutrition counseling session, from getting a patient to open up to empowering them with information and strategies for self-care.
- Strategies for the provider to address personal challenges such as cultivating empathy, implicit bias, and cultural competence.
- Routine eating patterns and challenges reported in nutrition counseling, such as night eating, emotional eating, and more.
- Common reasons for referral to a dietitian, and frequently asked questions on topics including diabetes, heart disease, kidney disease, irritable bowel syndrome, and weight counseling.
- Special issues in health education.

This book is appealing to both early nutrition professionals and experienced dietitians alike, providing a holistic toolkit for RDNs of all levels of experience.

Think Like a Dietitian
A Nutrition Counseling Starter Kit

J. Barretto Patterson

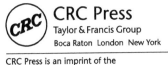

CRC Press
Taylor & Francis Group
Boca Raton London New York

CRC Press is an imprint of the
Taylor & Francis Group, an **informa** business

First edition published 2024
by CRC Press
2385 NW Executive Center Drive, Suite 320, Boca Raton FL 33431

and by CRC Press
4 Park Square, Milton Park, Abingdon, Oxon, OX14 4RN

CRC Press is an imprint of Taylor & Francis Group, LLC

© 2024 J. Barretto Patterson

ISBN: 9781032352466 (hbk)
ISBN: 9781032352459 (pbk)
ISBN: 9781003326038 (ebk)

DOI: 10.1201/9781003326038

Typeset in Times
by codeMantra

Access the Support Material: https://resourcecentre.routledge.com/books/9781032352459

To Elliot, for teaching me how to be a writer.
To Ken and Grant, for putting up with me being one.

Contents

Figures xi
Tables xv
Author xvii
Introduction xix

PART I SHARE

Chapter 1   SHARE — A Step-by-Step Approach to Nutrition Counseling 3

References 5

Chapter 2   Start with a Blank Sheet...6

Learning the Ropes...6
Breaking the Ice...9
What Do Patients *Want* to Know? 11
What Do Patients *Need* to Know? 12
What *You* Need to Know 12

Chapter 3   Hear and Understand..14

The Patient-Dietitian Relationship 15
Cultivating Empathy...17
Communicating Compassion 19
Compassion Starts from Within 20
Beneath the Surface..20
Implicit Bias 21
Limits and Boundaries 25
References 26

Chapter 4   Assess and Review 28

Understand the Science 28
Think Like a Dietitian 30
Speak Like a Person 32
References 34

Chapter 5   Empower the Patient...35

Goal Setting, Problem Solving, and Action Planning 36
References 41

PART II *Everyday Eating Routines: A Different EER*

Chapter 6 Motivations and Barriers...45

References 46

Chapter 7 A Different EER..47

Everybody Eats..47
Everyday Eating Routines: A Different EER 48

Chapter 8 Commonly Reported Eating Patterns 50

Night Snacking...50
Skipping Meals...51
Squeezing Calories and Chasing Hunger 56
Emotional Eating...57
All or Nothing 59
Grazing...59
Frequent Dining Out..60
Habit Cycling 61
A Multifactorial Pattern...63
References 64

PART III *Common Referrals and FAQs*

Chapter 9 Common Referrals 69

References 71

Chapter 10 Type 2 Diabetes and Prediabetes 72

What You Need to Know...74
  Key Assessment Questions for Diabetes Care...............................74
What Patients Want to Know...75
What Patients Need to Know 81
References 92

Chapter 11 Heart Disease Prevention and Management 94

Dyslipidemia 95
  What You Need to Know 95
  What Patients Want to Know..99
  What Patients Need to Know..105
Hypertension 108
  What You Need to Know 109
  What Patients Want to Know?..110
  What Patients Need to Know?..113
References 119

Chapter 12 Chronic Kidney Disease...122

    What You Need to Know 124
        Key Considerations for CKD.....................................124
    What Patients Want to Know...125
    What Patients Need to Know 129
    References 135

Chapter 13 IBS and the Low FODMAP Diet 137

    What You Need to Know 139
        Key Assessment Questions for Irritable Bowel Syndrome.......139
    What Patients Want to Know...142
    What Patients Need to Know 145
    References 149

Chapter 14 Weight Counseling 151

    Beyond Calories 152
        What You Need to Know 154
        What Patients Want to Know.....................................158
    What Patients Need to Know?...167
    References 172

PART IV *Putting It All Together*

Chapter 15 Health Literacy...179

    What Is Health Literacy?..179
    Know Your Audience..180
    Tailor the Education 180
    Consider Learning and Teaching Styles.............................180
    Use Various Teaching Modalities 181
    References 189

Chapter 16 Cultural Competence..192

    What Is Cultural Competence?..192
    References 197

Chapter 17 SHARE Your Screen – and Other Virtual Care Tips 198

    Lessons Learned..199
    Best Practices, Challenges, and Opportunities...................202
    References 206

Chapter 18 Making PLANS and Taking Action..207

Making PLANS..208
Turning PLANS into Action..209
Handouts for FAQs 210
Educational Slides 210
Counseling Handouts..210
Reference..211

Index..213

Figures

Figure 4.1 The best available evidence comes from the patients themselves. In addition to established guidelines, a thorough assessment of a person's medical history, lifestyle, barriers, and preferences will target the intervention.............. 32

Figure 8.1 To break a habit, identify the pattern, determine its purpose, and consider alternative ways to produce the same results. In this example, watching TV is a way of relaxing. However, watching TV is the cue to eat a snack, perpetuating a cycle of habit. To break the cycle, avoid the cue. In this case, reading a book achieves the purpose of relaxing, while the cue to snack is circumvented. 62

Figure 10.1 The diabetes plate method.. 77

Figure 10.2 MyPlate is the official symbol of the five food groups in the *Dietary Guidelines for Americans 2020–2025.* 78

Figure 10.3 The Diabetes Plate can be used when discussing the DASH Diet and the Mediterranean Diet. 79

Figure 10.4 Provide a description of which foods contain carbohydrates as well as their nutritional benefits.. 83

Figure 10.5 Comparing insulin to a key is a common analogy used to explain how insulin works. 84

Figure 10.6 Describing what causes insulin resistance can reinforce the recommendations for what can reverse insulin resistance, i.e., healthy diet, physical activity, and if applicable, weight loss...................................... 86

Figure 10.7 An explanation that type 2 diabetes is typically characterized by low insulin production helps people understand that medications are often required in addition to lifestyle changes. 87

Figure 10.8 Physical activity facilitates glucose transport into the muscle cells. Physical activity can also increase insulin sensitivity up to 24 hours after exercise (ADA n.d.). 88

Figure 10.9 Saturated fat has been shown to worsen insulin resistance. In a typical American diet, excessive intake of saturate fat comes from high fat meat, some processed meats, fast food, some deep-fried foods, and foods heavy with high fat dairy, e.g., pizza. 89

Figure 11.1 Ultra-processed foods have more than five ingredients, many of which are used to enhance texture or flavor, to disguise undesirable qualities, or to add or replace nutrients lost in processing. 96

Figure 11.2 For those with a sweet tooth, a comparison of fat and calories between fruit and their typical treat can demonstrate the benefits of choosing fruit for snacks........98

Figure 11.3 Identify the foods that the patient already enjoys that can fit into a heart healthy diet. 99

Figure 11.4   The 80/20 Rule is a popular concept that dietitians use to discuss healthy eating. This concept recognizes that 100% dietary compliance is impractical and difficult to maintain. On the other hand, flexibility can help prevent feelings of deprivation, thus making changes more sustainable. 100

Figure 11.5   For those motivated to lower LDL-C through diet, the information that fiber lowers cholesterol by blocking it from entering the body may be novel and motivating. 101

Figure 11.6   Demonstrate that all foods can fit into a healthy diet while emphasizing portion control, leaner choices, and balance. 104

Figure 11.7   A frequently asked question is, "What else can I have for breakfast?" Provide alternative protein choices to emphasize variety, maximal nutrition, and moderation. 104

Figure 11.8   A brief explanation of how food that is high in saturated fat affects LDL levels may enhance the patient's understanding—and acceptance—of nutrition recommendations... 106

Figure 11.9   Explain which types of food and drinks can increase triglycerides, and that high triglycerides are also associated with an increased risk for heart disease...107

Figure 11.10   To prevent a food rut, provide ideas and recipes for a variety of vegetable preparations. 111

Figure 11.11   When purchasing simple ingredients and sale items, cooking at home can be more affordable and much healthier than other seemingly "cheap" options...112

Figure 11.12   Provide quick and easy meal ideas that use time-saving tips like batch cooking, pre-prepping ingredients, and staple ingredients................................113

Figure 11.13   Relate blood pressure levels to the risk for complications............................... 114

Figure 11.14   Explain that the nutrients that are abundant in a DASH diet help to dilate blood vessels, reduce water retention, remove extra sodium through the kidneys, and overall protect the heart.. 117

Figure 12.1   Recent guidelines recognize that diets high in plant foods such as the Mediterranean Diet, DASH Diet, and plant-based diets are protective of the kidneys. 123

Figure 12.2   Due to differences in bioavailability, dietary counseling should focus more on food choices and portions rather than foods "high" in potassium or phosphorus... 129

Figure 12.3   Diabetes and hypertension are the leading causes of kidney damage and disease... 130

Figure 12.4   High potassium levels can be a result of inadequate insulin related to diabetes. Thus, correcting insulin doses or other diabetes medications can help manage potassium...131

Figure 12.5 Kidney disease, diabetes, and heart disease are closely related, which is why nutrition guidelines are more similar than different. 132

Figure 12.6 Due to inaccurate A1C values, some people with kidney disease believe their diabetes improved. Continued monitoring through fingersticks is important to prevent further damage from uncontrolled diabetes. 133

Figure 13.1 Use plain language and simple imagery to explain how FODMAPs cause symptoms. 142

Figure 13.2 Provide several meal and snack ideas showing how to enjoy a variety of foods. 144

Figure 13.3 Provide the patient with a description of each phase and an estimated timeline. 145

Figure 13.4 Each FODMAP challenge will last one to three days. Allow a two- to three-day washout period between each challenge. 146

Figure 14.1 An explanation about how different types of food affect blood sugar, insulin, and hunger reinforces the importance of balanced nutrition. 159

Figure 14.2 A brief explanation about the existence of hunger hormones helps explain why balanced meal planning helps prevent hunger and cravings. 160

Figure 14.3 A brief explanation about hunger hormones can help explain why skipping meals and/or unbalanced meals can lead to increased hunger at night. Learning about the existence of hunger hormones may help lessen the guilt about perceived "willpower." 161

Figure 14.4 Explain the benefits of balanced meal planning beyond calories. 162

Figure 14.5 Explaining that physical activity is not limited to formal exercise may help physical activity feel more attainable. 166

Figure 15.1 Health communications should engage the reader with eye-catching visuals, messages that resonate, and information that is easy to understand and actionable. 187

Figure 15.2 Define and frame measures of success. In the above weight tracking grid, the plotted points illustrate that incremental changes, occasional increases, and some plateaus can still be on track. 189

Tables

Table 3.1 Examples of Assumptions and Consequences in Nutrition Counseling 22

Table 4.1 Examples of Nutrition Guidelines for Various Conditions and Nutrition Diagnoses 31

Table 4.2 Examples of Targeted Education or Intervention 31

Table 8.1 Examples of Impact of Night Eating on Certain Conditions 51

Table 8.2 Possible Factors for Hunger and Cravings at Night 52

Table 8.3 SCOFF Questionnaire (Kutz et al. 2019; Morgan et al. 2000) 58

Table 9.1 Percentage of Physicians Who Refer to Dietitians for the Following Reasons (Sastre and Van Horn 2021) 70

Table 10.1 Risk Factors for Hyperglycemia or Hypoglycemia 76

Table 10.2 Common Diabetes Medications with Nutrition-Related Side Effects 85

Table 11.1 Sample Day with Heart Healthy Choices, Minimally Processed Foods, and Home-Prepared Meals 102

Table 11.2 Sample Day with Ultra-Processed and Restaurant Foods 103

Table 11.3 Blood Pressure Categories (Whelton et al. 2018) 115

Table 11.4 Relative Contributions of Dietary Sodium Sources (Mattes and Donnelly 1991) 116

Table 11.5 The Best Proven Diet and Lifestyle Interventions for Treating Hypertension (Whelton et al. 2018) 117

Table 12.1 Stages of Kidney Disease, eGFR, and Kidney Function (NKF 2022) 124

Table 12.2 Possible Causes for High Potassium or Phosphorus Levels (Pérez-Torres et al. 2022; NKF 2017) 126

Table 12.3 The 7-Point Subjective Global Assessment (Churchill et al. 1996; Lim et al. 2016) 126

Table 12.4 Examples of Food Additives Used in Food Manufacturing (NKF 2019; Sherman and Mehta 2009) 128

Table 12.5 Example Meals and Their Nutrient Content – Sample Day 1 133

Table 12.6 Example Meals and Their Nutrient Content – Sample Day 2 134

Table 15.1 Image Licenses, Terms of Use, and Available Resources 183

Author

J. Barretto Patterson, MPH, RDN, BC-ADM, CPT is a registered dietitian and a diabetes care and education specialist at Michigan Medicine in Ann Arbor. She also spent several years as a lifestyle coach for a CDC-recognized Diabetes Prevention Program. She is a recurring speaker for the Association of Diabetes Care and Education Specialists, where she has presented on topics including behavior change, weight management, physical activity, and telehealth. She also serves as the preceptor for dietetic interns who rotate through her clinic. She is a recurring guest lecturer for the clinical nutrition class at the University of Michigan School of Public Health.

She currently provides nutrition education and counseling for individuals with diabetes, obesity, hyperlipidemia, hypertension, and other nutrition-related conditions. She also provides group education to patients with diabetes and kidney disease. Prior to specializing in diabetes, she was a cardiovascular dietitian providing group education in cardiac rehab as well as individual counseling for patients with lipid disorders, hypertension, and other risk factors for heart disease.

Prior to becoming a registered dietitian, she spent several years working in marketing communications as an editor and a graphic designer. Having earned both her Master of Public Health and Bachelor of Arts degrees at the University of Michigan, she bleeds Maize and Blue. Her undergraduate degree is in English Language and Literature. She continues to write, frequently contributing to various blogs and publications including the *Food & Nutrition Magazine* Stone Soup blog, the University of Michigan's health blog, the *ADCES in Practice* journal, and her personal blog *thefeelingsnackyfix.com*. She is also the owner of *platemethodpics.com*, a stock photography website that specializes in royalty-free plate method images and educational materials.

Introduction

What this book is, what it is not, and why you need it.

Recently, near the end of a one-on-one diabetes education session, a patient said to me, "I'm glad I came. I was hesitant to see a dietitian at first, but I really learned something today."

I have been in the field for over ten years, and I must admit, I still feel a bit giddy when I receive feedback like this. It reminds me of why I became a dietitian in the first place: To help people learn that they can enjoy food healthfully.

As a student, I naively believed that once people understood how food affects their health, they would adopt the changes necessary to treat their conditions. I quickly learned, however, that nutrition counseling is not that simple. In a world full of messages to restrict, eliminate, and fast, gaining a patient's trust can be tricky if your advice runs contrary to mainstream trends. Or, if there are other challenges in their lives, dietary changes may seem like one more burden to bear. Sometimes, personality differences can make it difficult to connect, hindering an effective counseling session. Every day and every patient are different, and what resonates with one may fall flat with another.

It took several years in the field, hundreds of patients, a pandemic, and my own cultural awakening before I understood the intricacies of nutrition counseling, including:

1. How to get a person to open up and engage.
2. How to bridge the complexity of nutrition science with the equally complex realities of life.
3. How to keep myself present for each patient—even for those who do not make it easy.

However, before I could fine-tune my interactions with patients, I first had to understand their points of view. While I had submerged myself in the biochemistry and clinical application of dietetics in school, I had not anticipated the kinds of questions and challenges that patients would ask in practice. Patients do not ask about the Krebs Cycle or dietary reference intakes. The Mifflin St. Jeor equation does not solve the problem of stress eating. And the Mediterranean Diet, despite all of its benefits, cannot protect someone's time. While my motivational interviewing class taught me how to *ask* questions, I still needed to learn how to *answer* them.

In practice, my patients teach me what they really need to know. Their questions are more practical in nature–breakfast ideas, healthy snacks, and time-saving tips. Misconceptions related to diet trends are common, such as macronutrient or supplement needs. And difficulty losing weight is a common complaint, regardless of the reason for referral.

In the beginning, I found myself starting from scratch with each person. Never knowing what they were going to ask, I had to scramble for ideas on the spot. My sessions felt disorganized and ill-prepared. Sometimes the patient left with nothing more than my suggestions scribbled on a piece of paper, with very little else to refer to later. I knew I could not continue like this.

Eventually, I picked up on various patterns, everyday challenges, and frequently asked questions. There were enough recurring topics that I could develop a standing set of materials to have at the ready. I developed an arsenal of educational tools—anecdotal stories, clarifying analogies, and motivational conversation starters—available to quickly address the questions I encounter every day. The purpose of this book is to share these materials and experiences to assist other nutrition counselors in expanding their toolkit.

What this book is…

As an internship preceptor, I observe dietetic interns knowledgeably answer questions about food, meal planning, or individual nutrients like fat or potassium. But just as I experienced when I was starting out, they struggle through verbal explanations without educational tools to reinforce their messages. They are empty-handed and starting from scratch, brainstorming meal ideas on the fly, or ticking off foods from an invisible list. I feel their frustration as they want to provide something more, and I know that patients need something to refer to later.

This book aims to introduce the nutrition counseling professional to common scenarios and to provide insight into the patient's perspective. While every patient is different, there are common challenges, behaviors, questions, and situations that life presents. Whether the patient is referred for hyperlipidemia, diabetes, obesity, or other nutrition-related conditions, identifying and addressing their lifestyle patterns are critical to implementing nutrition therapy.

With this book, I offer ready-to-use educational tools for common questions and challenges encountered in outpatient care, from "I'm tired of oatmeal. What else can I have for breakfast?" to "I'm busy with my kids' activities, so we go to the drive-thru a lot." I also include easy-to-understand educational materials for complex conditions including diabetes, kidney disease, heart disease, and IBS; educational slides that can be used in virtual visits or group presentations; and behavior change tools such as food journals, physical activity logs, and goal setting sheets. I also guide readers to key resources including clinical guidelines, relevant studies, professional associations, training programs, recipe websites, and reliable online tools and apps.

What this book is not…

This book is not a comprehensive guide to medical nutrition therapy. The nutrition professional who picks up this book has already completed courses in the science and clinical application of dietetics. This book aims to prepare nutrition professionals for their personal interactions with patients.

Why you need it.

While courses in nutrition counseling teach providers to listen to their patients, this book gives registered dietitian nutritionists a heads-up on what to listen *for*, with educational materials that address the everyday challenges many people, hence many RDNs, face.

This toolkit is suitable for dietitians at all levels of experience. With these materials, dietetic interns can rotate through outpatient clinics equipped to deliver comprehensive education and counseling for the most common nutrition referrals. New nutrition professionals can start practicing with deeper insight into the patient's perspective. Experienced dietitians can expand their educational library and virtual tools.

Wherever you are in your dietetics career, keep this book handy. Your patients are in it.

In the following pages, the "Tales from the Field" and other anecdotal stories are based on real people, real conversations, and real outcomes. Names, health information, and other details have been modified to protect their privacy.

Access the Support Material at: https://resourcecentre.routledge.com/books/9781032352459

Part I

SHARE

1 SHARE — A Step-by-Step Approach to Nutrition Counseling

As a new dietitian, my first position was at a cardiovascular clinic. Starting out, I only had a few patients a day. But my days were full as I would spend as much time preparing for each patient as I spent with them. While my typical referrals at that time were for hyperlipidemia or hypertension, the patients often had other comorbidities. Coming out of school, I learned about medical nutrition therapy for various conditions. Going into practice, I wondered how on earth to put it all together. On top of that, there were often a host of medications that I was still getting to know. What was a general overview in school is now a critical component of my nutrition assessments. Patients taking Warfarin needed guidance on vitamin K. Grapefruit juice was contraindicated with statins. Patients using ACE inhibitors needed to be cautioned about salt substitutes and potassium chloride.

I was so nervous that I would miss something. A fluid restriction. An electrolyte imbalance. A food–drug interaction. Not to mention lab values. The off-the-chart numbers one sees regularly in a specialty clinic are not in the typical case studies presented in class. And if I am being honest, the numbers I once memorized from my flash cards needed review.

Over time, I learned how to zero in on the most pertinent points in a patient's record—the reason for referral, medications, lab values, and their previous medical history. According to the Centers for Disease Control and Prevention, heart disease, stroke, diabetes, and kidney disease are among the country's leading causes of death and disability (CDC 2022), and my patients' comorbidities reflected this. Gastrointestinal conditions like IBS and GERD are also increasingly encountered. While I became familiar with the details of various nutrition guidelines, I also picked up on common behaviors, beliefs, and lifestyle factors that contribute to the patients' symptoms and self-care.

Most importantly, I have learned that the most critical information comes from the patients themselves.

Where I used to spend excessive time poring over a patient record, I now turn to the patients to direct my assessment. Through ice-breaking banter, encouraging questions, and thoughtful listening, the patient's needs can become quite clear. An EMR becomes a person. Listening becomes learning—for both patient and provider. And, hopefully, nutrition guidelines become a lifestyle change.

Today, when a dietetic intern observes me with patients, it may appear as if I follow a script, from intro to education to counseling. Indeed, I have established a certain outline—or flow—to how I conduct a nutrition consult. However, within each segment, the patient directs the topics, thus individualizing the session for themselves. In turn, I assist the patient in putting the puzzle pieces together, seeing the bigger picture, and framing that information so it fits in the space of their lives.

DOI: 10.1201/9781003326038-2

The outline I follow can best be described by the acronym SHARE. This step-by-step approach leads me through a comprehensive nutrition consultation, from assessment to action plan. It embodies the concepts of shared decision-making and empowerment, in which the patient and provider work together to determine the treatment plan that is right for them (Tamhane et al. 2015; Funnell and Anderson 2004). The acronym is a simple reminder to:

S – Start with a blank page
H – Hear and understand
A – Assess learning needs
R – Review relevant information
E – Empower the patient.

With SHARE, the complicated details of the patient's medical record are put into the context of their everyday lives. Through an open exchange of information, you will learn how they spend their time, with whom they spend it, where and how they eat, their feelings about food, and other priorities in their lives. You will discover what they know about nutrition, what they don't, and from where they get their information. From this, you will glean the most important information they need to hear in that moment, and the action plan will develop based on what resonates most with them. Through information sharing, you empower the patient to decide what next steps are right for them, and why.

This bidirectional interaction not only clarifies the patient's case for you, but it can also foster a relationship of trust. The more engaged you appear, the more open the patient may be with you. In turn, you will have more information to personalize their education. If a patient feels heard and understood, they may be more receptive to your guidance and more willing to implement a plan. Upon seeing positive results, they are more likely to follow up with you. As return visits are a critical component of your practice, their success will also be yours. Furthermore, while person-centered care recognizes that people truly are the managers of their own health, a satisfied patient can reinforce your own sense of purpose, confidence, job satisfaction, and, subsequently, performance (Trzeciak et al. 2017).

To be fair, it will not always be this straightforward. Personalities vary, as do emotions—both the patient's and yours. Work overload can threaten person-centered care. Implicit bias can affect your judgment. While keeping a keen eye on your patient's body language, you must also be aware of your own. Some patients may have complications beyond your expertise. Others may be outright resistant to change. From empathizing with the patient to managing your own reactions, self-awareness will be as important as active listening.

The SHARE approach humanizes the nutrition care process[1] (Swan et al. 2017) by uncovering the *why* behind the assessment and diagnosis, *what* intervention is most relevant, and *how* the patient can reach their goals. SHARE recognizes that the person is not a diagnosis, nor is the provider a magician. Both are flawed, sentient beings with limitations and barriers, but by working together, change can be possible.

In the first part of this book, you will learn about challenges you may encounter in nutrition counseling and ways to navigate them. You will enhance your skills in active listening with a preview of what to listen *for*. And for the times that you do not have all the answers, you can find solace in the fact that the burden is not all on you. That it is not only okay—but it is typically better—to SHARE.

---

[1] The Nutrition Care Process is a systematic approach to medical nutrition therapy that includes assessment, diagnosis, intervention, monitoring, and evaluation.

REFERENCES

Centers for Disease Control and Prevention. Chronic diseases in America; 2022 December 13. Available from: https://www.cdc.gov/chronicdisease/resources/infographic/chronic-diseases.htm. Accessed 1/14/2023.

Funnell MM, Anderson RM. Empowerment and Self-Management of Diabetes. *Clin Diabetes.* 2004;22(3):123–127.

Swan WI, Vivanti A, Hakel-Smith NA, Hotson B, Orrevall Y, Trostler N, Beck Howarter K, Papoutsakis C. Nutrition Care Process and Model Update: Toward Realizing People-Centered Care and Outcomes Management. *J Acad Nutr Diet.* 2017 Dec;117(12):2003–2014. doi: 10.1016/j.jand.2017.07.015.

Tamhane S, Rodriguez-Gutierrez R, Hargraves I, Montori VM. Shared Decision Making in Diabetes Care. *Curr Diab Rep.* 2015;15:112.

Trzeciak S, Roberts BW, Mazzarelli AJ. Compassionomics: Hypothesis and experimental approach. *Med Hypotheses.* 2017 Sep;107:92–97. doi: 10.1016/j.mehy.2017.08.015.

2 Start with a Blank Sheet

At the start of my dietetic internship, I had the pleasure of working under Kathy, a highly respected dietitian who specialized in lipid management. I was in awe of the knowledge she had about lipid metabolism, genetic disorders, medication management, and, of course, medical nutrition therapy. However, what changed the course of my career was her interaction with patients.

On my first day observing her, I was struck by how much gratitude her patients showed her. More than one had said to me, "In all these years, she is the only person who has ever helped me lose weight." One patient, in particular, is forever cemented in my memory as the reason I pursued a career as an outpatient clinical dietitian.

I'll call this patient Marilyn. She was a returning patient who had seen Kathy twice before over the previous few months for weight management and hypertension. She was accompanied by her husband. As they settled into the visit, Kathy asked if she had brought food records with her.

"No, Kathy, I'm sorry," Marilyn replied. "To tell you the truth, I stopped tracking. A lot of the changes I've made have become more of a habit, so there's no point in writing it down anymore." Marilyn proceeded to describe her typical meals. She stated that her husband brings her snacks of sliced vegetables. Together, they walked daily.

As I listened quietly on the side, I was struck by how comfortable and proud Marilyn was as she talked about these lifestyle changes as well as how supportive her husband was for her. But it was the last part of her story, and my reaction to it, that I have never forgotten. When Marilyn said, "Since we started doing this, I've lost 15 lbs and my blood pressure medications have been cut in half."

This was the first time I saw medical nutrition therapy at work. I remember thinking, "Huh, this stuff really works."

While I had become a dietitian because I believed in healthy eating, I had foreseen myself pursuing a career in health communications. My field experience during graduate school was promoting nutrition messages for the USDA's Food and Nutrition Services. In my own personal life, where my husband and children have various food intolerances, I have observed the direct impact that food can have on health and the challenge of finding ways to enjoy food. Prior to this internship rotation, I had focused on good nutrition as a preventive health measure. I had not yet witnessed its therapeutic potential. Thus, when Marilyn reported that she needed less medication, the power of nutrition and lifestyle solidified for me. Further, Marilyn's gratitude toward Kathy was stunning. It was in that moment that I thought, "This is what I want to do." I wanted to be Kathy. I wanted to inspire people to make changes that would improve their health in ways that were tangible, measurable, and enjoyable.

As such, once you find passion and purpose, opportunities have a tendency to present themselves. At the end of my dietetic internship, Kathy hired me, and so I started my career as a clinical dietitian. However, getting the job and doing the job are two different things. Like anybody starting a new career, there is a learning curve, some growing pains, and a lot of trial and error before your expertise starts to develop.

LEARNING THE ROPES

I once heard somebody say, "It takes a full year to learn a job." To this day, I can understand the wisdom behind that statement. While procedures and protocols can be easily reviewed

DOI: 10.1201/9781003326038-3

during training, many jobs have seasonal variations, as does nutrition counseling. Patient load can vary based on holidays and vacation periods. Patient barriers can also change with the season. Cold weather and shorter days can affect people's appetite or physical activity. Holidays can make it difficult to resist temptation. Summer travel can also affect food intake and mindfulness. After the first year, you learn to anticipate those conversations and develop strategies to address them.

For dietitians, the skills learned in school include the nutrition care process, medical nutrition therapy, and various counseling approaches. However, mastering patient interactions can only be learned on the job by, obviously, interacting with patients.

For many people, a visit to an outpatient dietitian is one of the few times in healthcare where they are given a full hour to discuss their daily routines. While conducting a dietary recall, you will learn more than just what they eat. You will also hear about the schedule of their day, their work demands, their family obligations, their level of stress, and their coping mechanisms. Therefore, an hour can go fast trying to get to know somebody while still leaving time to provide education and counseling. As such, one of my first struggles in patient care was time management. However, I eventually realized that the root of my problem was how I was conducting my nutrition assessment.

In the clinic, we had a nutrition assessment form that we completed with each patient. The comprehensive form included questions about various nutrition-related concerns: food allergies, GI issues, appetite, energy level, stress, weight history, and, of course, food intake. As a new dietitian, I diligently completed this form at the beginning of each new encounter with a patient. People willingly obliged to not only answer the questions, but even expand on their answers. I soon learned that when given the chance, people are very willing to share their stories. On one hand, having your patients open up is the key to effective nutrition counseling. On the other hand, it can sometimes make time management difficult.

As a new dietitian, when your patient list is still ramping up, you might have a little extra time to give each patient. On the other hand, if you are in a busy clinic with back-to-back patients, efficiency is key to staying on schedule.

Thus, as I obediently filled out each section of that nutrition assessment, time was a-ticking. Kathy observed me mechanically going through the assessment form and struggling with time and said something that I have never forgotten:

"Think about why you are asking the question."

That's Kathy. She had a way of saying things that were thought-provoking without spelling out exactly what to do.

While dietitians are trained in the range of nutrition-related issues, not every issue can be addressed in the first visit. For example, knowing a person's food allergies and GI issues is important information when developing a meal plan. However, unless those are the reasons for the referral, that information is likely to come out organically when discussing meal ideas. For example, when recommending low-fat dairy as part of the DASH diet, a patient who is lactose-intolerant or allergic to cow's milk will quickly tell you that they do not drink milk. Or when talking about healthy fats like nuts, the patient will let you know if they have nut allergies. More often than not, a patient can already name some foods they can or cannot tolerate, and they will likely let you know. Therefore, taking the time to explicitly ask about food allergies during the assessment may not be necessary, unless it is the reason for referral.

Similarly, knowing the patient's current stress level and coping skills is certainly important in assessing barriers to change, but systematically filling out an assessment form may not be the best way to address that topic. Again, when allowed to freely share their stories, the patient is likely to offer that information up on their own.

TALES FROM THE FIELD: DRINK TO THAT!

Amy was a dietetic intern who recently received her master's degree in nutrition. She had been with the clinic for about a week. As with other rotations, she started off observing various group classes and individual counseling. She spent time with each dietitian and saw a variety of different teaching styles. After about a week, she was ready to lead a nutrition assessment.

As she conducted a 24-hour recall, Amy inquired about the patient's fluid intake.

Amy: How much water do you drink a day?

Patient: Oh, I'm bad about that. Maybe three or four glasses a day.

Amy: How big are the glasses?

Patient: About this big [The patient holds up his hands to demonstrate the glass size.]

Amy: About how much do you fill the glasses?

Patient: Oh, not all the way. Maybe two-thirds of the way. How much water am I supposed
            to drink per day?

Amy: For men, about 12 cups.

Patient: 12 cups of water!

Amy: Well, that can include other drinks, like milk or tea or coffee.

Patient: I thought coffee was dehydrating.

Amy: Um, not really, unless you drink a lot. Other liquids would count too, like soup.

Patient: How about juice?

Amy: Well, you have to be careful with juice because of the sugar.

Patient: So what are good things to drink?

[…]

This exchange lasted a few minutes. When time is limited, a few minutes here and there can easily add up. In this case, the patient was referred for hyperlipidemia. As important as hydration status is, there was no indication that the patient was clinically dehydrated. Therefore, valuable time was spent before getting to the heart of the matter.

While a detailed assessment is important in determining the intervention, and hydration is an important issue, some details are more pertinent than others during the visit. When time is an issue, think about *why* you are asking a question as well as if you need to. In this example, digging deeper to learn about the types of fat, the amount of fiber, and their overall food choices would take precedent.

When asking questions, think about why you are asking. What are you going to do with that information? Is it pertinent to what the patient needs to learn today? Which brings me to another gold nugget that Kathy instilled in me:

"You are not going to cover everything in the first visit."

And there might be a lot to cover. Often, in preparation for a patient, their chart lists a medical history so long and complicated that you wonder where to start. The doctor may have indicated obesity as the reason for referral, but when you see diabetes and Celiac Disease on the list, there is more for you—and the patient—to consider. You pull up your carbohydrate list and review the patient's medications. Are they insulin-dependent with risk of low blood sugar? Or maybe they just started Metformin, in which case they may be battling some diarrhea or other GI issues. Have they already seen a dietitian for Celiac Disease, or will you need your list of gluten-free foods?

With every patient, you never know where the visit will lead. Even after 10 years of practice, I still get nervous before picking up each patient from the waiting area. Working in specialty clinics, most of my patients are advanced in their disease or have developed multiple related complications. The butterflies in my stomach that I felt as an intern have been with me ever since. And for good reason. Nutrition is a complicated science. It is the fuel, the medicine, the toxin, and the recreational drug. The dietitian, then, is simultaneously a food expert, educator, health care provider, counselor, and life coach. Before you sit down with a patient, you never know which skill you will need most. Quite likely, you will need them all. To this day, I always recall Kathy's words:

"Your patient will tell you what they need."

As a new dietitian, I relied on that nutrition assessment form to thoroughly assess the patient's needs. While the form initially taught me which topics are generally pertinent to a nutrition assessment, I eventually realized that there was a quicker way to find the answers I needed for each specific visit.

Don't ask. Listen.

I will never forget the day when I was facing a patient and it hit me: *Start with a blank sheet.*

I turned that nutrition assessment form over to where it was blank on the other side. As I broke the ice with the patient, they started to open up about their day, how they eat, what they wanted to change, and what other aspects of their lives impacted their food choices. Knowing they were with a dietitian, they intuitively focused on how they ate. I found that if I just let them talk, they answered a lot of the questions that were on the assessment form. And if they didn't, I either (1) asked when I got the opportunity, or (2) realized that it was not a priority for that day.

By shifting the focus from the dietitian's to the patient's point of view, the needs of the patient became clear faster. While they might have multiple nutrition concerns, they will tell you what they want to know today. By addressing what is top of mind for them, they are more likely to be receptive to the information you provide. This is fundamental to person-centered care.

However, before you can answer any questions, you must overcome the first challenge in nutrition counseling: Getting the patient to open up in the first place.

I recall the first time I was charged to lead a nutrition consult as an intern. I was so nervous. I reviewed the lengthy details of their medical chart and wondered, "But how do I start?"

Now, as a preceptor, I see the same trepidation in the students who rotate through my clinic. Recently, when I offered an opportunity to a very sweet intern to lead a consult, she said, "But what do I say?"

I appreciated that she was open about her feelings. As I mentioned earlier, to this day, I still get a little nervous when I retrieve a patient from the waiting area. I never know where the conversation will lead. What questions will they ask me? Will I have the answers they need?

BREAKING THE ICE

When interns show they are a little nervous about taking the lead, I remind them, "It's just a conversation."

Imagine when you meet a friend for coffee. Like a good friend, you ask how they have been, and you listen intently as they update you on their lives. Sometimes you interject with a question if you need more clarification.

Also imagine when you are the one updating your friend. Recall how nice it is to have someone listening to you, validating you, and maybe even giving you some guidance.

Good conversations and strong relationships often result when both participants have a chance to share information and when each takes time to listen.

Nutrition counseling works the same way. Imagine how glad your patient may be to have someone listen to them. As you demonstrate that you are interested in learning more about them, they may warm toward you, feel comfortable opening up, and be willing to hear what you have to offer.

New patient visits are typically 60 minutes long. I have found that the first 20–30 minutes is sufficient time to assess the patient's learning needs, leaving the rest of the hour for education and action planning. While each conversation can take different directions, the ultimate goals of the assessment are to:

1. Break the ice. Encourage the patient to open up about themselves.
2. Find out what they want to know.
3. Find out what they need to know.

You must meet the first goal in order to reach the other goals. Once the patient starts opening up, the agenda for the visit starts to form. While the doctor may have listed a reason for referral, the patient will reveal which topics to focus on.

PRACTICE TIP: BREAK THE ICE IN THREE STEPS

In nutrition counseling, a key tenet is to ask open-ended questions, and to focus on the patient's personal goals. As such, a well-intentioned nutritionist may be inclined to start a visit by asking, "What brings you to this visit today?" or "How can I help you today?"

Those questions are certainly a step in the right direction and may elicit an eager response such as, "My A1C went up and I don't want to go on medication. I want to see how I can turn this around through diet first." On the other hand, it is also not uncommon for a patient to respond, "I don't know. My doctor told me I should come."

For some people, opening up about themselves to a stranger may be uncomfortable. A person's emotions and life situation are very personal. They may be feeling fear, anger, sadness, or denial about their diagnosis. Social or cultural constructs may inhibit them from exhibiting, admitting, or discussing their feelings. Some people may arrive feeling a little defensive. After all, a person's relationship with food can be quite complex. I have heard on more than one occasion, "I know you're going to take all my favorite food away."

Furthermore, most people have several other responsibilities beyond their own healthcare, such as caring for others around them—small children, a sick spouse, or elderly parents. Perhaps other stressors, like work or finances, have caused them to neglect their health. As life is complicated, it is not uncommon that somebody may be feeling overwhelmed with multiple concerns. While they are trying to manage their daily responsibilities, considering their health and future can be difficult to prioritize. Thus, at the beginning of a visit, expecting the patient to set the agenda may be asking too much. Where do they start?

Give them time. Let them first settle in and collect their thoughts. Just as you are assessing them, they are also assessing you. As a new patient, they do not know who you are, what you do, what your qualifications are, or maybe even what happens in a nutrition counseling session. In the first few minutes, break the ice with the following steps:

Step 1. Welcome them to their visit and thank them for coming. Likely, they had to make arrangements to accommodate this appointment, like taking time off work or hiring a babysitter. They may have driven a distance, or arranged transportation, or struggled through logging into a virtual visit. Acknowledge their time and their efforts.

Step 2. Introduce yourself and your specialty. Describe what services you and your department offer, especially the services that are relevant to the patient. For example, if your patient was referred for a FODMAP trial, you might say, "I specialize in nutrition therapy for food-related conditions like irritable bowel syndrome and food intolerances."

If possible, align yourself with their referring provider. Perhaps you work in the doctor's clinic or you are part of the same health system. If the patient followed up on this referral, they likely trust their doctor's recommendations and may therefore extend some of that trust your way.

Be brief in introducing yourself, as the visit is not about you, but do take the time to establish your credibility. As many people are bombarded with nutrition information from the Internet, family, friends, or non-nutrition health and fitness professionals, establishing yourself as a reliable source of information will be important when discussing competing messages. On the other hand, be careful not to delve into every letter after your name as you do not want to come off as arrogant or unrelatable.

Early in the visit, be sure to inform the patient how much time is set aside for this visit. This allows them to work with you in managing the time and prioritizing which topics to discuss.

Step 3. Acknowledge what you already know about the patient. Restate the reason listed on the referral. If you have access to the doctor's last chart note, reiterate some information that is relevant to the visit. For example, if the patient is referred for post-bariatric hypoglycemia, you might say, "I see from the doctor's note that you have been experiencing some symptoms of low blood sugar." As you shift the conversation back to the patient, you open the door for them to start sharing their concerns. At this point, an encouraging pause may be enough to cue the patient to expand on the reason for referral. If needed, a transition statement may be needed to turn it over to the patient, such as:

We have about an hour set aside, and there is some information that I think you will find helpful. However, I want to be sure I answer the questions that have been on your mind. What do you want to make sure we discuss today?

At this point, the patient now knows more about you, what you do, and what you know about them. They are starting to sense that the visit will be personalized to their situation and their questions. The ice is starting to break.

WHAT DO PATIENTS *WANT* TO KNOW?

Once the patient starts to share why they came for the visit, they are now in the driver's seat. Allow them to take the freeway, where they can speak with minimal interruption. Often, the more intently you appear to be listening, the more they are willing to divulge. In this way, I have found that most of my questions can be answered without even having to ask. Ultimately, the answers I am looking for are:

Does the problem they want to address match the reason for the referral? For example, they might be referred for prediabetes, but their main concern is losing weight. While much of the information for these separate conditions is similar, *how* I present the information might differ. Furthermore, by addressing their personal concerns, they will feel heard, an important factor in building trust.

How do they feel about their condition? If it is a new diagnosis, they may be feeling scared. Or in denial. Or resigned to it due to their family history or their lifestyle choices. Sometimes, they are angry. Some are ready to act and may have already started making changes. How they feel will affect the tone of the visit. Your role may be more as an educator sharing information, or as a counselor providing reassurance.

Are they ready or willing to make changes? Perhaps they have already started changing their diet or purchased recipe books for their condition. Or they started walking more or joined a gym. Or they started to research information on the Internet or joined an online support group. On the other hand, perhaps they have no intention to change due to competing priorities or interests. Maybe they simply enjoy their life as it is. Wherever they are on the readiness scale, describing the nature of their condition and actionable steps for treatment might either reinforce—or elicit—their motivation.

WHAT DO PATIENTS *NEED* TO KNOW?

What a person wants to know and what they need to know are not always the same things. While this information can be different, they are not necessarily mutually exclusive. For example, patients will often say, "I just need to know what to eat." They might expect—or ask for—a specific menu that they should follow. On the other hand, if you are able to provide more specific information about how food relates to their symptoms, they may understand better how to plan their own menu. While it was not the information they were expecting, they needed it to get the answer to their question.

WHAT *YOU* NEED TO KNOW

The *dietary recall* is a tool dietitians use to assess a person's nutrient intake. However, nutrition is a lifestyle issue. As such, RDNs must look beyond what a person eats. Dietitians are more effective when they understand why people plan their meals the way they do. Whether they are a busy mom shuttling their kids to various activities, or an empty nester who finds it hard to cook for one, these factors have as much—sometimes more—influence on a person's food choices than their nutrition knowledge.

While a dietary recall is subject to reporting bias, inaccuracies, or memory lapses, this portion of the encounter can reveal a lot about a person's lifestyle. Like a reporter researching a story, you are listening for the who, what, where, when, and why.

Who—Who does the cooking? With whom do they eat or live? Who supports them, or hinders them, in making healthy choices?

What—What foods do they eat and enjoy? What do they drink? What do they eat that is protective, and what is contributing to their symptoms?

Where—From where do they get most of their meals? Are they making it at home, or do they dine out often? Do they receive meal delivery, or are they provided meals in assisted living? Do they use food pantries?

When—Do they stick with breakfast, lunch and dinner, or do they graze throughout the day? Will they eat soon after waking? Or do they skip meals? Do they snack after dinner?

Why—How do their symptoms, work, family, finances, stress, exercise goals, or diet trends affect what, when, or where they eat?

How—How are their nutrition and lifestyle affecting their health?

Not all of the information above will come up during the assessment. However, as you follow the thread of their day, the information that matters most likely will.

PRACTICE TIP: THE DIETARY RECALL—GUIDING PROMPTS

For this part of the assessment, the following questions can help prompt the patient to describe their typical day in detail.

1. What time do you typically start your day?
2. What time is your first meal, snack, or beverage? What do you typically have at this time?
3. When is the next time you have a meal, snack, or beverage? Please provide examples.
4. Repeat Question 3 until you have covered a full day.
5. How often in a day or a week do you dine out or get takeout?
6. How many servings of alcohol do you have in a day or a week?
7. Do you use any nutrition supplements or vitamins?
8. What else, if anything, do you have regularly that has not yet been mentioned?

Allow the patient to respond freely with minimal interruption. At times, you may need to interject with clarifying questions, or to redirect the patient for time management.

Keep responses neutral and objective. Refrain from responding with positive or negative comments, either of which could influence how a patient responds. As positive comments can be pleasing, they may cause the responder to seek more affirmation. Conversely, negative comments may lead them to exclude some details to avoid further judgment.

Avoid the terms **breakfast, lunch,** *and* **dinner.** As people keep different schedules, these terms can be mildly distressing. For example, for shift workers, traditional eating times do not apply, and they are often unsure of how to schedule their meals. For those who sleep in, many believe they "skip breakfast," even if they have their first meal soon after waking. For some, "skipping breakfast" has a negative connotation and can evoke feelings of wrongdoing or failure.

Repeat questions as needed, or not at all. Traditionally, dietetic students learn about the multi-pass approach, where you might have the patient describe a typical day three or four times for measurement details and to improve their recall. This is important if you are assessing for nutrient deficiencies or sources of excess calories. In lifestyle counseling, one or two passes are often sufficient to assess what types of food a patient consumes and what they know about nutrition.

Throughout the dietary recall, people often include details about their work, their family, or how they feel about food. By allowing them time to speak freely, you will learn more about them than just the foods that they eat.

3 Hear and Understand

When I started this chapter, I intended to dive straight into various eating patterns that I have observed in nutrition counseling. From meal skipping to night snacking to yo-yo dieting, there are several patterns that repeatedly emerge. However, the more I recalled the conversations I have had over the years, the more I realized how emotional the topic of eating can be. While the dietary recall reveals *what* people do, an astute counselor may also uncover *why* people eat the way they do. In some cases, those reasons could fall outside of the RD's comfort zone and perhaps even outside of their scope of practice. Thus, it is important to understand the emotional aspects of eating, identify possible psychopathological barriers to lifestyle changes, screen for possible eating disorders, and know when and how to refer to the appropriate specialists or programs.

Many nutrition counselors do not have to stray too far to understand the complexity of eating behavior. One only has to stop and think about their own feelings about food. I know that my relationship with food impacts my daily routine and, in fact, has shaped my life. I can identify several events or moments when food influenced my feelings, self-image, health decisions, and parenting choices—all ultimately leading me to a career in nutrition.

The first memory that comes to mind occurred when I was about 14 years old. As adolescence is already an impressionable, delicate time of life, the moment is still vivid in my mind. I was at a family gathering. Like most Filipino parties, a buffet table was set up laden with traditional dishes and delicacies, all provided pot-luck style, mostly by the women of the family—grandmas, great aunts, aunties, and even older cousins learning how to cook. The party truly begins when the paper plates are handed out with plasticware rolled up in napkins. We line up and make our way around the buffet, scooping white rice, noodle dishes (*pancit*), egg rolls (*lumpia*), meat and vegetable stews, and stir fries—all traditional favorites. There is never enough room on the plate for everything, so multiple passes throughout the night are inevitable.

The dessert table is also ready and waiting. Little muffins called *puto*, sweet cassava cake, creamy leche flan, and other tantalizing sweets lay in abundance. But no Filipino party is complete without a mocha cake. I was always a sucker for the sprinkles, the dark chocolate shavings generously covering a silky, light brown frosting coating a light, fluffy sponge that sweetly dissolves on the tongue.

On this night, the cake was placed high on a cake stand. I remember spotting it from across the room. I neared the table, zeroing in on the object of my desire. Anticipation excited the pleasure centers of my brain. As I approached the table, I was vaguely aware of the eyes on me. In hushed tones and weakly concealed laughter, words were exchanged in tagalog, the language I have never acquired even to this day. Unaware of what the commotion was about, I proceeded to help myself to a hearty slice of the mocha cake. Dessert plate in hand, its delicate appearance caused my mouth to water. I could not wait to find a comfortable place to settle in and indulge.

Before I could steal away, one of my aunts appeared at my side, the one who played the role of the family matriarch. First in age, highest in station, she claimed her right to speak freely, advise unsolicitedly, and criticize profusely. As such, her approach filled me with dread, if only because she was keeping me from my dessert.

The twinkle in her eye and the grin on her face hinted at the joke that was yet to come. I braced myself for the punchline.

DOI: 10.1201/9781003326038-4

"You are maganda," she said. I was familiar with the tagalog word for "beautiful," so I smiled. "But," she continued, "you will be fat one day like your mom."

In one sentence, my aunt left an indelible impression on how I interact with food. I wish I could say that was it—the moment that defined my self-image and my relationship with food. But life is not that simple, and eating behavior is not that one-dimensional. Add to that the years I watched my father struggle with diabetes, heart disease, and kidney failure, only to lose him when I was 20 years old. Later, newly married, I noticed that my husband had significant food intolerances with symptoms that he had just learned to live with over the years. Once we were living together, he started to exhibit signs of nutrient deficiencies as I unknowingly prepared dishes that he could not tolerate. Then as a mother, I watched my first child suffer through food allergies that triggered rashes, hives, and open sores at its best, vomiting and shortness of breath at its worst. Then my second child ended up in the emergency room on Halloween night when he was 2 years old after eating chocolate candy with peanut butter. Coughing and crying, he repeated "Itchy! Itchy!" at a time when his vocabulary was still so limited.

These experiences left indelible impressions on how I eat and how I feed the people around me. I came to appreciate the direct impact food has on health. I was constantly searching for more information about how to take care of my family with their various food restrictions. The learning curve was often frustrating, exhausting, and emotional. I had to learn how to cook from scratch, modify recipes, and substitute ingredients. I was constantly on the lookout for products without offending ingredients, or brands that specialize in allergy-friendly foods. As my kids and my husband had different intolerances, there were times when I had to prepare different foods to accommodate them all and learn how to efficiently do so.

On one hand, the effort it took to feed my family sounds complex and burdensome. And so it was. But on the other hand, it was incredibly worth it. I will never forget when my son was 4 years old. I came home from the grocery store with a package of allergy-friendly cookies. When I showed them to him, he was so happy and squealed, "Wow! I can't eat anything, but you keep finding me things!"

Another time, after suffering the consequences of eating at a party where my husband was intolerant to much of the food, he said to me, "No one feeds me like you, dear."

Over time, we found staple ingredients, established go-to recipes, and learned how to plan meals efficiently. While there was plenty of trial and error, and there were still occasional challenges, the difference in my family's health made it worth the effort. It was this experience that led me to a career in dietetics. I wanted to help others find ways to enjoy food regardless of the food restrictions they may have.

The field of dietetics is wide and varied. From clinical nutrition to public health, from environmental to policy issues, and from nutrition science to health behavior, nutritionists specialize in different areas and hence have different skills, viewpoints, and passions. For nutrition counseling, the ability to recognize, empathize with, and/or relate to various psychosocial issues is essential for identifying effective therapeutic plans for each patient. Further, the ability to communicate empathy and compassion is critical in gaining the trust of each patient. Through mutual understanding, a productive working relationship can be established, allowing for better outcomes for the patient. Ultimately, the more success your patients see, the more work satisfaction you will enjoy.

THE PATIENT-DIETITIAN RELATIONSHIP

In school, dietitians are trained in nutrition diagnoses, health behavior theory, and techniques like motivational interviewing, active listening, goal setting, action planning, and patient-centered care. We are simultaneously healthcare providers, educators, and counselors. We often see ourselves as coaches or cheerleaders for our patients. In fact, the Academy of Nutrition and Dietetics includes coaching in their 2017 Scope of Practice document (Academy Quality Management Committee, 2018), which states:

> RDNs work as health and wellness coaches in health care facilities, private practices, wellness businesses (eg, in-person or via telehealth), nonprofit organizations, and corporate wellness. RDNs:
>
> - Educate and guide clients to achieve health goals through lifestyle and behavior adjustments.
> - Have thorough knowledge and advanced understanding of behavior change, culture, social determinants of health, disease self-management, and evidence-based health education research.
> - Empower clients to achieve self-determined goals related to health and wellness.

Our patients may view our role in different ways. Minimally, they may consider us simply as nutritionists who will provide them with meal plans and recipes. "I just need somebody to tell me what to eat," they might say. Some might not even expect that much, saying, "I know what to do. I'm just not doing it."

Referring doctors may also not understand the complexity of nutrition counseling. Their referral notes may include comments such as "instruct on calorie counting" or "needs low-carb meal plan" or "start partial meal replacement." When I was new to the field, I might have followed the doctor's instructions in deference. Or I might have systematically pulled up a Mifflin St. Jeor calculator to determine energy needs, then develop guidelines suggesting numbers of servings per food group. Nutrition departments often have sample meal plans or handouts with lists of food. While these types of educational tools can be useful in guiding a patient toward implementation of a plan, they may not be helpful in developing the plan in the first place. Regardless of the doctor's referral instructions, upon meeting a patient for the first time, the plan itself is yet to be determined. While the patient, doctor, and dietitian may share outcome goals, the strategies to reach those goals will vary per person. Ultimately, these strategies are determined by the patient themselves. After all, it is the patient who is responsible for planning their meals, accommodating their schedules, managing their social interactions, and facing their feelings. The role of the dietitian is to explain how certain behaviors affect health, to explore the motivations and barriers that affect their decisions, and to guide the patient in identifying opportunities to address their health concerns.

While a prescriptive approach to nutrition counseling is certainly easier on the dietitian, patient-centered care is well established as the more effective approach (Swan et al., 2017). When the patient and dietitian collaborate together, the patient may find the resulting plan to be more acceptable and achievable, increasing the likelihood of not only implementation but also long-term change (Tamhane et al., 2015).

For the dietitian, this process is not easy. It requires an adept application of nutrition science knowledge, health behavior theory, communication skills, and emotional sensitivity. While the former two components are obtained through academic study, the latter two are also dependent on the innate characteristics of the dietitian, personal experiences, professional training, and factors influencing their current state of mind. Moreover, just as the patient must be aware of how their experiences and feelings affect their health behaviors, so too must a dietitian be aware of their own thoughts and feelings during a counseling session.

A patient's story may evoke memories or feelings in a dietitian that can either elicit empathy or trigger bias. The patient themselves may act in ways that provoke certain emotions within the dietitian. In some cases, the dietitian may find themselves emotionally distant from the patient and leaning toward a more prescriptive demeanor. These fluctuations can vary day to day or patient to patient. The challenges for the dietitian are to recognize how their inner state—whether conscious or unconscious—may be affecting their patient care; to harness their emotions in a way to relate to the patient; to protect themselves from becoming negatively impacted by the emotional aspect of the job; and to identify when training or intervention is needed.

CULTIVATING EMPATHY

As discussed in the previous chapter, breaking the ice and active listening can encourage a patient to open up. However, true rapport can only be established when the counselor, too, develops genuine interest in—and empathy for—the patient. Further, just as a good counselor can tune in to a patient's feelings, so too can a patient pick up on a counselor's compassion—or lack thereof.

Empathy is defined as "understanding, being aware of, being sensitive to, and vicariously experiencing the feelings, thoughts, and experience of another" (Empathy 2023). It is one thing to hear a patient's words, but it is another to imagine their experience, a key component in patient-centered care (Moudatsou et al. 2020). By understanding the patient's perspective, the provider can better identify the therapeutic approaches that will be most acceptable to—and therefore effective for—the patient (Hojat et al. 2011, 2013; Del Canale et al. 2012).

I recall a woman who was referred for nutrition counseling. For this visit, I was accompanied by a dietetic intern. The patient stated that a barrier to meal planning was her child's food allergies. As with my experience, she struggled with either preparing meals that are appropriate for the whole family or preparing separate meals to accommodate multiple needs. She described several episodes where her child was brought to the emergency room for anaphylactic reactions. Thus, for her child's safety, she was very careful about the foods and ingredients that were brought into the home.

In this example, my level of empathy was naturally high as I, also, have two children with food allergies. However, after the patient left, the intern exhibited a different response to the patient's experience. The intern asked me, "Do you think she is just overreacting?"

Clearly, in this scenario, I had the advantage of having a similar experience. While the patient told her story, I recalled the helplessness I felt watching my children struggle with bloody rashes and difficulty breathing. I remembered the emergency room team surrounding my baby to administer injections, breathing equipment, and monitors. I can still hear the fear in my baby's cries as the team poked and prodded him.

Having had a similar experience to the patient, my response was different from that of the intern. Regardless, neither of us were in a position to judge the patient's feelings or behaviors. As healthcare providers, it is not for us to determine how a person should react to their life experiences. Our job is to understand what they feel and why, then guide the patient in developing health behavior plans that will accommodate their concerns.

Obviously, we will not always have similar experiences to our patients. Throughout any given day, we will meet people of various ages, races, health conditions, or socioeconomic status, each with a different life history, culture, and upbringing. They will have situations that do not have even a remote similarity to anything you have experienced. They may have an advanced disease state, or a disability, or a financial hardship that you have never endured. Perhaps their cultural or religious traditions are completely different from those in which you were raised. They may have had a past trauma that you could never fully comprehend.

While we may not truly feel *what* the patient is suffering, we must appreciate *that* they are suffering. In turn, as a patient detects empathy and understanding in their provider, a relationship of trust may develop.

The ability to empathize varies for each clinician depending on their innate characteristics, family and social influences, and personal and professional experiences (Yu et al. 2022). While some providers feel that their life and work experiences increase their ability to relate to their patients, studies show that empathy can decline with age and experience (Yu et al. 2022; Spraggins et al. 1990). Factors such as work stress, desensitization, and burnout may contribute to the decline in empathy for experienced clinicians (Yu et al. 2022; Wagaman et al. 2015).

However, empathy can be developed and protected. While Yu et al. state that born character-istics and early-life experiences cannot be changed, they found that empathy may be enhanced through training, practice, and reinforcement of a clinician's identity as a healthcare provider (Yu et al. 2022). Further, clinical organizations can help prevent the decline in empathy by taking actions to minimize workplace stress and prevent burnout (Yu et al. 2022).

For you as a clinician, staying aware of the fluctuations in your ability to empathize, and the factors behind those fluctuations, can allow you to nurture and protect that ability, thus enhancing your job performance, patient satisfaction, and ultimately your own personal fulfillment (Yu et al. 2022; Hojat et al. 2013).

Understanding the various components of empathy can help identify the areas of develop-ment. Mark H. Davis from the University of Texas identified four areas of the empathic process: (1) *fantasy*, or the ability to imagine oneself in a fictional situation such as movies or books; (2) *perspective taking*, or the ability to imagine oneself in another person's real-life situation; (3) *empathic concern*, or the tendency to feel warmth, compassion, and concern for a person expe-riencing a negative situation; and (4) *personal distress*, or the tendency to feel anxiety, apprehen-sion, or discomfort when observing another person in a negative situation (Davis 1980). Among dietitians and dietetic interns, Spraggins et al. found that fantasy and empathic concern are higher among interns, indicating that these qualities may decline with experience (Spraggins et al. 1990). Again, repeated patient exposure, overloaded schedules, and overall work stress may lead to desensitization.

With each patient, you may find yourself reacting in different ways. When meeting people who are similar to you, you may develop an immediate rapport. On the other hand, you may have little in common with your patient and find it more difficult to relate to them. In some cases, you and your patient may have conflicting personality traits, or their emotional state may pose a challenge during counseling. Moreover, your own emotional state may also affect your approach with the patient.

Throughout your encounter with each patient, you may need to frequently perform a self-check to remain engaged. While you are interviewing them, you may sense yourself processing certain thoughts, feelings, judgments, or conclusions about the patient. Practicing mindfulness during these situations can help you to remain present for your patients, work productively with them, and successfully fulfill your role as a healthcare provider.

Mindfulness is "the practice of maintaining a nonjudgmental state of heightened or com-plete awareness of one's thoughts, emotions, or experiences on a moment-to-moment basis" (Mindfulness 2022). It allows you to recognize—without judgment—that you are experiencing reactions to your patient. The practice of mindfulness has been shown to help clinicians foster empathy for their patients as well as for themselves (Tement et al. 2021). By accepting your own state of mind, you minimize the impact of any conflict you may have between how you feel and your role as a healthcare provider, thus minimizing the stress that can contribute to work-related burnout.

PRACTICE TIP: CULTIVATE MINDFULNESS AND EMPATHY

If you sense yourself disengaging from a patient, below are some questions you might ask yourself:

- What am I feeling in response to the patient?
- Why am I feeling this way?

- What feelings are the patient exhibiting? (e.g., fear, anger, sadness, ambivalence, enthusiasm, motivation)
- Why might they be feeling this way?
- If I were in the patient's situation, how would I feel?
- If a loved one were in this patient's situation, how would I feel?
- What experiences have I had that are similar?

The questions above not only help to raise awareness about your feelings during a session, but they also help to understand the perspective of the patient. While you may not share in the experiences of your patient, you may develop empathy by imagining yourself or a loved one in a similar situation. If possible, you might draw from a similar experience of your own so as to appreciate the reasons behind the patient's behaviors. As you mindfully attend to the patient, they are likely to sense that you are engaged. As mentioned earlier, the more they perceive your empathy, the more trust they will develop in you.

COMMUNICATING COMPASSION

The actions and body language you employ to communicate compassion not only demonstrate empathy to the patient, but can also help you thoroughly engage with the patient. Patel et al. (2019) identified the behaviors that may improve patient perceptions of provider empathy and compassion:

- sitting (versus standing) during the interview
- detecting patients' facial expressions and non-verbal cues of emotion
- recognizing and responding to opportunities for compassion
- non-verbal communication of caring (e.g., facing the patient, eye contact)
- verbal statements of acknowledgment, validation, and support.

Most of the behaviors above require that the provider listens closely to the patient so that they can respond appropriately. Mindful listening alone would allow the provider to better understand the patient's point of view.

Effective patient-centered care requires focus, intention, and active engagement. It is no small effort. Communicating compassion while managing your own feelings can be challenging, especially with a difficult patient. It is no wonder that clinicians are at risk of work-related burnout, especially when health care organizations require high patient loads. As such, the energy required to effectively cultivate and communicate empathy can be exhausting.

On the other hand, with each patient that demonstrates improvement, the effort is worth it. Just as you shared their experience through empathy, so can you share in the celebration of their progress. As you observe the impact you make on the lives of others, your sense of fulfillment as a healthcare provider is enhanced, which may minimize the risk of burnout (Trzeciak et al., 2017).

PRACTICE TIP: LISTEN MINDFULLY

Listening will be the hardest part of your job.

In counseling classes, "active listening" is frequently discussed. In a nutshell, active listening involves attentive body language, reflective responses, clarifying questions, and paraphrasing. The more you convey interest and compassion, the more information your patient may be willing to share.

Mindful listening requires that you are also cultivating empathy for their situation, filtering competing thoughts, and being aware of your own feelings and reactions. While being present for the patient, you are simultaneously analyzing the information you are hearing and planning your intervention.

This cognitive balancing act is no small task. It can be physically, mentally, and sometimes emotionally draining. You may feel exhausted at the end of the workday, even though you have spent most of the time sitting in an office.

Some days are better than others. But when done well, you will know it. The most reliable evidence that you are doing your job will come from the patients themselves:

"Thank you. You really listened to me. It really helps me be motivated when I feel heard and understood." *64 year old female, diabetes education participant*

COMPASSION STARTS FROM WITHIN

As outpatient dietitians counsel as much on lifestyle as they do on nutrition, stress management is a common topic of discussion. However, just as our patients may struggle with self-care, so may healthcare professionals. We experience the same life challenges as our patients—busy work schedules, family commitments, health concerns, to name a few. For our patients, we remind them that they will be less able to care for others if they do not take care of themselves first. This same point applies to us as healthcare providers.

If you feel your stress level is impacting your ability to care for your patients, you must consider if you are able to manage it on your own, or if you might require support from a mental health provider. Studies have shown that mindfulness-based interventions can also prevent or relieve burnout among healthcare professionals, as well as foster empathy and compassion (Del Canale et al. 2012; Shapiro et al. 2005). For example, Shapiro et al. (2005) demonstrated that an intervention based on Jon Kabat-Zinn's Mindfulness-Based Stress Reduction program (Kabat-Zinn 1982) was a cost-effective program that could easily be implemented in a healthcare setting. The eight-week intervention provided training in meditation practices emphasizing emotional and cognitive awareness, physical awareness and strengthening, and compassion for self and others.

As burnout prevention is an ongoing concern in health care, discuss with your supervisor or management if such interventions are available through your organization.

BENEATH THE SURFACE

As mentioned earlier, patients may arrive with predisposed notions of what a dietitian can—or cannot—do for them. Further, other past experiences may affect how they respond to you. As counselors, our intent is to provide support and encouragement in response to the patient's concerns. However, the very qualities that make up an empathetic listener can also cause even the most experienced counselor to feel emotional toward a patient. Your own reactions—conscious or subconscious—can influence the direction of the visit.

In researching this chapter, I came across the terms "transference" and "countertransference." Transference was first coined by Sigmund Freud and refers to when a patient directs feelings they once had for an influential individual from their early lives toward their therapist during counseling (Reidbord 2010; Parth et al. 2017). Countertransference, in turn, refers to the counselor's own emotional response to the patient, a phenomenon that can also occur in nutrition counseling (Watts 2001).

In their review, Parth et al. (2017) summarize various views on countertransference, where several theorists emphasize the importance of the therapist in recognizing their emotional responses. They cite Freud's recommendation that therapists themselves undergo analysis to prevent interference in their work. In her article, Watts (2001) further recommends seeking support or advice from trusted colleagues and other team members, as well as a mental health professional, to develop strategies to recognize and manage countertransference. She further states the possibility that, due to personal values, beliefs, or experiences, there may be certain patients or populations for whom the counselor might not be suited. On the other hand, Reidbord (2010) writes that countertransference can occur in direct response to the patient, or in response to a person or event encountered just prior to seeing that patient.

Regardless of the trigger of your emotions, the general consensus is that self-awareness is key. Further, if you notice a recurring pattern of countertransferrence, you may benefit from consulting with a therapist to learn management strategies—not only to prevent interference with your patient care but also to help prevent these emotions from negatively impacting your own mental health.

IMPLICIT BIAS

Just as patients may come to the visit with underlying assumptions and emotions, so too can healthcare providers. These assumptions may be based on implicit bias. As many clinicians enter the field with the intent to help people, many have strong feelings against prejudice in patient care. However, despite our best efforts, it is possible that unconscious stereotyping can affect how we deliver care.

Implicit bias can be defined as unconscious associations, prejudice, or judgments of others based on race, age, gender, weight, or some other characteristics (FitzGerald et al. 2017). The effects of bias in healthcare—both implicit and explicit—are of particular concern to patients who are already most vulnerable (FitzGerald et al. 2017). In their review, FitzGerald et al. (2017) demonstrated that bias can affect how diagnoses are made, how medications are prescribed, or how many tests are ordered. For example, in the review, they cite one study (Burgess et al. 2008) showing that physicians were more likely to prescribe higher doses of opioids to black patients exhibiting belligerent behavior compared to white patients exhibiting the same behavior, possibly due to racial stereotype. Another study (Maserejian et al. 2009) in the review showed that physicians were less likely to diagnose coronary heart disease in women compared to men, but women were more likely to be diagnosed with a mental health condition.

For the RDN, implicit bias may affect how they talk about food or meal planning, how they assess learning needs, what or how much education is provided, level of patient-centered approach, how many behavior change techniques are employed, or how often follow-up visits are scheduled.

In nutrition counseling, body weight is a frequently recurring topic. In some cases, patients will initiate care with an intrinsic motivation to lose weight. In others, they may come on the recommendation of their doctor. There are also cases where neither their complaint nor their referral includes body weight, but it may be a contributing factor. In any case, the impact of stigma and weight bias affects both the patient and the provider. As nutrition is a primary target of weight management, RDNs are often a key component in the intervention. However, one study suggests that about 60% of RDNs have a moderate or strong preference for "thin people over fat people" (Wijayatunga et al. 2021). Thus, developing awareness about—and strategies for—implicit bias is essential.

To learn more about your own tendencies for implicit bias, free self-assessment tools are available online through Project Implicit®, https://implicit.harvard.edu/implicit/. On this site, assessments are available for weight, age, race, gender, disabilities, and more. Project Implicit® is a research collaboration developed by scientists from Harvard, the University of Washington, and the University of Virginia. Their mission is to raise awareness about implicit bias and to collect data to learn more about it. The online assessments are brief and provide results upon completion. It is worthwhile completing some of these assessments as the results can help you think more critically about how you interact with patients. Table 3.1 provides examples of the assumptions that can occur due to implicit bias and how they can detract from the nutrition counseling session.

I wish I could say that I wrote this book because I am so good at what I do, that I can write about bias because I have mastered its impact on myself and my work. But if I am being honest, this book is much more about what I have learned from my mistakes. One thing I have learned is that implicit bias can sneak up on you in surprising ways.

While the topic of implicit bias tends to elicit images of interactions between people of different backgrounds, it should be noted that underlying assumptions can also be based on similarities. As a Filipina-American, I often find myself recalling my own personal experiences when I meet Filipino patients. The moment I encounter somebody whose features are oh-so-identifiable, and whose accent is so comfortably familiar, I am instantly triggered to think about the people who surrounded me all of my life. Images of large families gathered around buffet tables come to mind. In their hands, paper plates sag under the generous weight of saucy stews and stir fries. Aunties force their food onto nieces and nephews, while the uncles are happy to oblige. The elders laugh as they compare A1C levels while they scoop white rice onto their spoons.

Obviously, not all families are the same, regardless of their culture. Thus, these reactions have only enlightened me as to how susceptible we all are to implicit bias. In these cases, I find myself assuming that their intent and motivations are the same as those of my family. Such assumptions might affect how—or if—I apply behavior change strategies.

Ironically, implicit bias does not discriminate. Anyone can be negatively affected. I recall the first time a doctor came to me as a patient. I was still new to the field and learning what people know—and don't know—about nutrition. Moreover, I was accustomed to presenting information in ways that oversimplified the science. When the doctor entered my office, I felt compelled to minimize the information I usually provide, as I assumed he was already familiar with the concepts. To be honest, I was working with a common tendency toward reverence and the belief that doctors are omniscient. As the visit progressed, I came to realize that a detailed review was necessary. After all, if it were not necessary, he would not have come. Unfortunately, valuable time was wasted as I worked through my implicit bias, and the doctor was not receiving my best care.

Over the years, these scenarios, among others, have taught me that when I make assumptions, I am often wrong. The patient who does not appear to be listening ends up applying all of your

---

TABLE 3.1

Examples of Assumptions and Consequences in Nutrition Counseling

Assumptions	Possible Consequences
They will not understand the science	You will not give them a compelling reason to apply your recommendations
They already know the information	You withhold information and they will not learn anything new or worthwhile
They are not interested in the information	You miss an opportunity to tell them something that may appeal to their motivation
They are unable to change	You fail to show them how

recommendations. The person who only wants to be told what to eat ends up grateful for the physiological information. The birthday celebrant who is adamant to indulge all month long ends up celebrating mindfully. The patient, who was initially inactive due to joint pain, reports that exercise actually helped him feel better. And the doctor who asks for help expresses gratitude for a professional and informative visit.

Just as with empathy and compassion, managing bias requires a constant and conscious effort. With each patient, you will find yourself making decisions about what educational strategies you will use or what information you will share. These decisions will be based on the judgments you make while assessing the patient. If you sense yourself holding back your effort, or feeling doubts about the patient, you may be acting on implicit bias. Again, mindfulness is key. Tune in to each hesitation you feel, then question if your hesitation is justified. Some signs that you are acting on implicit bias might be:

- ***You are withholding information.*** Perhaps you are not explaining the physiology of their condition. Or addressing barriers. Or discussing strategies for change. If so, why not? Some assumptions you may have include:

  You think they will not understand it.

  You think they will not apply it.

  You think they do not want it.

  You think they already know it.

  Whatever your reason, do you have evidence that this is true? Did they explicitly decline the information?

  If not, remember that they came to the visit for a reason. Be sure you are asking enough questions to understand the root of their concerns, then make every effort to thoroughly address it.

- ***You are talking more than listening.*** Perhaps you are frequently interrupting the patient. Or not asking enough clarifying questions. Or not allowing time for the patient to ask questions. If your patient has not had a chance to speak in a while, pause and turn it over to them. Encourage them to respond by asking open-ended questions, such as

  "What questions do you have about this information?"

  "Based on this information, what might you do differently?"

  "What, if anything, might keep you from applying this information?"

  Based on their answers, you will learn more about their point of view.

- ***You are feeling impatient with or irritated by the patient.*** If so, why? Perhaps their personality conflicts with yours. Or maybe they are expressing their own irritation. Is this causing you to reduce your education or counseling efforts? If so, remind yourself of your role as a healthcare provider. Ask yourself:

  Will the patient be better off having met me today?

  If not, rethink your assessment. Did you ask enough questions to get to know the patient as a person? Try to learn the patient's point of view. Perhaps ask

  "What motivated you to make this appointment?"

"How does this condition affect your daily life?"

"How will your life be different if this condition improves?"

"What do you hope to accomplish from this visit today?"

By humanizing your patient, you may rediscover your purpose in your work, as well as your responsibility to the patient. When they leave your office, will they

Have a better understanding about their condition?

Feel empowered to take action to protect their health?

Have a plan for what changes to make and how to make them?

- **You are not offering a return visit.** Some reasons you might not offer a return visit include:

  You believe they understood everything.

  You think they will successfully make change without further support.

  You do not think they will make change.

  You feel that you have nothing new to add.

  You did not like them.

If you are making assumptions about what the patient knows, understands, or is willing to do, also assume that you could be wrong. Unless the patient explicitly says they do not want another visit, most people will benefit from follow up. Whether it is to provide more information, answer new questions, reassess their condition, or reinforce their motivation, it is your responsibility to the patient to ensure that your recommendations are effective. The only way you will know is if you follow up with them.

If your personal feelings are impacting your ability to provide ongoing support, you still have an ethical responsibility to provide follow up care to the patient. Arrange for them to follow up with another dietitian in your department. If you struggle with separating your personal feelings from your professional role, consider consulting with a therapist. You may need assistance in developing strategies to identify and overcome any emotional barriers to providing appropriate patient care.

PRACTICE TIP: STRATEGIES TO REDUCE IMPLICIT BIAS

Stereotype replacement. Identify and accept when your response is based on stereotypes, then replace it with a non-stereotypic response.

Counter-stereotypic imaging. Imagine people (such as famous figures or people you know) who break the stereotype. This strategy helps to challenge the stereotypes validity.

Individuation. Focus on the person's individual characteristics, as opposed to stereotypic characteristics.

Perspective taking. Take the perspective of the stigmatized group or stereotype.

Increasing opportunities for contact. Seek ways to interact more often with stigmatized groups to allow for direct evaluation and positive experiences.

Source: Devine et al. (2012)

LIMITS AND BOUNDARIES

I won't lie. Some days are better than others. There will be some patients who are resistant to you, no matter how mindful or compassionate you try to be. Or there may be things you are dealing with yourself that distract you from the moment. Maintaining awareness of both you and your patients' limitations will be key to objectively managing each situation.

If you are struggling to connect with a patient, I have found that the following points may help you stay on task throughout the encounter:

- *Listen and acknowledge.* Whatever feelings your patient may be exhibiting, they are expressing them for a reason. They want to be heard. Acknowledging their feelings will go a lot further than ignoring or debating them. Phrases like, "This must have been hard for you," or "Anyone in your position would be upset" communicates to the patient that you recognize and understand how they feel (Yu et al. 2022; Boissy et al. 2016). Allowing them to vent will release some of their stress in the moment, which may help them become more comfortable during the session. By showing that you care to listen and understand their feelings, they may develop more trust in you and become more receptive to your counsel.

  For you, by listening closely, you will identify what information will be most meaningful for them in that moment, and also rule out which information may fall on deaf ears. You will save valuable time by pinpointing one or two actionable items that directly address the patient's concerns and feelings rather than trying to squeeze in a systematic overview of a topic.

- *You cannot control how they feel, but you can control how you react.* Once you remember the first point, you may be able to focus on the purpose of the visit: to provide education. Sometimes, the anger or resistance that a patient expresses is based on the fear of the unknown, especially if they do not fully understand their condition. By providing them with a better understanding of their condition, with information specific to their concerns, as well as actionable tips that can be reasonably implemented by them, they may be reassured that there are actions still within their control. Moreover, by empowering them with information, they are positioned to take responsibility for their self-care.

  Too often, nutrition counselors feel the pressure to take responsibility for their patients' progress. However, in doing so, we set ourselves up to question our professional competence, which can increase our susceptibility to stress and burnout. By delineating the patient's responsibility in self-care from your role as educator and coach, you can protect yourself from feelings of self-doubt related to your patient's actions or inactions.

- *It's rarely personal.* It is not uncommon for a clinician to feel defensive if a patient expresses negativity during a visit. If your patient exhibits resistance or negativity early in the visit, it likely has nothing to do with you. At that point, they have not known you long enough to develop an opinion of you personally. Their behavior may be based on other feelings. For example, they may be expressing emotions they have regarding their health concerns. Or perhaps they had previously negative healthcare experiences. Maybe they experienced something stressful before arriving.

  On the other hand, if you notice them becoming more resistant to you as the visit progresses, then you may have to consider why they are reacting in such a way. In that case, consider first bullet point.

The opposite can also be true, where a patient may become attached to you beyond the scope of your role. I recall one patient early in my career who requested continued follow-up and dutifully came to each visit. Our interactions were friendly, and we felt warmly toward each other. However, after a few meetings, her visits became more about emotional support and less about nutrition and lifestyle change. On one hand, ongoing support is part of our role as counselors. However, in this case, I noticed that a lot of our discussions were about personal issues surrounding her relationships and other emotional topics. I realized that our visits had gone beyond my expertise. When I suggested that her nutrition education needs had been met, her immediate reaction was, "But I don't have anyone else to talk to."

As I said, we both felt warmly toward each other. Personally, I was glad to provide a listening ear. I knew she appreciated it. However, professionally and ethically, I knew that her needs were not within my scope of practice. To continue seeing her would withhold the type of help she actually needed and would be a misuse of her healthcare funds. Thus, I offered her a referral to a social worker, which she accepted. Later, she reported to me how pleased she was to have the social worker, and I knew that she was in good hands.

By recognizing our limits and boundaries as providers, we can enhance care for our patients by directing them toward the support that will benefit them most, even if it means letting them go.

REFERENCES

Academy Quality Management Committee. Academy of Nutrition and Dietetics: Revised 2017 Scope of Practice for the Registered Dietitian Nutritionist. *J Acad Nutr Diet*. 2018 Jan;118(1):141–165. doi: 10.1016/j.jand.2017.10.002.

Boissy A, Windover AK, Bokar D, Karafa M, Neuendorf K, Frankel RM, Merlino J, Rothberg MB. Communication Skills Training for Physicians Improves Patient Satisfaction. *J Gen Intern Med*. 2016 Jul;31(7):755–761. doi: 10.1007/s11606-016-3597-2.

Burgess DJ, Crowley-Matoka M, Phelan S, Dovidio JF, Kerns R, Roth C, Saha S, van Ryn M. Patient Race and Physicians' Decisions to Prescribe Opioids for Chronic Low Back Pain. *Soc Sci Med*. 2008 Dec;67(11):1852–1860. doi: 10.1016/j.socscimed.2008.09.009.

Davis MH. A Multidimensional Approach to Individual Differences in Empathy. *J Pers Soc Psychol*. 1980;10:85.

Del Canale S, Louis DZ, Maio V, Wang X, Rossi G, Hojat M, Gonnella JS. The Relationship between Physician Empathy and Disease Complications: An Empirical Study of Primary Care Physicians and Their Diabetic Patients in Parma, Italy. *Acad Med*. 2012 Sep;87(9):1243–1249. doi: 10.1097/ACM.0b013e3182628fbf.

Devine PG, Forscher PS, Austin AJ, Cox WT. Long-Term Reduction in Implicit Race Bias: A Prejudice Habit-Breaking Intervention. *J Exp Soc Psychol*. 2012 Nov;48(6):1267–1278. doi: 10.1016/j.jesp.2012.06.003.

Empathy. In Merriam-Webster.com; 2022. Retrieved May 27, 2022 from: https://www.merriam-webster.com/dictionary/empathy.

FitzGerald C, Hurst S. Implicit Bias in Healthcare Professionals: A Systematic Review. *BMC Med Ethics*. 2017 Mar;18(1):19. doi: 10.1186/s12910-017-0179-8.

Hojat M, Louis DZ, Maio V, Gonnella JS. Empathy and Health Care Quality. *Am J Med Qual*. 2013 Jan-Feb;28(1):6–7. doi: 10.1177/1062860612464731.

Hojat M, Louis DZ, Markham FW, Wender R, Rabinowitz C, Gonnella JS. Physician Empathy and Clinical Outcomes for Diabetic Patients. *Acad Med*. 2011;86:359–364.

Kabat-Zinn J. An Outpatient Program in Behavioral Medicine for Chronic Pain Patients Based on the Practice of Mindfulness Meditation: Theoretical Considerations and Preliminary Results. *Gen Hosp Psychiatry*. 1982 Apr;4(1):33–47. doi: 10.1016/0163-8343(82)90026-3.

Maserejian NN, Link CL, Lutfey KL, Marceau LD, McKinlay JB. Disparities in Physicians' Interpretations of Heart Disease Symptoms by Patient Gender: Results of a Video Vignette Factorial Experiment. *J Womens Health*. 2009;18:1661–1667.

Mindfulness. In Merriam-Webster.com; 2022. Retrieved June 5, 2022 from: https://www.merriam-webster.com/dictionary/mindfulness.

Moudatsou M, Stavropoulou A, Philalithis A, Koukouli S. The Role of Empathy in Health and Social Care Professionals. *Healthcare (Basel)*. 2020 Jan;8(1):26. doi: 10.3390/healthcare8010026.

Parth K, Datz F, Seidman C, Löffler-Stastka H. Transference and Countertransference: A Review. *Bull Menninger Clin*. 2017 Spring;81(2):167–211. doi: 10.1521/bumc.2017.81.2.167.

Patel S, Pelletier-Bui A, Smith S, Roberts MB, Kilgannon H, Trzeciak S, Roberts BW. Curricula for Empathy and Compassion Training in Medical Education: A Systematic Review. *PLoS One*. 2019 Aug;14(8):e0221412. doi: 10.1371/journal.pone.0221412.

Project Implicit(r). Available from: https://implicit.harvard.edu/implicit/aboutus.html. Accessed 6/12/2022.

Reidbord, S. An overview of countertransference: What is countertransference? [Internet]. *Psychology Today*. 2010 March 24. Available from: https://www.psychologytoday.com/us/blog/sacramento-street-psychiatry/201003/overview-countertransference. Accessed 1/15/2023.

Shapiro SL, Astin JA, Bishop SR, Cordova M. Mindfulness-Based Stress Reduction for Health Care Professionals: Results from a Randomized Trial. *Int J Stress Manag*. 2005;12(2):164–176. doi: 10.1037/1072-5245.12.2.164. Accessed 6/11/2022.

Spraggins EF, Fox EA, Carey JC. Empathy in Clinical Dietitians and Dietetic Interns. *J Am Diet Assoc*. 1990 Feb;90(2):244–249.

Swan WI, Vivanti A, Hakel-Smith NA, Hotson B, Orrevall Y, Trostler N, Beck Howarter K, Papoutsakis C. Nutrition Care Process and Model Update: Toward Realizing People-Centered Care and Outcomes Management. *J Acad Nutr Diet*. 2017 Dec;117(12):2003–2014. doi: 10.1016/j.jand.2017.07.015.

Tamhane S, Rodriguez-Gutierrez R, Hargraves I, Montori VM. Shared Decision Making in Diabetes Care. *Curr Diab Rep*. 2015;15:112.

Tement S, Ketiš ZK, Miroševič Š, Selič-Zupančič P. The Impact of Psychological Interventions with Elements of Mindfulness (PIM) on Empathy, Well-Being, and Reduction of Burnout in Physicians: A Systematic Review. *Int J Environ Res Public Health*. 2021;18:11181. doi:10.3390/ijerph182111181.

Trzeciak S, Roberts BW, Mazzarelli AJ. Compassionomics: Hypothesis and Experimental Approach. *Med Hypotheses*. 2017 Sep;107:92–97. doi: 10.1016/j.mehy.2017.08.015.

Wagaman MA, Geiger JM, Shockley C, Segal EA. The Role of Empathy in Burnout, Compassion Satisfaction, and Secondary Traumatic Stress among Social Workers. *Soc Work*. 2015 Jul;60(3):201–209. doi: 10.1093/sw/swv014.

Watts LM. Countertransference: A Psychological Aspect of Nutritional Counseling [Internet]. *Eating Disorders Review*. 2001 May/Jun;12(3). Available from: https://eatingdisordersreview.com/counter-transference-a-psychological-aspect-of-nutritional-counseling. Accessed 5/9/2022.

Wijayatunga NN, Bailey D, Klobodu SS, Dawson JA, Knight K, Dhurandhar EJ. A Short, Attribution Theory-Based Video Intervention Does Not Reduce Weight Bias in a Nationally Representative Sample of Registered Dietitians: A Randomized Trial. *Int J Obes (Lond)*. 2021 Apr;45(4):787–794. doi: 10.1038/s41366-021-00740-6.

Yu CC, Tan L, LE MK, Tang B, Liaw SY, Tierney T, Ho YY, Lim BEE, Lim D, Ng R, Chia SC, Low JA. The Development of Empathy in the Healthcare Setting: A Qualitative Approach. *BMC Med Educ*. 2022 Apr;22(1):245. doi: 10.1186/s12909-022-03312-y.

4 Assess and Review

Coming out of school, I was well versed in the science of nutrition. From the Kreb cycle to the pathophysiology of various diseases, I still geek out over scientific illustrations of cell metabolism.

However, I quickly found that there is a learning curve to transitioning from nutrition nerd to nutrition educator.

I am forever grateful to the amazing dietitians who trained me. Experts in their field, their knowledge is deep and always at the ready. The way they deliver information is engaging. They present themselves professionally and credibly. To this day, I am inspired by the practical ideas that they share with their patients.

Starting out, I watched and listened. I took note of the facts that they shared, the analogies that they used, and the tools they employed. I did my best to emulate them. I reiterated their messages and borrowed their techniques. And that is how you learn.

However, with time comes growth. Eventually, it felt like I was borrowing a uniform that was not my size. I looked the part, but I was not fully comfortable. As I learned more about what patients experience, their questions, and their influences, I knew it was time to develop my own style.

What is so engaging about my mentors is their individuality. With their knowledge and experience, they confidently express themselves in their own way. And I realized that I had to do so as well. Just as we aim to provide patient-centered care, so too should educators be true to themselves. After all, relatability goes both ways. The more we get to know our patients, the better we can tailor the intervention. In turn, the better they get to know us, the more confidence they will have in our credibility. Ultimately, you develop a true exchange of information, making for a more productive encounter and hopefully a more positive outcome for the patient.

Once I found my voice, I noticed the difference immediately. Where before my patients were passively listening, I now notice them leaning in. Through their facial expressions and body language, they demonstrate not just understanding, but resonance. They interact more openly with me and actively participate in problem solving. I learned that patient-centered care is not just about customizing the education for the patient, but personalizing it for the educator as well.

From that point, my patients more frequently expressed satisfaction with their care. In turn, I found more purpose in my work and subsequently, more job satisfaction. As previously discussed, professional fulfillment is essential for clinicians to provide compassionate care.

Therefore, developing an effective education experience involves not just the patient's perspective, but yours as well. Tailoring your message will require you to:

> **Understand the science.**
> **Think like a dietitian.**
> **Speak like a person.**

In other words, BE REAL.

UNDERSTAND THE SCIENCE

Upon finishing a dietetics program, graduates have studied an overview of various diseases and related nutrition guidelines. Yet nutrition information continues to evolve. Since I passed my RDN exam over a decade ago, food restrictions in CKD have loosened, the war wages on over fats

DOI: 10.1201/9781003326038-5

versus carbs, and eggs come in and out of favor every couple of years. It is as frustrating to nutrition professionals as it is to patients.

It is important for dietitians to continue to learn, be curious, and stay up to date on the latest guidelines. Read new research with a critical eye, but be open to new information. There is certainly still more to discover.

You will also learn a lot from your patients. They will often ask about popular diets, supplements, and media reports. They will describe various meal plans they have tried. Become familiar with commercial programs and online tools—not necessarily to discredit them, but to understand if or how they work. In my experience, I find that many diet trends are effective not because they are novel, but because they are similar. Whether somebody is watching calories, carbs, fat, protein or points, these key concepts are commonly upheld:

1. Limit added sugars and ultra-processed foods.
2. Eat plenty of plant foods.
3. Control portions.

Whichever condition your patient is concerned with, these concepts are critical in guiding both the nutrition assessment, the education, and the action planning.

A recent patient comes to mind who demonstrates exactly this point. Like many referral notes, the doctor indicated a specific nutrition plan that he wanted the patient to follow. In this case, the doctor was recommending partial meal replacement (PMR). This young man has type 1 diabetes coupled with obesity, but no other complications. He manages his blood glucose with an insulin pump and continuous glucose monitor. His A1C was above goal at 7.4%. His primary goal was to lose weight. However, barriers included a demanding work schedule as he balanced his full-time job with a side hustle. In both jobs, he was mostly sedentary. Due to limited time and meal prep skills, most of his meals came from restaurants of various cuisines in the typical American fashion of large portions and high fat foods.

On one hand, a PMR plan addresses several of his barriers and concerns. They are quick and convenient, requiring little preparation. Medical grade products are highly fortified with protein, vitamins, and minerals, while being low in calories. The carbohydrates are consumed in controlled amounts, spread out throughout the day. On the other hand, it requires the purchase of high-quality products and limits variety day to day.

During the first visit, the patient received a description of his personalized plan, which included two to three PMR products, two to three healthy snacks as needed for hunger or to prevent hypoglycemia, plus one balanced meal, with a calorie goal of about 1,600–1,800 kcal per day. He also received instructions on how to order the PMR products. The patient verbalized understanding and intent to follow the plan.

At the two-week follow-up visit, the patient had already achieved a significant amount of weight loss. However, he was not yet using the PMR products. In fact, he was still getting most of his meals from restaurants. However, he had changed the type of foods that he ordered, choosing mostly salads and protein for meals, plus fruit for snacks. His continuous glucose monitor indicated that his blood sugar was within the target range over 90% of the time with almost no episodes of hypoglycemia. The patient denied frequent hunger, low energy, or any other complaints with his nutrition changes. He also indicated that he found the nutrition changes sustainable.

While PMR is an evidence-based approach to weight loss, the patient's experience demonstrated some key factors that help to reduce weight independent of PMR. By changing the types of food he ordered from restaurants, focusing on healthier choices with more vegetables and fruit, he lowered his overall calorie intake while also improving his intake of vitamins, minerals, and fiber. Not only had he reduced his calories, but he was eating more foods that support metabolism and less foods that hinder it. These choices resulted in improved glycemic patterns that reduced his insulin needs, which also benefits weight loss. Also, by focusing more on fresh, minimally processed foods, he reduced his sodium intake, further reducing weight from water retention.

This case is just one example of how the key concepts of healthy eating can be applied effectively through mindful choices, with or without a specified meal plan, nutrition prescription, or supplement. For the dietitian, these results are not a surprise. However, the challenge is not in understanding which diet approaches work and why. The true challenge is in demonstrating how these concepts can be applied in ways that fit a person's lifestyle, which need not be as complicated as some of these diet plans make it seem. Therefore, nutrition counselors must think beyond the science of nutrition. They must understand behavior and lifestyle factors as well.

THINK LIKE A DIETITIAN

A common expectation among both patients and referring providers is that all dietitians teach specific eating patterns and then *prescribe* meal plans with specific calorie counts, nutrient amounts, or numbers of servings. In turn, the patient would be required to read labels, calculate nutrients, and/or track food throughout the day. However, outpatient dietitians often find that this approach is not always suitable. While some people initially indicate that they are ready to measure and record their foods, the sustainability of this practice is limited, no matter how effective it proves to be. When the initial motivation succumbs to other demands of life, the food log is often one of the first things to go. For some, reading and numeracy skills can be a limiting factor. For others, the effort or emotional burden of counting and tracking prevents them from following a plan.

Another expectation is that dietitians provide specific menus for the patient to follow. In reality, creating ready-to-go meal plans that would appeal to everybody is not feasible, as food preferences, cultural differences, food accessibility, and meal prep skills vary widely. Nor could a dietitian produce a personalized menu for each individual during a 30- or 60-minute session.

When specific meal plans or menus are used, patients commonly report that they are unsure how to adhere to the plan when they are dining out, attending social gatherings, or traveling. The practicality of a specific plan quickly dissipates when a person is taken out of their regular routine or environment, which can occur frequently throughout the year.

Furthermore, when a meal plan becomes tiresome, people often do not understand how to apply the underlying concepts to their own meal planning. Hence, overall efforts at nutrition changes are often discontinued completely. As people commonly say, "I just returned to my old habits."

While dietitians working in a hospital or research setting use meal plans—often with food provisions—to assist patients during the duration of their care, outpatient counseling for lifestyle change often requires a different approach. Dietitians must think beyond calorie counts and serving sizes and consider other factors that affect the patient's choices.

Established guidelines for various conditions provide a framework that guides nutrition therapy, but counseling for behavior change requires more information. In practice, the best available evidence comes from the patients themselves. While research guides us in what to look for (see Table 4.1), the patients show us what else is there (see Table 4.2). From their medical history to their lifestyle choices to their beliefs and barriers, the dietitian can develop a hypothesis—and therefore a targeted intervention—for each individual patient (see Figure 4.1).

For example, if a patient with hyperlipidemia is referred for education about the Mediterranean diet, a description of healthy fats may not be a priority if the patient exhibits emotional eating tendencies. Or carbohydrate counting may not be relevant if a person with diabetes is rationing their insulin. Or the person who frequently socializes over food and drinks may not be able to follow a structured meal plan. For the dietitian, uncovering these factors and having strategies to address them are as important as keeping up with the latest nutrition findings.

TABLE 4.1

Examples of Nutrition Guidelines for Various Conditions and Nutrition Diagnoses

Reason for Referral	Nutrition Diagnosis	Relevant Nutrition Guidelines	Reference
Hypertension	Excessive intake of sodium	Low sodium DASH diet	Whelton et al. (2018)
Hypercholesterolemia	Excessive intake of saturated fat	American Heart Association diet recommendations or Mediterranean diet	Grundy et al. (2019)
Hyperglycemia	Excessive intake of added or refined sugar	American Diabetes Association, Nutrition Therapy for Adults with Diabetes or Prediabetes: A Consensus Report	Evert et al. (2019)
Unintended weight gain	Excessive calorie intake	Obesity in Adults: A Clinical Practice Guideline	Wharton et al. (2020)

TABLE 4.2

Examples of Targeted Education or Intervention

Reason for Referral	Nutrition Diagnosis	Related Lifestyle Behaviors	Patient Reasoning	Targeted Education
Hypertension	Excessive intake of sodium	Frequent dining out	No time to cook	Common sources of excess sodium, i.e., restaurant foods Effect of sodium on blood pressure Time-saving meal planning tips Dining out strategies
Hypercholesterolemia	Excessive intake of saturated fat	Large portions of high fat meat and/or high fat dairy	Following a high protein, low carb diet	Effect of saturated fat on LDL-cholesterol Examples of lean protein Benefits of carbs and fiber Heart healthy fats Balanced meal planning and portion control Mediterranean diet
Hyperglycemia	Excessive intake of added or refined sugar	Regular consumption of fruit juice	Juice is natural and healthy	Effect of various types of carbohydrates on blood sugar Amount of sugar in juice Benefits of fiber and whole fruit
Unintended weight gain	Excessive calorie intake	Inadequate intake during the day (i.e., skipped or inadequate meals), leading to increased hunger and overconsumption in the evening	"Saving calories" in effort to lose weight	Role of nutrients and calories Benefits of balanced meals on hunger, satiety, and cravings Meal timing Daytime versus nighttime metabolism

Typically, upon completion of the nutrition assessment, a person's individual risk factors and behaviors become apparent. Targeting the education toward those factors will resonate more than a general description of nutrition guidelines. Whether they need dining out strategies or tips on meal planning, understanding the person's lifestyle is as important as knowing the science.

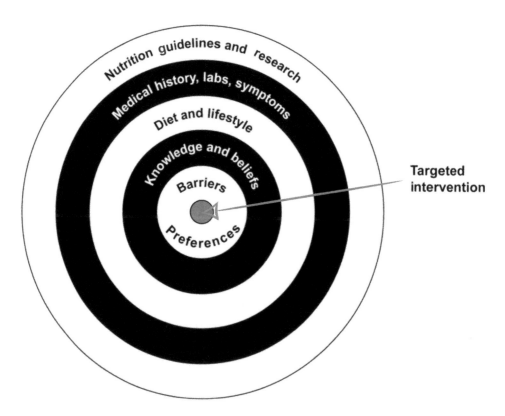

FIGURE 4.1   The best available evidence comes from the patients themselves. In addition to established guidelines, a thorough assessment of a person's medical history, lifestyle, barriers, and preferences will target the intervention.

SPEAK LIKE A PERSON

Communicating with a patient goes beyond using plain language. While the words that we use, the speed in which we speak, and the imagery that we invoke can transfer knowledge, true understanding will also come from relatability.

I recall a dietetic intern who assisted me with a group education session. She was discussing yogurt and recommended to sweeten plain, non-fat yogurt with fresh berries, which is certainly a delicious and healthy choice. However, during our lunch break after class, I noticed that she had a flavored yogurt packed in her lunch—as I have seen many dietitians do, including myself. For these dietitians, convenience is as much a factor in their meal planning as it is for our patients. Like others, we also have to rush in the morning to throw our lunch together or have healthy choices easily accessible when hunger hits. In other words, we are not just dietitians. We are people too. Further, we understand that our health is determined not by any one product, but by our overall eating pattern. As such, our recommendations should reflect that. For example, in addition to recommending plain yogurt sweetened with berries, a discussion about how to select healthier convenience products would also be beneficial.

To suggest strategies that we do not ourselves employ may not only be impractical for our patients, but may also impact our credibility. At best, the patient may perceive the educator as unrelatable. At worst, the patient may find healthy eating an unattainable goal, reinforcing any resistance to change they already have. This is especially probable for those with an "all or nothing" mindset—which, unfortunately, is a common attitude in diet culture.

On more than one occasion, I have heard a patient begin a nutrition assessment by saying, "I know you're going to take everything good away from me." While they may be referring to some of their favorite foods, dietitians must be mindful not to disregard their overall quality of life. Factors such as convenience, enjoyment, social interactions, and other issues must be incorporated into the education and counseling.

Many dietitians promote the "80/20 rule," which acknowledges that dietary perfection is an impractical approach. Specifically, this rule of thumb suggests that people follow dietary recommendations 80% of the time, and not to worry about the other 20%. Dietitians can further illustrate this concept by sharing some of their own challenges, demonstrating their understanding about the everyday barriers that life can impose. While it is important to display your knowledge as a nutrition educator, establishing relatability may enhance your influence as a nutrition counselor. In some ways, you might serve as one of the initial role models for change. After all, dietitians themselves face similar challenges—work schedules, family matters, financial budgets, and social activities. Dietitians can draw from these experiences to relate to their patients.

One of the most important experiences that a dietitian can share is that perfection is not only unattainable but also unnecessary. Even centenarians often admit to some lifelong indulgences. Hail to those who preserve their own vegetables and make their own sourdough. But if your patient is not already doing that, a focus on mindfulness for overall balance will suffice.

Health literacy refers not only to understanding information but also to applying that information in everyday life. Therefore, while you should think like a dietitian, be sure to speak like a person—imperfections and all. Your patients will hear you better that way.

PRACTICE TIP: IF YOU WANT THEM TO COME BACK, TELL THEM SOMETHING NEW

When I first started as a health coach for a lifestyle change program, I faithfully followed the curriculum, but struggled with early attrition. While the program materials were practical and well designed, the information was not new. For many of the participants, this was not their first rodeo. They had heard the "size of a deck of cards" speech before. They had tracked food, calories, or points before. They learned to "shop the perimeter of the grocery store" before.

I realized that in order to get them to come back, I needed to give them something they had not heard before. Something generally not covered in a commercial weight loss program or health app.

I recalled how I felt the first time I started learning about nutrition. All of a sudden, things started to make sense, like why some foods helped me to feel full longer, while others made me shaky and starving within an hour or two. Or why I struggled with weight loss, even though I was exercising. Or why I craved junk food when my stress was high.

The *science* of nutrition resonated because it shed light on everyday experiences.

It is not uncommon for some nutrition counselors to jump right into nutrition guidelines or meal planning. Many shy away from explaining the science, assuming that it may be too confusing or uninteresting for the patient. However, I argue that it is foundational for empowering the patient.

The sheer number of products and programs claiming to "reset your metabolism" or "cleanse" your system indicates that many people are indeed interested in the science.

But few receive comprehensive and reliable nutrition education and are unable to discern between marketing ploys and good science. They are making food choices and purchase decisions based on minimal or misleading information. Therefore, when they come to us for help, it is our duty to provide that education.

And the more new information you can give them, the more likely they will see value in coming back.

More about health literacy and teaching strategies are covered later in this book.

REFERENCES

Evert AB, Dennison M, Gardner CD, Garvey WT, Lau KHK, MacLeod J, Mitri J, Pereira RF, Rawlings K, Robinson S, Saslow L, Uelmen S, Urbanski PB, Yancy WS Jr. Nutrition Therapy for Adults with Diabetes or Prediabetes: A Consensus Report. *Diabetes Care.* 2019 May;42(5):731–754. doi: 10.2337/dci19-0014.

Grundy SM, Stone NJ, Bailey AL, Beam C, Birtcher KK, Blumenthal RS, Braun LT, de Ferranti S, Faiella-Tommasino J, Forman DE, Goldberg R, Heidenreich PA, Hlatky MA, Jones DW, Lloyd-Jones D, Lopez-Pajares N, Ndumele CE, Orringer CE, Peralta CA, Saseen JJ, Smith SC Jr, Sperling L, Virani SS, Yeboah J. 2018 AHA/ACC/AACVPR/AAPA/ABC/ACPM/ADA/AGS/APhA/ASPC/NLA/PCNA Guideline on the Management of Blood Cholesterol: A Report of the American College of Cardiology/American Heart Association Task Force on Clinical Practice Guidelines. *Circulation.* 2019 Jun;139(25):e1082–e1143. doi: 10.1161/CIR.0000000000000625. Epub 2018 Nov 10. Erratum in: Circulation. 2019 Jun 18;139(25):e1182–e1186.

Wharton S, Lau DCW, Vallis M, Sharma AM, Biertho L, Campbell-Scherer D, Adamo K, Alberga A, Bell R, Boulé N, Boyling E, Brown J, Calam B, Clarke C, Crowshoe L, Divalentino D, Forhan M, Freedhoff Y, Gagner M, Glazer S, Grand C, Green M, Hahn M, Hawa R, Henderson R, Hong D, Hung P, Janssen I, Jacklin K, Johnson-Stoklossa C, Kemp A, Kirk S, Kuk J, Langlois MF, Lear S, McInnes A, Macklin D, Naji L, Manjoo P, Morin MP, Nerenberg K, Patton I, Pedersen S, Pereira L, Piccinini-Vallis H, Poddar M, Poirier P, Prud'homme D, Salas XR, Rueda-Clausen C, Russell-Mayhew S, Shiau J, Sherifali D, Sievenpiper J, Sockalingam S, Taylor V, Toth E, Twells L, Tytus R, Walji S, Walker L, Wicklum S. Obesity in Adults: A Clinical Practice Guideline. *CMAJ.* 2020 Aug;192(31):E875–E891. doi: 10.1503/cmaj.191707.

Whelton PK, Carey RM, Aronow WS, Casey DE Jr, Collins KJ, Dennison Himmelfarb C, DePalma SM, Gidding S, Jamerson KA, Jones DW, MacLaughlin EJ, Muntner P, Ovbiagele B, Smith SC Jr, Spencer CC, Stafford RS, Taler SJ, Thomas RJ, Williams KA Sr, Williamson JD, Wright JT Jr. 2017 ACC/AHA/AAPA/ABC/ACPM/AGS/APhA/ASH/ASPC/NMA/PCNA Guideline for the Prevention, Detection, Evaluation, and Management of High Blood Pressure in Adults: Executive Summary: A Report of the American College of Cardiology/American Heart Association Task Force on Clinical Practice Guidelines. *Hypertension.* 2018 Jun;71(6):1269–1324. doi: 10.1161/HYP.0000000000000066. Erratum in: Hypertension. 2018 Jun;71(6):e136–e139. Erratum in: *Hypertension.* 2018 Sep;72(3):e33.

5 Empower the Patient

Throughout an encounter, your patient will nod along, verbalize understanding, and hopefully ask engaged questions. You will feel assured that you are delivering information in ways that are comprehensible and, hopefully, practical. Perhaps you use pictures, models, or Internet resources to illustrate your points. As you near the finish line, you feel confident that the education you are providing is clear, and maybe even motivating.

And then a funny thing happens.

After dropping all of that eye-opening nutrition knowledge, you ask them what goal they are ready to set for themselves. You wait in anticipation for them to validate your skills as a nutrition educator. You expect to hear a goal to increase vegetables, or avoid the drive-thru, or cut back on sweets.

But then they say, "I'm going to start exercising more."

After 45 minutes of talking about food, and perhaps only five minutes spent on physical activity, the piece that often resonates is exercise. This is a phenomenon I have observed over and over again, and I almost laugh because it happens so often. When I first encountered this response, I felt compelled to redirect them and to consider changes in their meal planning. I wondered if I had been unconvincing in my delivery, or if I failed to demonstrate the direct impact of food on their symptoms. Or perhaps they were simply resistant to changing their eating habits.

But then I remember the lessons I learned in patient empowerment training at the University of Michigan and I realize that my job is not to define the patients' goals for them, but to assist them in making informed decisions about managing their own health (Funnell and Anderson, 1991). Martha Funnell MS, RN, CDCES, FAAN and colleagues introduced the *philosophy of empowerment* to diabetes education, recognizing that "people have an inherent drive towards health and growth, and…the fundamental right … to have the power to control their own healthcare behavior" (Funnell and Anderson, 1991). Together with Robert M. Anderson, EdD and their team, they posited that "if given the freedom to choose and the opportunity to reflect on their lives, [patients] would be willing and able to select appropriate goals related to living with and caring for their diabetes" (Anderson et al., 1995). Their research not only supported that assumption but also resulted in improved glucose control (Anderson et al., 1995).

In my own practice, I have observed similar outcomes in nutrition and lifestyle counseling. As such, I no longer worry when a patient seemingly excludes nutrition changes from their goals. In fact, I have observed another recurring phenomenon that has given me solace on these occasions: a domino effect. When a person makes one healthy change, they often make others as well. In other words, when those patients who set a goal around physical activity return, they often report healthful nutrition changes as well. I have also observed the opposite, where those who planned to make dietary changes also report increases to physical activity. Furthermore, similar to the findings of Anderson et al., clinical improvements are often observed with these changes, even if clinical management was not the focus of the goal-setting exercise (Anderson et al., 1995).

The philosophy of patient empowerment aligns with the principles of *evidence-based medicine*, in which clinical decisions are made based on the best available evidence, together with the values and preferences of the patient (Djulbegovic and Guyatt, 2017; Tamhane et al., 2015). EBM also encourages *shared decision-making*, where the patient is informed of their treatment options, efficacy, risks, and benefits, and then are included in the decision-making process (Djulbegovic and Guyatt, 2017; Tamhane et al., 2015).

DOI: 10.1201/9781003326038-6

GOAL SETTING, PROBLEM SOLVING, AND ACTION PLANNING

Ideally, by the end of the encounter, the SHARE process will result in an action plan—a tangible outline of what the patient is willing and able to do about something that is important to them.

To be fair, some will be ready to implement a plan right away. Others may need to think about it some more. Some may decide that they are not willing to do anything at all. These levels of readiness, or stages of change, are described by Prochaska and DiClemente's *Transtheoretical Model of Change* (1983), a behavior change theory that is commonly applied in lifestyle change interventions (as cited by Prochaska et al., 2008). The theory posits that people's intent to change increases with their stage of readiness, and that the intervention should be tailored to their current stage, with the goal of advancing them to the next stage. However, moving from one stage to another is a dynamic process that can progress or regress. The stages include:

1. Pre-contemplation - No intention to change.
2. Contemplation - Intends to take action within six months.
3. Preparation - Intends to take action within 30 days.
4. Action - Changed within the last six months.
5. Maintenance - Changed for over six months.
6. Termination - No relapse and 100% confidence.

While this theory has some criticisms for its arbitrary timelines and seemingly obvious association between readiness and intention (West, 2005), it would be remiss to deny that each person will present at a different stage. Some will already have implemented healthy changes. And yes, there will be others who came just "because my doctor told me to." Others may want to change, but do not know how.

There is also the possibility that the counselor could misread the person. A person may appear resistant and ambivalent when in fact they actually lack confidence, or self-efficacy, because they are unsure of what to do or how to do it. Conversely, someone could exude motivation and confidence, but might not truly understand the severity of the situation, and therefore their motivation might easily wane. Either of these scenarios might cause a counselor to withhold information or exclude the action planning process—either because they think the person does not want it or does not need it.

PRACTICE TIP: MAKE NO ASSUMPTIONS

One concern with the Transtheoretical Model of Change is that counselors may be dismissive of someone who appears not ready, and therefore make a weaker attempt at intervention (West, 2005).

Be cautious not to equate "readiness" with "ability" to change.

Both factors could be affected by any or all the following:

Lack of information (e.g., what, why, and how).
Lack of self-efficacy.
Lack of social support or role models.
Lack of resources.

As discussed in the section on implicit bias (Chapter 3), make no assumptions, withhold nothing. SHARE knowledge equitably and without judgment. You just might provide the one thing they need to hear to consider or make change.

In most cases, a counselor cannot go wrong in providing education. From there, the person is equipped to decide what course of action they are ready and willing to take. As Ryan and Deci (2000) proposed with the *Self-Determination Theory* (as cited in Street and Epstein, 2008), autonomy and competence (also known as self-efficacy) are key components in eliciting intrinsic motivation (Legault, 2016). As the counselor, you can empower your patient with information and guide them in the action planning process. But ultimately, the likelihood of long-term success is increased when they select the actions that are important and enjoyable to them.

Motivational interviewing is an evidence-based approach designed to guide a patient in exploring how their values align with their behaviors (Miller and Rollnick, 2013; Motivational Interviewing Network of Trainers, 2021). The approach is ubiquitously discussed in behavior change and counseling courses and provides a framework for communication for the counselor that emphasizes open-ended questions, active and reflective listening, and information exchange. As with empowerment and shared decision-making, a compassionate, respectful, and collaborative discussion can encourage a patient to open up about the underlying thoughts and feelings that impact their health decisions. Again, uncovering a person's intrinsic motivation will be critical to behavior change.

TALES FROM THE FIELD: LONELY AT THE TOP

Kevin, age 61, suffered from osteoarthritis in his knees. His doctor advised him that weight loss would help relieve some of the pressure on his joints. They had also discussed the possibility of knee replacement surgery. In that case, the doctor also advised that weight loss would help minimize complications after surgery.

Like many people, Kevin's weight had slowly crept up over the years. As his knee pain developed, he restricted physical activity, which further contributed to weight gain. Unfortunately, the extra weight only worsened his knee condition, resulting in a vicious cycle.

One day, he was on vacation with his daughter's family. While exploring a state park, they came upon a long set of stairs that led down to a lake. While his grandchildren were excited to run down to the beach, he was unable to join them. Instead, he stayed behind and watched them from the top of the stairs.

As he relayed his story in nutrition counseling, his eyes brimmed with tears. "I want to be able to enjoy time with my grandchildren. I don't ever want to wait at the top again. Next time, I want to go down to that beach with them."

Kevin had identified a long-term goal that was rooted deeply in his values: Family time and togetherness. His knee pain had affected him not only physically, but emotionally and socially as well.

He envisioned an outcome that went beyond pain relief, but also a quality of life that was deeply important to him.

Change for the sake of change is generally not enough. Sometimes, change for the sake of health is difficult to grasp as well. But when a person can recognize a deeper benefit, that vision may serve as the driving force to initiate, and hopefully maintain, change.

As with everybody, motivation comes in different ways, at different times, and with different intensities. But no matter what, it can only come from one place: From within.

The practice of *goal setting* repeatedly shows efficacy in behavior change (Bailey, 2017; Samdal et al., 2017), therefore is often incorporated into intervention programs or counseling approaches. Throughout the years, I have encountered various goal sheets designed to guide self-reflection and invoke intrinsic motivation. They often aim to elicit the following information:

A long-term goal.
A short-term goal.
An action plan.
A back up plan.

Kevin's story is an example of a *long-term goal*, a vision for what he wants for himself in the future. This type of goal encapsulates the patient's personal values and desires and may provide the foundation that upholds their motivation.

The second type of goal is a *short-term goal*, or a measurable objective that can help the patient move closer towards their long-term goal. Commonly referred to as "incremental steps," research supports that performing achievable tasks with progressive difficulty can lead to behavior change (Samdal et al., 2017). However, determining which short-term goals to set will require a deeper investigation into which factors have been undermining the patient's health behaviors in the first place.

Therefore, guiding the patient through the problem-solving process is a worthwhile exercise. While there are several variations of the problem-solving process, the main points generally include:

1. Identify the root problem.
2. Brainstorm several solutions to the problem.
3. Select one solution to try.
4. Develop an action plan to test the solution.
5. Implement the plan.
6. Evaluate the outcome.
7. Decide next steps—either continue the plan or repeat the problem-solving process to create a new plan.

TALES FROM THE FIELD: THE ROOT PROBLEM

Michelle, 44, was a participant in a group weight loss program. She was a mother of three children in elementary school. Like most parents, her mornings were hectic as she helped them get ready for school each day. From getting them dressed to feeding them breakfast to driving them to school on time, her own needs were not the priority at that time of day. As such, she often left the house without having breakfast.

For Michelle, once she left the house, her mornings were filled with school events, errands, or appointments. Without breakfast, she often found herself starving while she was out and about. As she learned more about balanced meal planning and managing hunger, she decided she wanted to include breakfast more often. However, she struggled with ideas, so at one meeting, she asked, "What are some good breakfasts I can have in the car while I drive my kids to school?"

Her question triggered a group discussion about breakfast ideas. Suggestions ranged from protein bars to trail mix to mini frittatas made in muffin tins. She nodded to some suggestions, wrinkled her nose at others. But after bouncing around some ideas, Michelle blurted out, "But I don't have time in the morning. That's the real problem!"

At that point, Michelle had stumbled upon the first step in the problem-solving process: *Identify the root problem*. Initially, she thought she needed breakfast ideas. But in reality, before she could put those ideas to work, what she really needed was to find ways to carve out time to plan and prepare—which would require its own brainstorm of ideas.

For Michelle, possible solutions included prepping breakfast the night before, preparing several ready-to-go meals at the start of the week, or waking up earlier to eat before leaving. Throughout the program, she continued to try new things, make different choices, and become more mindful about meal planning. As for many people, some weeks were better than others, but she continued to strive towards change.

Problem solving is a dynamic process. It involves trial and error and is subject to motivation and intent. But the process addresses some key tenets of behavior change: awareness, autonomy, skill building, and self-efficacy. Therefore, problem-solving is a worthwhile exercise to include with each patient encounter.

For the counselor, developing an *action plan* is the ultimate goal of the encounter. This final exercise appeals to the patient's autonomy and self-efficacy by encouraging them to determine what steps they are willing and able to take next. When implementing the plan, they further bolster their self-efficacy through hands-on experience and practice (Lawrance and McLeroy, 1986). Taking action also builds the relevant skills needed to achieve mastery of these behaviors. Through the plan, the patient can test the information they received and evaluate their efficacy for themselves.

TALES FROM THE FIELD: SEEING IS BELIEVING

At 70 years old, Lola had not previously worried about her diet. In retirement, she enjoyed an active social life, frequently dining out or attending parties with her friends. Although she took medications for blood pressure and lipid management, she did not have cardiovascular complications. Despite her food choices, low physical activity, and higher weight, she did not have diabetes or any other chronic disease. With few health concerns, she had no compelling reason to worry about nutrition. As such, her diet was excessive in sodium from dining out and processed foods; high in simple sugar as she had a weakness for sweets; and also high in refined carbs due to the white rice and noodles that are staples in her Asian cuisine.

On occasion, Lola would experience symptoms of hypoglycemia, typically after a prolonged fast or missed meal. When this happened, her tendency was to reach for soda or sweets, often together, and without regard to portion.

In speaking to a dietitian, at first, Lola was jovial and courteous throughout the discussion, albeit ambivalent about the information. However, as the discussion progressed, she became more thoughtful and her countenance became more serious. As it turned out, both her mother and older sister had suffered massive, debilitating strokes that resulted in long-term suffering before ultimately passing. As she learned more about how nutrition affected her personal risk for stroke, there was a visible change in her demeanor. One might say that in that moment, she moved from pre-contemplation to contemplation.

Over the next several weeks, she started trying new things. First, she mixed brown rice and white rice in her rice cooker. After a couple of weeks, she switched completely to brown rice and easily adjusted to the change. She also reduced how much rice she ate with each meal.

At breakfast, instead of four pieces of toast, she cut back to two pieces with peanut butter and added an orange.

At lunch, she included a salad.

She even started walking in the neighborhood. At first, she started with one block, but then progressively started walking farther.

Within a few months, her clothing size went from 1x to size 12. She was glowing with pride and welcomed the compliments.

Most notably, she stated, "If these changes didn't work, I wouldn't keep doing it. But they work, so I do it."

Wise words.

An important part of action planning is *preparing for obstacles*. Obstacles may be logistical and/ or emotional. For example, logistically, if a person planned to walk in the neighborhood, weather conditions might affect their plan. Therefore, having an alternative plan lined up can help keep the person on track. Perhaps they can go to an indoor location like a mall or recreation center instead. Or maybe they have access to online walking videos that they can do in the living room. Having these ideas ready can help sustain a person's sense of empowerment when the unexpected occurs.

There will be times, of course, when alternatives are not available, and these may have emotional consequences. An urgent matter may come up at work or at home. Or there might be a last-minute invitation from a friend. Or a bad night's sleep may affect their energy level or appetite or both. Life happens. And it will happen again and again. These are perhaps the most impactful challenges that people encounter because they are recurring and inevitable. They may be accompanied by an emotional burden such as stress or worry. Or the episode may be followed by feelings of guilt or failure, especially for those whose self-efficacy was low in the first place. If it happens repeatedly, the cost of the effort may seem to outweigh the benefit, leading to a complete cessation of action. All too often, this cycle of regression repeats itself.

Therefore, a self-reflection on *coping skills* is also critical in the action planning stage. Anticipating how setbacks may make one *feel* is as important as planning what someone can *do*. For many of your patients, this will not be their first rodeo. In fact, many will tell you about past experiences that worked and did not work for them. Exploring these past experiences can help them uncover what thoughts and feelings impacted the outcome of those efforts and consider ways to reframe similar situations in the future.

Every person has a story. Through SHARE, their story will unfold in ways you cannot predict. From their past experiences with food, to their current challenges, to where they want to be in the future, people will reveal quite a bit when they are given the space to speak, and when they feel they are being heard. The more you learn about their lives, the more you see what is contributing to their symptoms and lab values. When you help them see those connections, many will respond with relief. What was once puzzling becomes clear. Effective solutions become apparent. In many cases, people learn that their struggles are not their fault, but that the pathophysiology of their disease is the underlying culprit. For example, for a woman with PCOS, learning about the effects of hyperinsulinemia on blood sugar and fat production finally explains why she craves sweets and has trouble losing weight, whereas before she blamed her lack of willpower. In other cases, people become more amenable to applying recommendations as they learn *why* those recommendations are made. For example, the person newly diagnosed with diabetes who has been avoiding carbohydrates will better understand why they are fatigued with recurring headaches when they learn about the role of glucose, then may be less leery of including carbohydrates in their diet. Most people will find that the changes that will help them are not as extreme or restrictive as they had believed.

Information is power. Sharing that power helps both the provider and patient. By listening to their story, you are empowered to guide them. By providing education, you empower them to take the lead.

In classes and in training, I was ingrained with the strategies and approaches for patient-centered care. Going into practice, however, I was not sure where to begin. In preparation for my first job, I pulled out my textbooks and journal articles on motivational interviewing. I tried to memorize open-ended questions and conversation starters. I even created assessment sheets to guide myself in guiding the patient. But in practice, I found it easier just to engage the person in open dialogue and get to know them.

To SHARE is to respect.

REFERENCES

Anderson RM, Funnell MM, Butler PM, Arnold MS, Fitzgerald JT, Feste CC. Patient Empowerment. Results of a Randomized Controlled Trial. *Diabetes Care*. 1995 Jul;18(7):943–949. doi: 10.2337/diacare.18.7.943.

Bailey RR. Goal Setting and Action Planning for Health Behavior Change. *Am J Lifestyle Med*. 2017 Sep;13(6):615–618. doi: 10.1177/1559827617729634.

Djulbegovic B, Guyatt GH. Progress in Evidence-Based Medicine: A Quarter Century on. *Lancet*. 2017 Jul;390(10092):415–423. doi: 10.1016/S0140-6736(16)31592-6. Epub 2017 Feb 17.

Funnell MM, Anderson RM, Arnold MS, Barr PA, Donnelly M, Johnson PD, Taylor-Moon D, White NH. Empowerment: An Idea Whose Time Has Come in Diabetes Education. *Diabetes Educ*. 1991 Jan-Feb;17(1):37–41. doi: 10.1177/014572179101700108.

Lawrance L, McLeroy KR. Self Efficacy and Health Education. *J Sch Health*. 1986;56(8):317–321.

Legault L. "Intrinsic and Extrinsic Motivation." In: Ziegler-Hill V, Shackelford TK. (eds) *Encyclopedia of Personality and Individual Differences*. Cham: Springer-; 2016. pp. 1–4. doi: 10.1007/978-3-319-28099-8_1139-1.

Miller, WR, Rollnick S. *Motivational Interviewing*: *Helping People Change* (3rd Edition). New York NY: The Guilford Press; 2013.

Motivational Interviewing Network of Trainers. Understanding Motivational Interviewing [Internet]. Alexandria, VA: MINT; 2021. Available from: https://motivationalinterviewing.org/understanding-motivational-interviewing. Accessed 5/9/2023.

Prochaska JO, DiClemente CC. Stages and Process of Self-Change of Smoking: Toward and Integrative Model of Change. *J Consult Clin Psychol*. 1983;51:390–395.

Prochaska JO, Redding CA, Evers KE. "The Transtheoretical Model and Stages of Change." In: Glanz K, Rimer BK, Viswanath K. (eds) *Health Behavior and Health Education*: *Theory, Research, and Practice*. San Francisco, CA: Jossey-Bass; 2008. pp. 97–121.

Ryan RM, Deci EL. Self-determination Theory and the Facilitation of Intrinsic Motivation, Social Development, and Well-Being. *Am Psychol*. 2000;55(1):68–78.

Samdal GB, Eide GE, Barth T, Williams G, Meland E. Effective Behaviour Change Techniques for Physical Activity and Healthy Eating in Overweight and Obese Adults; Systematic Review and Meta-Regression Analyses. *Int J Behav Nutr Phys Act*. 2017 Mar;14(1):42. doi: 10.1186/s12966-017-0494-y.

Street RL, Epstein RM. "Key Interpersonal Functions and Health Outcomes: Lessons from Theory and Research on Clinician-Patient Communication." In: Glanz K, Rimer BK, Viswanath K. (eds) *Health Behavior and Health Education: Theory, Research, and Practice*. San Francisco, CA: Jossey-Bass; 2008. pp. 237–269.

Tamhane S, Rodriguez-Gutierrez R, Hargraves I, Montori VM. Shared Decision-Making in Diabetes Care. *Curr Diab Rep*. 2015 Dec;15(12):112. doi: 10.1007/s11892-015-0688-0.

West R. Time for a Change: Putting the Transtheoretical (Stages of Change) Model to Rest. *Addiction*. 2005 Aug;100(8):1036–1039. doi: 10.1111/j.1360-0443.2005.01139.x.

Part II

Everyday Eating Routines

A Different EER

6 Motivations and Barriers

At the start of any lifestyle change program, a survey of the room will reveal a common experience: a health scare.

In many group programs, it is a common practice to ask each participant to introduce themselves and share why they joined the program. The sentiments are often so similar, that by the last person, they start answering, "Just as everybody else said…I want to turn this around."

Whether in a group or individual setting, for many, a meeting with a dietitian will not be their first foray into diet and lifestyle change. Many have counted calories, joined commercial weight loss programs, worked with personal trainers, or tried other strategies. And indeed, most would testify that they were effective, "…until I stopped." Subsequently, they returned to old habits, the results diminished, and they found themselves starting over, stating, "I know what to do. I'm just not doing it."

Indeed, the basic concepts of a healthy lifestyle are well accepted by most people. Portion control. Eat vegetables. Don't eat junk food. Exercise. Few people argue the merits of these concepts. Even less aspire to develop a chronic disease.

And yet, maintaining motivation continues to be the holy grail.

While many people experience this vicious cycle, with each individual, the challenge for the dietitian is to pinpoint *why*. Why do people make—or not make—the changes that could keep them healthier longer? Identifying a patient's personal barriers is the first step in determining which educational points will resonate most for that person. Rarely is a discussion about calories the impetus for change. Instead, a deeper investigation is required to uncover whether a person's challenges are logistical, emotional, social, informational—or some hierarchical combination of them all. Thus, developing insight into how life influences behavior is key for nutrition counseling.

A few years into my career, I had the opportunity to facilitate a CDC-recognized Diabetes Prevention Program. I found this experience to be the best training for nutrition counseling. Over the course of a year, health coaches witness first-hand the efficacy of evidence-based strategies such as goal setting, action planning, food and exercise tracking and self-monitoring (Samdal et al. 2017). While the program itself has its criticisms—from its focus on weight to its downplay of healthy fats to its requirements for Medicare reimbursement—the personal interactions with and among the participants are deeply affecting. Experiences are shared. Friendships form. There are a lot of laughs. Participants share their struggles as well as their successes. They learn from each other, and the health coach learns from them. Over the year, the participants demonstrate the seasonality of people's lifestyles, and how food preferences, energy levels, social influences, and motivational factors can differ with the weather or around holidays. They reveal how friends and family can help, or hurt, their efforts, and how some barriers may be simply insurmountable. Overall, coaches develop a clearer view of how health behaviors intersect with the daily realities of life.

With the Health Belief Model (HBM), Hochbaum and colleagues (1958) suggested that the decision to change behavior follows a cue to action (as cited in Champion and Skinner 2008). Many of the introductions at the start of a lifestyle change program demonstrate that theory. Some common sentiments include:

"I was diagnosed with prediabetes and I knew I had to do something."
"I saw what it did to my [*dad/mom/other*] and I don't want to go through that."

DOI: 10.1201/9781003326038-8

"I don't want to start any medications."

"I want to turn this around."

However, while there may be a trigger to take action, HBM also recognizes that there are several other factors that influence the change process. While a sense of severity and susceptibility may bring a person to a lifestyle change program or nutrition counseling, overcoming barriers and building self-efficacy will be important in making and maintaining change.

While each person has their own unique situation and perspective, there are some common factors that result in certain eating patterns. While the first part of this book focused on the importance of listening to your patient, the next part of this book describes some of the things you will hear, including various barriers, concerns, frequently asked questions, and everyday eating patterns that come up in nutrition counseling.

COMMON FACTORS THAT AFFECT EATING PATTERNS

Time constraints

Family responsibilities

Work demands

Stress

Mental and emotional health

Comorbidities

Lack of social support

Lack of access

Misinformation

REFERENCES

Champion VL, Skinner CS. "The Health Belief Model." In: Glanz K, Rimer BK, Viswanath K. (eds) *Health Behavior and Health Education: Theory, Research, and Practice.* San Francisco, CA: Jossey-Bass; 2008. p 45–65.

Hochbaum GM. *Public Participation in Medical Screening Programs: A Socio-Psychological Study.* Washington, DC: US Dept. of Health, Education, and Welfare; 1958.

Samdal GB, Eide GE, Barth T, Williams G, Meland E. Effective Behaviour Change Techniques for Physical Activity and Healthy Eating in Overweight and Obese Adults; Systematic Review and Meta-Regression Analyses. *Int J Behav Nutr Phys Act.* 2017 Mar;14(1):42. doi: 10.1186/s12966-017-0494-y. PMID: 28351367; PMCID: PMC5370453.

7 A Different EER

Twenty years ago, at a summer barbeque, I watched a friend wrap a hot dog in a slice of American cheese. "I'm doing Atkins," he said, adding, "I already lost five pounds since last week."

Around that same period, my office mate grumbled about a headache. She was a few days into South Beach, another very low carb diet.

These low carb diets came on the heels of the low-fat years, when people believed they could consume fat-free cookies without limitation.

Those were certainly not the first diet trends to sweep the nation, and certainly they would not be the last. As a child, I watched my mom stock up on Slim Fast shakes. I recall my aunt being hospitalized for following the cabbage soup diet for too long. In more recent years, Paleo has come and gone, rivaled by 30-day resets, 1-week juice cleanses, and eventually trumped by the Ketogenic Diet. Intermittent fasting of various formats is currently heralded by both the fitness industry and researchers, and it is not uncommon to see people doing IF and Keto concurrently.

In each instance, the coveted prize is often weight loss, which can be, unfortunately, as inconstant as the diet trends themselves. The same could be said for the motivation that drives these goals, which can also wax and wane with time.

Even for those who are not working on weight loss, these diet trends may still impact their food choices. For example, with the popularity of low carb diets, many get the impression that carbs are generally unhealthy and then avoid them unnecessarily. At one point, the gluten-free diet gained traction, leading people to believe that gluten was universally harmful. Or in the case of the Ketogenic Diet, the pendulum swung in favor of fats, causing many people to relax their fat choices. Protein is another commonly misunderstood nutrient, and many people supplement with protein powder or protein bars when they are not truly deficient.

EVERYBODY EATS

Whether people are concerned with weight, chronic disease, exercise performance, or general wellness, the topic of nutrition is ubiquitous. From the workplace to family parties to social media, people are often talking about eating clean, cutting carbs, or cleansing. People spend hundreds of dollars on supplements, diet programs, and packaged foods "free" of one thing or another.

However, many people struggle with prioritizing their nutrition. In some cases, lifelong habits, family influences, and/or cultural traditions may run counter to dietary guidelines. Or the perceived cost of healthy eating may drive some to choose cheaper, ultra-processed foods and discourage them from consuming more vegetables, fruits, and other healthy choices. Another common barrier is time. From planning ahead to grocery shopping to meal prep, the effort of healthy eating can seem insurmountable when other time-consuming priorities exist.

There are also some who are under-informed about the direct relationship between health and nutrition. While most people can distinguish between healthy and unhealthy foods, many may not understand the extent to which foods or beverages affect disease risk. Unlike food allergies, intolerances, or blood sugar levels, the effect of food on the body is not always immediate. It can take years before someone sees the impact of an unhealthy diet. Without immediate feedback, it can be difficult for someone to find the motivation to make healthy choices.

For many, the knowledge of how or why to eat healthy is overshadowed by their emotional relationship with food. The emotional effect could be transient, like when somebody wants to

DOI: 10.1201/9781003326038-9

celebrate something special. Or the impact could be more habitual, like winding down at the end of the workday with a snack in front of the TV. For some, emotional eating may be indicative of negative coping skills, where food has evolved into a source of comfort, fleeting as it may be.

COMMONLY REPORTED BARRIERS TO HEALTHY EATING

"I don't have time to cook."
"Healthy eating is expensive."
"It's just a bad habit."
"The food of my culture is not healthy."
"I've had a lot of stress lately."
"I don't know what I can eat."
"I'm an emotional eater."
"I know what to do. I'm just not doing it."
"I just can't stay motivated."
"I don't have the willpower."
"I love sweets. I think it's an addiction."

Health behaviors are not influenced by knowledge and education alone. The everyday challenges of life will also be primary targets of health counseling. Whether your patient is a busy parent, an overbooked executive, or an empty-nester, challenges are present at every stage of life. Recognizing and addressing an individual's personal barriers will have more long-term impact than providing a diet and exercise plan that can easily become tiresome. As such, there is no one-size-fits-all prescription for diet and physical activity.

While everybody's story is different, the barriers listed above often lead to similar eating patterns.

EVERYDAY EATING ROUTINES: A DIFFERENT EER

Upon graduating from my nutrition program, I was prepared to calculate estimated energy requirements (EER), protein needs, and exchange plans. However, in the outpatient setting, I found that EERs, Dietary Reference Intakes, and serving sizes were rarely the information that patients needed. In fact, that information often confuses people. It turns eating into a math problem, which poses so many challenges. For one, numeracy is not a skill with which everybody is comfortable. Measuring food and applying Nutrition Facts information can be confusing, burdensome, and for some, outright irritating. Not to mention the common misconception that all calories are equal, evidenced by the common proclamation, "I'm saving my calories for later!"

It is true that many patients will ask, "How many calories do I need?" And certainly, it is respectful to provide that information. However, a deeper discussion about the person's eating pattern will often bring to light that they can meet their goals without having to count a thing.

Therefore, instead of pulling up a Mifflin St. Jeor calculator, I first assess *a different EER–their everyday eating routine*. Their personal eating pattern is often revealed during their dietary recall. While some will argue that the dietary recall is subject to underreport or poor recall, I have found that a comprehensive interview is sufficient for assessing learning needs. While I may or may not be able to accurately assess their nutrient intake, what a person reports reveals a lot about what they know or believe about nutrition. Even if they are reporting their best day or only healthy foods, they will often demonstrate some knowledge gaps—and filling in those gaps often turns out to be the information they needed in the first place.

During the nutrition assessment, RDNs are investigating the following:

1. How are their eating patterns and lifestyle affecting their symptoms, biomarkers, or other indicators of health?
2. How are their lives affecting their food choices or lifestyle?
3. What do they already understand about their nutrition?
4. What would they benefit from learning?
5. How do they feel about their current condition?
6. How do they feel about lifestyle changes?

With this insight, the RDN can provide the nutrition answers that people are seeking and also the information they did not realize they needed. While many people can identify the behaviors that contribute to their health concerns, a dietitian is uniquely trained to explain some of the driving forces behind those behaviors. From physiological fluctuations to emotional factors to misinformation, proper nutrition education teaches people not only how their choices affect their health but also why they make the choices that they do, and ultimately, how they can change.

The following pages will describe some of the eating patterns you will frequently encounter in counseling, and the conversations you might have to address them.

8 Commonly Reported Eating Patterns

For many health conditions, there are established nutrition guidelines that can help. For example, a patient with high blood pressure would benefit from the DASH Diet. Or someone with IBS might find solutions with a FODMAP elimination approach. The Mediterranean Diet continues to show benefits for heart health and many other conditions.

However, for many people, applying these guidelines will require addressing some other hurdles first. For example, a focus on vegetables and healthy fats may be ineffective for someone who struggles with emotional eating. Or a low-sodium diet may feel unattainable for someone who relies on restaurant meals.

Therefore, it is imperative to understand a patient's eating pattern before a counselor can provide nutrition education. In doing so, not only will you use time efficiently by focusing on the most relevant information, but you will also be able to personalize the education in a way that will be most relevant and—hopefully—motivating.

NIGHT SNACKING

"Night is my hardest time." I hear this statement so frequently that it is one of the things I listen for during a dietary recall. The stories are similar. After coming home from work, or settling in after a hectic day, they say they are starving by dinner. But then they do not stop there. Soon afterward, they will have dessert or an evening snack, maybe both. Some say, "It's like I'm hungry all night." Others admit that they are not truly hungry at these times and chalk it up to a bad habit. Either way, they often qualify the routine by saying something like, "I know it's bad to eat after a certain time."

While not all nighttime eating is problematic, there can be some negative consequences when the food choices are poor or the portions are excessive (Kinsey and Ormsbee 2015). Table 8.1 lists how night eating may impact certain conditions.

Like many diet approaches, a person motivated to change might attempt abstinence and "cut out the night snacks," and successfully do so for a time. In fact, some well-meaning nutrition advisors might guide their patients to set goals around either eliminating the snack or choosing a healthier alternative—the celery and carrot stick solution. "It satisfies the need for that crunch!" they might say. Not to say that celery and carrot sticks are not a fine suggestion. They just might not be the only solution required.

For some people, there may be physiological causes for their evening cravings, either independently or in addition to psychological or emotional reasons. Whether those physiological causes are the result of medications, unbalanced meal planning, or misguided approaches to weight loss, addressing the physiology of cravings is a skill unique to dietitians. Dietitians are trained to understand how physiology drives eating patterns. From the impact of hunger and satiety hormones and the undulations in glucose levels to the biomechanical workings of gastric emptying, digestion, and absorption, the RDN can help the patient plan meals in a way to manage and prevent hunger.

The psychology of cravings, on the other hand, can range in severity. From common emotional eating behaviors to eating disorders, the dietitian will need to gauge whether they can counsel the patient on their own or if they need to refer the patient to eating disorder specialists.

DOI: 10.1201/9781003326038-10

TABLE 8.1

Examples of Impact of Night Eating on Certain Conditions

Reason for Referral	Impact of Night Eating[a]
Diabetes	Hyperglycemia before bed and overnight
	Possibility of excessive calorie intake, weight gain, and insulin resistance
	Note: For those at risk of nocturnal hypoglycemia, a bedtime snack may help reduce that risk
Other metabolic disorders (e.g., metabolic syndrome, dyslipidemia, prediabetes, and PCOS)	Possibility of excessive intake of foods high in fat, refined sugars, and/or total calories contributing to abnormal lipid values, weight gain, and insulin resistance
GERD	GI discomfort at bedtime
	Delayed or disrupted sleep
Weight management	Excessive calorie intake coupled with lower energy expenditure at night (Sharma and Kavuru 2010)
General health, disease prevention	Possibility of excessive intake of ultra-processed, nutrient-deficient foods
	Possibility of excessive intake of total calories, unintended weight gain and related disease risks
Night eating syndrome[b]	Possibility of excessive calorie intake and increased risk for obesity
Binge eating disorder[b]	Excessive calorie intake and increased risk of obesity and weight-related conditions

[a] The negative impact of night eating may be related to the types or amount of food eaten at night and may be mitigated with smaller portions of nutrient dense foods (Kinsey and Ormsbee 2015).

[b] The treatment of eating disorders will require advanced training for the RDN and collaboration with a multidisciplinary team of ED specialists.

Table 8.2 lists some factors that can contribute to hunger and cravings at night.

The answer to night snacking might lie in a person's daytime routine. Or their blood sugar. Or nutrition beliefs. Or coping skills. Or it could be a long-standing habit that is tied to other evening activities. Thus, when a person poses a specific question like, "How do I stop snacking at night," completing the nutrition assessment is the first step in problem solving.

The dietary recall can reveal how people plan and consume their meals throughout the day, and why they make the decisions that they do. During the education portion of your session, you can help them connect the dots between their eating routine and hunger patterns.

While the solution may not be simple in its implementation, empowering your patient with this information can be a great relief to them. I once had a patient cry with gratitude after I provided a brief explanation about the rise and fall of hunger hormones. Like others, she had spent years blaming herself. Many people chalk up their night snacks to a lack of willpower or a bad habit. They repeatedly try to solve the problem by changing their actions in the evening—using smaller dinner plates, swapping potato chips for cucumbers, or committing to abstinence—only to regress to old patterns because they did not address the true cause of their cravings—whether physiological, emotional, or both.

With absolution comes empowerment.

SKIPPING MEALS

On one hand, it is commonly espoused among nutrition professionals that skipping meals can lead to increased hunger later in the day. On the other hand, the recent rise in intermittent fasting calls that theory into question.

TABLE 8.2

Possible Factors for Hunger and Cravings at Night

Possible Factors	Contributing Behaviors or Situations	Reasons for Behaviors or Situations
Inadequate energy intake during the day, leading to lower glucose levels in the evening and increased hunger hormones	Inadequate portions at breakfast and/or lunch Skipped meals Long duration since last meal or snack Nutrient or calorie restriction for the purpose of weight management Inadequate fueling before or after daytime physical activity	Knowledge deficit or time constraint regarding meal planning Too busy to stop to eat Knowledge deficit regarding energy requirements Knowledge deficit regarding meal timing, blood glucose levels, and satiety
Lower blood glucose related to diabetes medication	Long duration between meals in the setting of hypoglycemic medication Inadequate carbohydrate intake in the setting of hypoglycemic medication Inadequate blood glucose monitoring in the setting of hypoglycemic medication Improper use of hypoglycemic medications Excessive doses of hypoglycemic medication—consult with doctor for medication adjustment Physical activity in the setting of excessive hypoglycemic medication doses—consult with doctor for medication adjustment	Knowledge deficit regarding medication action in relation to nutrient intake and physical activity
Inadequate balance in meals leading to increased rate of gastric emptying (i.e., low protein, low fiber, low fat)	Restricted portions of protein, fat, or carbohydrates for the purpose of weight management Dislike of high fiber foods like vegetables or whole grains	Knowledge deficit regarding balanced meal planning and the effects of food on satiety
Excessive intake of refined carbs in meals or snacks, leading to hyperinsulinemia and rapid drop in blood sugar	Excessive consumption of meals, snacks or beverages high in refined carbs or added sugars	Knowledge deficit regarding the effects of food on blood sugar and satiety

(Continued)

TABLE 8.2 (*Continued*)

Possible Factors for Hunger and Cravings at Night

Possible Factors	Contributing Behaviors or Situations	Reasons for Behaviors or Situations
Increased cortisol levels related to chronic stress, increasing appetite and pleasure-seeking behavior	High stress related to psychosocial or socioeconomic factors	Multifactorial Lack of support A referral to a social worker may be required
Mild stress leading to pleasure-seeking behavior	Everyday responsibilities at work and/or at home	Lack of awareness regarding emotional eating and coping skills
Alcohol intake leading to lower blood glucose and increased appetite	Habitual behavior Social behavior Stress and coping behavior Alcohol abuse	Knowledge deficit regarding effect of alcohol on blood sugar and, subsequently, hunger and cravings Negative coping skills Alcohol addiction A referral to a social worker and/or addiction counselor may be required
Financial constraints limiting food access for adequate energy intake and balanced meals	Socioeconomic factors including employment, educational access, and lack of social support	Possible knowledge deficit regarding nutrition assistance programs and/or low cost options for healthy meal planning A referral to a social worker may be required
Inadequate hydration	Low intake of water and other hydrating fluids Excessive intake of dehydrating fluids like sugary beverages, caffeine, energy drinks, or alcohol	Knowledge deficit regarding fluid requirements and good sources of hydration
Binge eating disorder, bulimia nervosa, or night eating syndrome	Underlying mental illness related to genetics, trauma, depression, anxiety, social pressure, or idiopathic etiology	Requires treatment by eating disorder specialists including medical, mental health, and nutrition interventions

Or does it?

While diet debates will forever impact the dialogue of nutrition, patient-centered care provides a space that is sound-proofed against the noise. In counseling, the strongest evidence you have comes from the patient themselves. Once they describe their symptoms, feelings, daily routines—combined with their lab values and other measurements—the RDN can draw from their knowledge of physiology, metabolism, and research to hypothesize possible contributors to a person's individual experience.

For example, unless skipping breakfast is purposefully intended to reduce calories or "burn more fat" as in intermittent fasting, those who skip breakfast—or any meal—do not necessarily consume a third-less calories than those who have three meals a day. Instead, dietary recalls often reveal that they merely shift their calorie intake later in the day and into the evening hours. Moreover, food choices in the evening are more likely to be larger in portion and/or energy-dense snacks or sweets.

Another common scenario reported during a dietary recall is missing lunch. Perhaps they are so consumed by their responsibilities that they do not feel hungry. Or their daily schedules do not allow for a break. Or they are on the road throughout the day, unable to stop for a meal. Whatever the reason, they say that by evening, they are "starving."

Having completed thousands of dietary recalls, I have found that dinner is the meal that is most consistently consumed. Dinner is often the biggest meal of the day, at least on weeknights. In composition, it is often the most complete, and people are more likely to include vegetables, protein, and starch with their meal. However, for those who eat little during the day, the challenge at this point is controlling portions or limiting additional servings.

Which makes physiological sense. At that point, grehlin—typically referred to as the "hunger hormone"—has been building up. With higher levels of grehlin and lower levels of glucose, the drive to food is stronger and the onset of satiety takes longer, making it harder to be mindful about food choices or portion control. Eager to reach satiation, they may find themselves eating faster than their satiety signals work, perhaps reaching for seconds before leptin and other satiety hormones kick in, subsequently eating more than they actually need. In fact, studies have shown that leptin-to-grehlin ratios can take at least two hours to peak (Adamska-Patruno et al. 2018). Hence, the sense of hunger may be prolonged even after consuming a full meal.

The regulation of appetite involves a complex interplay of metabolic hormones that is beyond the scope of this text. However, the take-home point is that the impact of meal timing can affect people in different ways.

A NOTE ABOUT DIET TRENDS

While many popular diets are based on minimal scientific evidence, others are highly studied and debated among nutrition researchers and clinicians. Among those are the **Ketogenic Diet (KD)** and **Intermittent Fasting (IF)**.

The KD is a treatment often used to treat epilepsy and seizures in children. Further research has also shown benefits in rapid weight loss, metabolic disorders including diabetes and dyslipidemia, as well as improvements in other disease states (Zhu et al. 2022). While long-term studies are still needed to determine the long-term safety of KD, the observed short-term benefits have piqued interest in this dietary pattern in clinical practice.

Similarly, the various forms of intermittent fasting have also shown potential as treatments for obesity and cardiometabolic disorders (Varady et al. 2021). In time-restricted feeding, one form of IF, it does not limit, nor promote excess of, specific nutrients, thus may be generally safe in regard to nutrient intake. For alternate-day fasting or prolonged fasts, more studies are needed to assess the long-term safety of these approaches.

When certain diets show promising findings in research, many well-meaning, non-nutrition clinicians will be quick to recommend these approaches. And if adhering to diet prescriptions were as straightforward as medication regimens, perhaps such recommendations would be more effective.

However, in practice, RDNs will frequently encounter the following patterns:

Inconsistent practice. Consistency is particularly challenging for KD, where the benefits found in research are associated with reaching and maintaining ketogenesis. Outside of the research setting, many people find it difficult to limit their carb intake consistently—either because it is difficult to maintain or because they are not fully informed on how to implement KD. As such, they periodically indulge in carbohydrate foods, either preventing or withdrawing from the ketogenic state. This cycling undermines not just the metabolic purpose of KD but also the presumption of benefit. Furthermore, those who "cut carbs" without actually following KD often suffer prolonged side effects like headaches and low energy, which further limits the sustainability of this approach.

Inconsistent glycemic response. In both KD and IF, patients on certain diabetes medications (e.g., sulfonylureas or insulin) may be at risk for *hypoglycemia*. Not only can this be life threatening for people with diabetes, frequent treatment with fast-acting carbs can also offset ketogenesis—not to mention lead to *hyperglycemic rebounds* and possibly excessive calorie intake. Therefore, while there may be benefits for people with diabetes (PWD), medication adjustments and close monitoring would be required. Although KD and IF are often promoted to PWD, various outcomes have been observed in practice. For those with a pattern of *dawn phenomenon*, or elevated fasting blood sugar, some PWD will notice a rise in their FBG after starting IF. While this is not the case for everybody, close monitoring will be required to determine if IF is appropriate for each individual.

Similar results can occur in PWD who are limiting carbs. Again, if the person does not consistently restrict carbohydrates to enter ketogenesis, gluconeogenesis may lead to *hyperglycemia*. This can also occur in those who use mealtime insulin. When restricting carbohydrates, they will reduce—or exclude—their fast-acting insulin with meals. Thus, lower circulating insulin may lead to gluconeogenesis and/or inadequate metabolism of glycerol from triglycerides. In these cases, KD can undermine the proposed benefits. Low insulin levels can also lead to diabetic ketoacidosis, another life-threatening complication in diabetes. Of note, PWD using SGLT-2 inhibitors also have an increased risk for DKA. Therefore, KD should not be implemented with these patients.

Concurrent IF and KD. Frequently, people who follow IF may also be leery of carbohydrates, which may further exacerbate the risks and side effects discussed above. At the time of this writing, there is limited research to support this combined approach in terms of safety and long-term outcomes.

Yo-yo dieting. Often, KD and IF are among the diet approaches that people report they tried, worked, but then stopped. While the efficacy and safety will continue to be researched and debated, the nutrition counselor will more often have to address the sustainability of these, and any, diet trends.

Overall, an overview of the risks and benefits of any approach should be presented comprehensively and objectively. Trust your ability to educate as well as your patient's ability to learn. In the end, respecting your patient's autonomy will enhance their trust in you. Thus, if they decide to try an alternative diet, they will be more amenable to follow up with you for monitoring and ongoing support.

SQUEEZING CALORIES AND CHASING HUNGER

Not all patients push nutrition down the priority list. In fact, some are so aware of their choices that they control themselves straight into hunger. They know their way around a grocery store and leave no package unturned, scanning and comparing nutrition labels. They have found their lowest calorie go-to brands, but still double check the label every time. They believe that calories-in-versus-calories-out are rule number one in weight loss. On top of that, they may also be leery of carbs and choose the lowest carb options they can find. Breakfast might be a light yogurt, and lunch may be no more than a vegetable salad.

However, the tendency to squeeze calories throughout the day can keep them in the hunger zone. They may find themselves frequently snacking or constantly thinking about their next meal.

Or they might end up ravenous by dinner. Perhaps they leave work so hungry that they cannot wait to get home to eat, so they hit a drive-thru on the way. Or they find themselves snacking before dinner or while cooking. Sometimes it can feel like an eating marathon. After dinner, they find themselves reaching for sweets or snacks. By the end of the day, all the calories and carbs they avoided early in the day pile up at night, just when their metabolism is preparing for the overnight fast.

While mindfulness is a key tenet in healthy eating, calories and certain food groups have been vilified by diet culture. Whether people are counting calories, carbs, fat, sodium, or other nutrients, the interpretation is often "less is more." Instead of focusing on healthy food choices and overall balance, some people get caught up in the minutiae of nutrients. They feel food is something to be avoided, as opposed to being the fuel that provides power, strength, and protection. On the one hand, they might set a goal of 1,200 calories per day. But when you suggest a 400-calorie breakfast, their eyes pop, as that number seems excessive, even though it allows for an equally balanced lunch and dinner. Similarly, for those who are avoiding sugar, they go as far as cutting fruit from their diet—disregarding the vitamins, antioxidants, and fiber that fruit provides. For some people, fat has retained some stigma, where they will squeeze lemon onto a salad in lieu of oil-based dressing, unaware of the benefits of healthy fats and their role in absorbing fat-soluble vitamins.

For many, diet culture has shaped their relationship with food throughout their lives. From the parental influences of their childhood to the virality of social media today, these beliefs can be deeply ingrained. Addressing long-standing values in ways that are respectful and empathetic is critical in reassuring the patient that it will be okay to try something new.

TALES FROM THE FIELD: CHASING HUNGER

The concept of "chasing hunger" brings to mind a participant in a lifestyle change program whom I will call May, age 61. Upon introductions, she described herself as someone who has "tried it all" for weight loss. Like many, her weight had cycled up and down with every start and stop of a diet, finding each strategy unsustainable.

Early in the program, the National Diabetes Prevention Program curriculum covers the Plate Method and healthy eating (Centers for Disease Control and Prevention, 2022). By itself, the information is straightforward and easy to understand. The handouts provide lists of healthy choices for each food group, beautiful images of appetizing foods, and engaging worksheets for meal planning. For some, that information is sufficient to start planning healthier meals. However, for those who have become accustomed to minimizing the amount of food on their plates, or are hesitant to eat certain food groups, the Plate Method can actually look like too much food, or even the wrong food. Some responses I have heard include, "That's a lot of food!" or "I thought you weren't supposed to eat carbs."

May was among those who were hesitant. However, during this session, I augmented the curriculum with information about the role of carbohydrates and glucose; the effect of fat, fiber, and protein on digestion and glycemic response; the timing of meals in conjunction with blood sugar patterns. With that information, I provided the *what* with the *why*.

Thus, for those in the group who "just want to be told what to eat," a simple description of the Plate Method may be sufficient. But for those who have spent years following diet trends, they may need more information.

For May, she decided to apply this new information. After a few weeks of adding more balance to her meals, May was all smiles as she reported:

"I just can't believe it. I'm losing weight and I'm eating more."

EMOTIONAL EATING

The term "emotional eating" has been widely used to refer to the tendency to eat in response to negative emotions, with the chosen foods being primarily energy-dense and highly palatable (Konttinen 2020). The concept of emotional eating often conjures images of uncontrolled episodes that include high levels of anxiety. And justifiably so, as emotional eating has certainly been associated with binge eating disorder (BED) (Masheb and Grilo 2006; Meule et al. 2014).

However, quite often, patients will describe themselves as emotional eaters or state that they engage in "stress eating," without otherwise meeting criteria for BED. Further, emotional eating is not limited to negative emotions. The term could also be applied to eating in response to positive emotions or boredom, although these scenarios have not been as thoroughly investigated (Braden et al. 2018).

In practice, when a person reveals a recurring snack time, a thought-provoking question for the patient may be, "When you reach for this snack, are you physically hungry at this time?"

This question is often followed by a pause as the patient considers the question. For some, this may be the first time they have thought about it. Some people will attribute the pattern to boredom or habit and admit that they are not truly hungry at those times.

When eating is a form of entertainment or relaxation, a discussion about mindfulness and alternative strategies may suffice.

However, for those who describe themselves as *"stress eaters,"* a deeper investigation into their level of stress will be needed. For some, their stress may be mild to moderate and related to everyday concerns of work demands, family responsibilities, or scheduling issues. In these cases, brainstorming basic stress management strategies may be sufficient. For others, stress may be more chronic, rooted in situations that are not easily resolved, such as financial distress, health concerns, relationship issues, or other complex situations that require professional support beyond medical nutrition therapy. In these cases, a referral back to the PCP, a social worker, and/or other mental health professionals would be required.

A NOTE ABOUT EATING DISORDERS

While eating disorders are not common, there will be times when a patient presents with signs or symptoms. In these cases, the RDN must consider the differences between skipped meals and anorexia nervosa; or fad dieting and food avoidance; or stress eating and BED; or night snacking and night eating syndrome.

The presence of an eating disorder may not always be obvious. A clinician may have implicit weight bias, associating eating disorders only with undernutrition and severe weight loss. Thus, someone of normal or higher weight may slip under the radar. Or a person with obesity may be dismissed as simply overeating and being sedentary. Or a patient who exercises excessively might be commended for their active lifestyle when they are actually engaging in compensatory behavior.

According to the Academy of Nutrition and Dietetics, dietitians of all levels are considered competent to identify signs and symptoms of ED (Hackert et al. 2020). However, not all dietitians are qualified to provide treatment. The Academy recommends advanced training through the International Association of Eating Disorders Professionals (iaedp) for the Certified Eating Disorders Registered Dietitian credential (CEDRD) (Hackert et al. 2020). The requirements to obtain this credential include 2,500 clinical practice hours under the supervision of a CEDRD supervisor (CEDRD-S), at least 2 years of experience practicing within ED, and successful completion of the qualifying exam (Hackert et al. 2020). Thus, for RDNs who are not credentialed to treat patients with ED, it is essential to have a referral system in place to coordinate care with ED experts. Treatment of ED requires a multidisciplinary team that includes medical, mental health, and nutrition specialists. Treatment options include inpatient, partial inpatient, and outpatient care, depending on the needs of the patient.

Dietitians in all areas are likely to encounter patients with ED at some time or another, regardless of their specialty. The National Institute of Mental Health lists BED and bulimia nervosa (BN) as common types of ED (NIMH n.d.). They list lifetime prevalence of BED in adults at 2.8% and BN at 1.0%, and lifetime prevalence of anorexia nervosa (AN) at 0.6% of adults (NIMH n.d.; Hudson et al. 2012).

Screening. A commonly used screening tool used for ED is the SCOFF questionnaire (Kutz et al. 2020). Originally developed by Morgan and colleagues in screening young women for AN or bulimia, the tool provides a brief, easy-to-remember, and simple-to-use questionnaire for nonspecialists (Morgan et al. 2000). While the SCOFF questionnaire has not yet been validated for identifying all types of eating disorders, it has been deemed adequate for use in screening ED in adults (Feltner et al. 2022). The questions are listed in Table 8.3.

TABLE 8.3

SCOFF Questionnaire (Kutz et al. 2019; Morgan et al. 2000)

	Question	Answer	
Sick	Do you make yourself sick because you feel uncomfortably full?	Yes	No
Control	Do you worry that you have lost control over how much you eat?	Yes	No
One stone (14 lbs)	Have you recently lost more than one stone (14 lb) in a 3-month period?	Yes	No
Fat	Do you believe yourself to be fat when others say you are too thin?	Yes	No
Food	Would you say that food dominates your life?	Yes	No

Each "yes" equals 1 point. A score of 2 indicates a likely diagnosis of an eating disorder

---

ALL OR NOTHING

Another statement you can expect to hear again and again is, "I lost a lot of weight doing *[insert diet plan here]*, but then I gained it all back again."

Many people are pretty savvy when it comes to diet trends. They keep up with the latest trends and are willing to try new things. They become familiar with terms like "macros" or "alkalinity" or "ketones." When they put their minds to it, they are able to lose weight rather quickly. They know how to slim down for a wedding or a cruise or a beach vacation. When they're ready, they dive right in and see results.

Many exhibit an "all or nothing" mentality, where they describe a similar pattern: They were highly motivated and followed a diet to a T. Plus they were exercising. Maybe they were going to the gym or working with a trainer. But then something happened. Another priority took precedent—work, family, a health concern. Or in many cases, they hit the inevitable plateau, became frustrated, and thought, "What's the point?" Whatever the reason, they found old habits creeping back, and whatever results they were seeing slipped away.

TALES FROM THE FIELD: ALL OR NOTHING

"Andrea," age 49, had been active as a gymnast throughout her youth and early adulthood. However, a knee injury caused her to give up her sport. While she was able to coach others, she herself became less active. As she got older, her weight had crept up. At one point, she was motivated to get some of the pounds off, at which point she started a very low carb diet. "I was able to cut out carbs for three or four months," she said, "and it worked! I lost about 35 pounds." She said she was feeling great and was pleased with the results. Then she shook her head as she continued, "but one day, I remember I was feeling upset—I can't remember why. But I went to a drive-thru and ordered fries. And I ate them. All of them. That was it. I thought, 'I ruined it,' and just gave up the whole thing. Then I gained back the weight and even more."

Andrea's experience—and pattern of thinking—is quite common. While extreme diets are appealing for rapid weight loss, most can be difficult to maintain.

For many, depriving oneself of their favorite foods can lead to feelings of resentment and anxiety about eating. When faced with higher stress situations, they may find themselves turning to food for comfort and rebelling against the anxiety they have had about food, thinking, "I don't care. I'm eating it!" For those with an "all or nothing" mentality, what often follows is a complete cessation of the diet, a relief to start eating their favorite foods again, and another turn on the diet roller coaster.

For Andrea, enhancing her knowledge about metabolism and balanced meal planning helped her reframe her approach not just to nutrition but also to setbacks. Instead of "all in, all of the time" she was able to accept "mostly in, most of the time," and achieved a healthier relationship with food.

GRAZING

During the dietary recall, a patient might report frequent snacks throughout the day. For example, they may have a light breakfast, followed by a midmorning snack. They may have a simple lunch and/or several snacks throughout the day. Perhaps they keep a package of nuts or snack mix near their favorite chair, grabbing a handful here and there, continuing the pattern after dinner as well. Some people keep snacks in a drawer at work. Or share snacks with their kids throughout the day.

On one hand, small meals and snacks can be a healthy approach to eating. On the other hand, if left unchecked, mindless snacking can often lead to excessive calorie intake. For those whose snacks are high in refined carbs or simple sugars, they may exacerbate the cycle of cravings by spiking insulin levels, followed by rapid drops in blood sugar.

The tendency to graze may result from a variety of reasons:

A general lack of nutrition knowledge might prevent someone from building balanced, satisfying meals, leading to frequent hunger.

Inadequate meals. As mentioned earlier, a preoccupation with calories and over restriction might prevent somebody from achieving true satiety from their meals, leaving them hungry between meals.

Lack of time for planning. Busy schedules can push meal planning down the priority list. Without go-to recipes or a stock of staple ingredients, people may find themselves grabbing whatever is available whenever, and however, they can.

Avoiding carbs. While many people report less hunger and cravings on a KD, those who inconsistently limit their carbs are less able to rely on ketones as a steady fuel source. Without ketogenesis or adequate carbs, they may find themselves in a low fuel state, hence increased hunger. For those who experience low blood sugar, low carb intake may lead to frequent treatment with fast-acting carbs, triggering a cycle of blood sugar spikes and drops.

Emotional or stress eating could play a role. As discussed previously, whether they are coping with a busy day or breaking up their boredom, many people consume food without physiological need.

FREQUENT DINING OUT

"I eat out a lot."

From high fat ingredients to large portions, restaurant foods are often fat, sodium, and calorie bombs. With restaurants ranging from fast food to fast casual to fine dining, eating out is a common and frequent American experience.

TALES FROM THE FIELD: DINING OUT IN AMERICA

My mother grew up in the Philippines. Though a typical Filipino diet is high in white rice and high fat meats, growing up, most of her meals were made at home or purchased locally. Food was not wasted, but not abundant either.

She followed my father to the States as he pursued his lifelong dream to be a doctor in America. As they built their life together, they enjoyed the life of plenty that they imagined. Compared to the small town where she grew up, the American landscape was lit with golden arches and 24-hour-open signs, and we were living the dream. My own childhood memories include a lot of restaurant meals. Burger King, Olive Garden, Big Boy, "Pizza!Pizza" with Crazy Bread and a 2-L. Every Sunday after Church. Sometimes after midnight, my mom would come home from her night shift laden with takeout. It will not be a surprise to say that my mom became part of the 67% of Americans who are overweight or obese (CDC n.d.), leading to much ribbing from friends and family in the Philippines.

Years later, after becoming a dietitian, I asked my mother why she thought she gained weight after moving to America. She summed it up rather succinctly when she said:

"In America, you can eat a lot of good food for cheap."

Indeed, dining out makes up a large portion of food expenditures in this country. The United States Department of Agriculture Economic Research Service reported that in 2020, foods away from home made up about 48% of total U.S. food expenditures, and over 50% prior to the COVID-19 pandemic (USDA ERS 2020). From 2013–2016, approximately 37% of adults consumed fast food on a given day (Fryar et al. 2018).

Dining out will continue to be part of the American experience. From relaxing with friends and family to socializing with coworkers to exploring various cuisines, the occasional meal out is not problematic in and of itself. However, if restaurant foods make up a large portion of a patient's nutrient intake, the types, portions, or frequency may need addressing. But first, you must identify the reason someone relies on restaurant food.

No time to cook. Many people have so much on their plate that they cannot find time for meal planning. Perhaps work is very demanding. Or family keeps them busy with school, sports, and other activities. Perhaps it is both. They are the go-to person for the people around them, and they do not want to let anybody down.

For them, preparing a meal for themselves or their family can be a struggle. To buy time, it is often easier to eat out. They might grab lunch in the work cafeteria, hit a drive-thru on the way home from work, or pick up a pizza for the family when the events of the day are done. Time constraints can often result in higher stress levels, which may also affect the type and amount of foods they order. Even when there are healthy choices on the menu, they may still gravitate toward foods they find more comforting.

Limited cooking skills or interest. Some people may have little experience with meal prep. Perhaps they have had little need or interest to learn their way around a kitchen. While they can assemble a simple sandwich or microwave a frozen meal, it is just as easy and perhaps more satisfying to go to a nearby restaurant.

With limited cooking skills, even simple meals may feel time-consuming and overwhelming. With only a few meal ideas up their sleeve, they may struggle with variety. For example, breakfast ideas can be especially challenging on a busy morning. For some, oatmeal is the healthiest idea they have, and anything else may seem like a big production when they are trying to get out the door. Thus, picking up a breakfast sandwich or two on the way to work is an easier solution. Packing a lunch or preparing dinner at the end of a day can feel similarly unattainable.

Active social life. From happy hours to weekend get-togethers to family celebrations, going out to eat is a fun and festive way to socialize. However, in addition to the usual challenges of dining out, the social context adds another layer of complexity to making healthy choices. Some find it difficult to resist poor food choices when the people around them are indulging. Moreover, they may feel pressure to participate in extras like shared appetizers or desserts for fear of making their companions uncomfortable. Conversely, sometimes friends or family overtly exert pressure, insisting that "this one time won't hurt you." If alcoholic beverages are involved, disinhibition may weaken one's resolve.

HABIT CYCLING

In the absence of physiological need, emotional eating, or eating disorders, the impact of habit cannot be underestimated. In *The Power of Habit: Why We Do What We Do in Life and Business,* author Charles Duhigg describes a cycle that includes a cue, a routine, and reward (Duhigg 2014). He writes:

> First, there is a cue, a trigger that tells your brain to go into automatic mode and which habit to use. Then there is a routine, which can be physical or mental or emotional. Finally, there is a reward, which helps your brain figure out if this particular loop is worth remembering for the future.

I observed this cycle of habit in my own nighttime routine. Like many people, I found myself relaxing at the end of the night with a snack. The routine was always the same. With dinner done and the kids settled in their bedrooms, I would sit in front of the TV. Despite the balanced dinner that I finished just a couple of hours prior, my mind would wander toward savory snacks. Whether it is exposure to fast food commercials, or the content of the cooking shows I enjoy, or simply the routine itself, as a nutrition counselor, I became fully aware of what was occurring. I was especially aware that I use that time as "me time," and am typically trying to shake off the stress of the day. I was indulging in a mild—yet common—form of emotional eating, wrapped up in a cycle of habit.

I found myself trying to resist, to employ "willpower," to simply tell myself that I am not hungry and I do not need a snack. However, the association between watching TV and eating is so ingrained that I eventually give in, make my way to the kitchen, then indulge in my favorite snack. Fleeting as it may be, the reward is enough to establish the routine for the next time I expose myself to the cue—namely the TV. I had learned that no matter how good my intentions were, the routine of watching TV and snacking was set in stone.

Identifying the habit and finding where to break the cycle can require some trial and error. And if it was difficult for me, how much more for somebody without formal nutrition training? In my example, the link between the cue and routine was so strong that, after repeated attempts at resistance, I found the connection too hard to break, despite my awareness of the situation. Eventually, I realized that to cut back on my evening snack, I simply would have to avoid the cue. As I have counseled many times, I had to find alternative ways to relax at night. In my case, I found that retreating with a good book was equally effective in relaxing at the end of the day, an activity that I did not associate with eating (Figure 8.1).

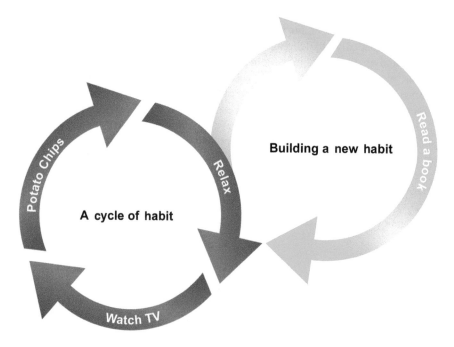

FIGURE 8.1 To break a habit, identify the pattern, determine its purpose, and consider alternative ways to produce the same results. In this example, watching TV is a way of relaxing. However, watching TV is the cue to eat a snack, perpetuating a cycle of habit. To break the cycle, avoid the cue. In this case, reading a book achieves the purpose of relaxing, while the cue to snack is circumvented.

While seemingly simple and straightforward, breaking the cycle requires a deeper dive into motivation and behavior change. While I describe my own scenario as a fully intentional, stepwise approach to habit breaking, make no mistake that several levels of emotion underlie my motivation to change. Familial pressures around weight and appearance during childhood, the loss of my father to diabetes at an early age, the education and training I have received about nutrition and disease, and my daily interactions with patients have all shaped my relationship with food and influence my lifestyle choices. For patients, their relationship with food may be equally—if not more—complex.

However, every small change can have a significant impact.

TALES FROM THE FIELD: PROBLEM SOLVING A HABIT

Identify the problem. On the way to work each day, Dan, age 52, would stop at the gas station to pick up a coffee. Near the coffee station, there was also a display of donuts. Unable to resist, he would purchase a couple of donuts and bring them to work with him for his breakfast.

State the goal. When Dan was diagnosed with prediabetes, he was determined to cut back on sweets.

Identify the root, or trigger, of the problem. One day it hit him. If he did not stop at the gas station, he would not be cued to buy and eat the donuts.

Brainstorm solutions and make a plan. Avoid the gas station. He decided to invest in a single serve coffee maker for home. With that, he was able to make his coffee before leaving for work and did not have to stop at the gas station.

Evaluate the result. It was a slight change to his routine, but with big results. He was able to cut about 500 calories and 60 g of refined carbs from his morning.

While Dan had embraced several other changes to help prevent diabetes, this particular story demonstrates how the problem solving process can help identify—and break—an unwanted habit.

A MULTIFACTORIAL PATTERN

While the above scenarios of skipping meals, squeezing calories, emotional eating, frequent dining out, or habit loops can individually be problematic, you may find that many people exhibit a combination of patterns. For example, someone who is too busy to eat lunch may be physiologically disadvantaged in managing their stress eating at night. Or someone who grazes throughout the day might further exceed their calorie needs if they frequently dine out for meals.

As discussed earlier in this book, the basic steps in problem solving include identifying the root problem, brainstorming solutions, then developing an action plan to test a solution. However, just as the determinants of health can be complex and multifactorial, so too is the problem-solving process. For many people, the initial step of identifying a root problem may reveal that there are several challenges to overcome, each equally impactful. Thus, the initial step will be to determine (1) which issues are modifiable and (2) what information the person needs to feel ready and able to take action.

For the counselor, the actionable solutions may appear quite clear. However, people may be more likely to act on something that *they* identify as important, not what the counselor proposes. Therefore, providing an impartial, objective, and comprehensible education may be more effective than advising on which behaviors need changing. With enough information, the person can decide for themselves which changes will be right for them.

TALES FROM THE FIELD: PRESSURE RELIEF

Maya's birthday was coming up. She was turning 49 and planning a trip to Vegas with a girlfriend. Prior to the trip, she said to her dietitian, "I intend to fully celebrate my birthday. There will be lots of drinks. There will be lots of food. I don't want to miss out on anything."

Up to that point, Maya had complained about a weight loss plateau. While she had made some progress, her active social life had prevented her from seeing progress as quickly as she wanted. Her upcoming birthday would seemingly be no exception. Like many, she associated celebration with food and drinks. However, to honor her goal to enjoy her birthday, the dietitian took a different approach to action planning. Instead of brainstorming mindfulness strategies or discussing travel tips, she shifted the discussion to expectations. "When it comes to travel and special occasions, *maintaining* weight is as much an achievement as losing weight." With that, Maya decided to reframe her goal for that month. She would not worry about weight loss during the trip.

One month later, when Maya logged into her video visit with the dietitian, she proudly reported that she lost weight during her trip, despite the initial goal to maintain weight. "My friend and I did a lot of walking. Sometimes I ordered healthier foods like salads. I won't lie, not everything I ordered was healthy, but I found that I could enjoy things without overdoing it. When I wanted something sweet, my friend and I would share it."

What was most noteworthy about her report was not what she did, but how she felt. "Once we decided that weight loss was not the goal for the trip, it's like all of this pressure was lifted off me. I found I did not have to deprive myself, but I could still have fun and enjoy different things, as long as it was in moderation."

Maya came back refreshed and ready to continue toward her goals. In fact, she exhibited a more energized motivation than before her trip. She had left with a plan that aligned with her values and felt empowered to make choices that were important to her. In turn, she came back with an enhanced self-efficacy in handling social occasions, and a better understanding about her emotional relationship with food.

No EER equation could have calculated that.

REFERENCES

Adamska-Patruno E, Ostrowska L, Goscik J, et al. The Relationship between the Leptin/Ghrelin Ratio and Meals with Various Macronutrient Contents in Men with Different Nutritional Status: A Randomized Crossover Study. *Nutr J.* 2018;17:118. doi: 10.1186/s12937-018-0427-x.

Braden A, Musher-Eizenman D, Watford T, Emley E. Eating When Depressed, Anxious, Bored, or Happy: Are Emotional Eating Types Associated with Unique Psychological and Physical Health Correlates? *Appetite.* 2018 Jun;125:410–417. doi: 10.1016/j.appet.2018.02.022.

Centers for Disease Control and Prevention. National Center for Chronic Disease Prevention and Health Promotion, Division of Nutrition, Physical Activity, and Obesity. Data, Trend and Maps [Internet]. Centers for Disease Control and Prevention. [cited 2023 May 12]. Available from: https://www.cdc.gov/nccdphp/dnpao/data-trends-maps/index.html.

Centers for Disease Control and Prevention. National Diabetes Prevention Program Curricula and Handouts [Internet]. Centers for Disease Control and Prevention; 2022 [cited 2023 January 1]. Available from: https://www.cdc.gov/diabetes/prevention/resources/curriculum.html.

Duhigg C. *The Power of Habit: Why We Do What We Do in Life and Business.* New York: Random House Trade Paperbacks; 2014.

Feltner C, Peat C, Reddy S, Riley S, Berkman N, Middleton JC, Balio C, Coker-Schwimmer M, Jonas DE. Screening for Eating Disorders in Adolescents and Adults: Evidence Report and Systematic Review for the US Preventive Services Task Force. *JAMA*. 2022 Mar;327(11):1068–1082. doi: 10.1001/jama.2022.1807.

Fryar CD, Hughes JP, Herrick KA, Ahluwalia N. Fast Food Consumption among Adults in the United States, 2013-2016. *NCHS Data Brief*. 2018 Oct;322:1–8.

Hackert AN, Kniskern MA, Beasley TM. Academy of Nutrition and Dietetics: Revised 2020 Standards of Practice and Standards of Professional Performance for Registered Dietitian Nutritionists (Competent, Proficient, and Expert) in Eating Disorders. *J Acad Nutr Diet*. 2020 Nov;120(11):1902–1919.e54. doi: 10.1016/j.jand.2020.07.014.

Hudson JI, Hiripi E, Pope HG Jr, Kessler RC. The Prevalence and Correlates of Eating Disorders in the National Comorbidity Survey Replication. *Biol Psychiatry*. 2007 Feb;61(3):348–358. doi: 10.1016/j.biopsych.2006.03.040. Epub 2006 Jul 3. Erratum in: *Biol Psychiatry*. 2012 Jul 15;72(2):164.

Kinsey AW, Ormsbee MJ. The Health Impact of Nighttime Eating: Old and New Perspectives. *Nutrients*. 2015 Apr;7(4):2648–2662. doi: 10.3390/nu7042648.

Konttinen H. Emotional Eating and Obesity in Adults: The Role of Depression, Sleep and Genes. *Proc Nutr Soc*. 2020 Aug;79(3):283–289. doi: 10.1017/S0029665120000166.

Kutz AM, Marsh AG, Gunderson CG, Maguen S, Masheb RM. Eating Disorder Screening: A Systematic Review and Meta-analysis of Diagnostic Test Characteristics of the SCOFF. *J Gen Intern Med*. 2020 Mar;35(3):885–893. doi: 10.1007/s11606-019-05478-6.

Masheb RM, Grilo CM. Emotional Overeating and Its Associations with Eating Disorder Psychopathology among Overweight Patients with Binge Eating Disorder. *Int J Eat Disord*. 2006 Mar;39(2):141–146. doi: 10.1002/eat.20221.

Meule A, Allison KC, Platte P. Emotional Eating Moderates the Relationship of Night Eating with Binge Eating and Body Mass. *Eur Eat Disord Rev*. 2014 Mar;22(2):147–151. doi: 10.1002/erv.2272. Epub 2013 Dec 2.

Morgan JF, Reid F, Lacey JH. The SCOFF Questionnaire: A New Screening Tool for Eating Disorders. *West J Med*. 2000 Mar;172(3):164–165. doi: 10.1136/ewjm.172.3.164.

National Institute of Mental Health. Eating Disorders [Internet]. Bethesda, MD: National Institutes of Health; [cited 7/2/2022]. Available from: https://www.nimh.nih.gov/health/statistics/eating-disorders.

Sharma S, Kavuru M. Sleep and Metabolism: An Overview. *Int J Endocrinol*. 2010;2010:270832. doi: 10.1155/2010/270832.

United States Department of Agriculture Economic Research Service. Food prices and spending [Internet]. United States Department of Agriculture; 2020 [cited 4/24/2022]. Available from: https://www.ers.usda.gov/data-products/ag-and-food-statistics-charting-the-essentials/food-prices-and-spending/.

Varady KA, Cienfuegos S, Ezpeleta M, Gabel K. Cardiometabolic Benefits of Intermittent Fasting. *Annu Rev Nutr*. 2021 Oct;41:333–361. doi: 10.1146/annurev-nutr-052020-041327.

Zhu H, Bi D, Zhang Y, Kong C, Du J, Wu X, Wei Q, Qin H. Ketogenic Diet for Human Diseases: The Underlying Mechanisms and Potential for Clinical Implementations. *Signal Transduct Target Ther*. 2022 Jan;7(1):11. doi: 10.1038/s41392-021-00831-w.

Part III

Common Referrals and FAQs

9 Common Referrals

When I was in high school, my father had a quadruple bypass. I wish I could say that was the hardest time in his life, but actually, that was just the beginning. Soon after that, I learned that he had diabetes. Later, I came to find out that he had known about his diabetes for a long time, but when I was a child, that was not discussed around me.

After his heart surgery, his health steadily declined, and there was no hiding it. As I was older, I drove him to doctors appointments. At home, I helped him test his blood sugar. As he lost much of his vision, I would help read things to him.

He also developed end-stage renal disease and went to hemodialysis three times a week. I have a brief memory of him hooked up to a big machine while sitting in a cushy hospital chair, covered in a blanket.

During that period, I thought that he was just dealt a bad hand. The heart disease, the kidney failure, and the vision loss. I had no idea that they were all related. I did not understand that diabetes was the underlying cause of his problems.

As a matter of fact, it was not until my mid-30s, 15 years after his passing, that I finally understood my father's final cause of death, which was heart failure.

I was a dietetic intern, rotating through a dialysis unit, observing my preceptor counsel a young man whose potassium levels were elevated. Despite my physiology, biochemistry, and micronutrient classes, I had not yet put all the puzzle pieces together in terms of how the fine details added up to the whole person. In class, we look at illustrations of cellular components like receptors and transporters. We discuss how electrolytes interact to send signals, innervate actions, and maintain homeostasis. We view photos of diseased organs with close-ups of damaged tissue. For a science nerd, I thought it was fascinating.

However, on that day in the dialysis center, the dietitian said something to that young man that reframed my understanding of nutrition and disease, as well as what may have happened to my dad. She said, "High potassium levels can stop your heart."

In that moment, my dad's "bad deck of cards" finally made sense to me. For the first time, I realized that my father's cause of death was not just that his heart failed, but likely because his kidneys had failed, and his kidneys failed because of his diabetes.

In the classroom, I had learned about each of these conditions individually, but did not fully appreciate their interconnectedness. Once in practice, the illustrations and photos and close-ups now came together and took shape as a person, a patient, my dad.

Today, as a diabetes care and education specialist, the memory of my dad is with me at the start of every program I teach. I remember how little my family understood about diabetes, heart disease, and kidney failure at that time, and how limited access to nutrition education was 30 years ago. Even today, I feel bad when I explain the development of diabetes and its complications, knowing how preventable they can be. If only people were referred for nutrition education sooner, many might not develop a metabolic disease in the first place. Regardless, I feel honored to help people learn about how nutrition is related to their health and to provide them with the information that I wish my family had received. To help them prevent the debilitating complications that I witnessed in my father.

Today, heart disease is still the leading cause of death in America, with diabetes and kidney disease not far behind (Xu et al. 2022). The majority of cases are considered preventable through good nutrition, physical activity, and other lifestyle choices. Unfortunately, at this time, only 36%

TABLE 9.1

Percentage of Physicians Who Refer to Dietitians for the Following Reasons (Sastre and Van Horn 2021)

Reason for Referral	% of Physicians Who Refer to Dietitians
Diabetes	81
Weight management	78
Chronic disease prevention	42
Cardiovascular disease or hypertension	35
Renal disease	25
General health and prevention	25
Other	10

of family practitioners report having a dietitian at their practice, even though the majority of them are affiliated with a large health care system (Sastre and Van Horn 2021). Of those who do have access to dietitians, they do not always refer. The reasons for referral to a dietitian are listed in Table 9.1.

The most common referrals I receive are consistent with the findings above. In addition, increasing evidence for the low FODMAP diet in treating irritable bowel syndrome is triggering more referrals as well (Bellini et al. 2020). The American College of Gastroenterology estimates that about 1 in 20 Americans suffer from IBS (ACG n.d.), for whom the condition greatly reduces their quality of life. Surprisingly, a small percentage of primary care physicians and GI specialists refer their patients to a dietitian for GI conditions. Regardless, as patients find that food directly impacts their symptoms, it is prudent for dietitians to be prepared for the most common questions asked in these encounters and to have educational materials on hand.

With or without the presence of metabolic or GI disorders, weight management is also a frequently discussed topic in nutrition counseling. At the time of this writing, the prevalence of obesity among adults in the United States was 41.9% (CDC 2021). As mentioned earlier, if physicians have access to a dietitian, a majority of them will refer for weight counseling. Indeed, obesity is associated with an increased risk for many of the conditions listed above. However, weight bias can negatively affect how clinicians counsel patients and therefore how patients respond to treatment. As such, understanding the perspective of the patient is critical in addressing weight concerns, if indeed they are seeking weight management support. In some cases, patients may be resistant to weight counseling. In others, they may themselves initiate the conversation. Either way, a patient-centered approach that allows the patient to set the agenda for the visit allows the clinician to identify which topics will best resonate with the patient at that visit. Whatever their preference, a focus on healthy behaviors and disease management will address their concerns.

The following pages will highlight some of the frequently asked questions and misconceptions about the conditions listed above, and the key messages that help clarify that information. Further, as many patients are diagnosed with multiple comorbidities, they often feel that the nutrition guidelines for different conditions contradict each other. The materials and messages discussed in this book will help to lessen that confusion. Again, an objective presentation of information often answers the questions that patients initially ask at the start of a visit and can also discredit the misinformation they may have previously received.

While some conditions and intolerances may require specific food restrictions, an emphasis on overall balanced nutrition not only benefits most nutrition-related disorders but is often better accepted and more easily implemented by people. Often, when a person arrives for nutrition counseling, they are expecting to be told to avoid certain foods and make difficult sacrifices. Some may already be restricting their diets, and many will report trying and failing popular diets in the past. By understanding each patient's personal eating pattern as discussed earlier in this book, a dietitian can provide people with a better understanding of what can work, what might not, and why past efforts were so difficult to sustain.

Where the rest of the world sends messages of "don't eat this" and "never eat that," dietitians provide the insight that people need to make changes that work, and just as important, changes that last. While barriers to referrals still need addressing, those who do see a dietitian often see improvements to clinical indicators (e.g., blood pressure, lipids, blood glucose), dietary intake, and weight management (Mitchell et al. 2017). Furthermore, patients report a better understanding of nutrition, improvements to how they feel physically and emotionally, and they feel more in control of their condition (Schiller et al. 1998).

But one of my favorite outcomes is when the patient says, "Oh thank goodness. I can eat again!"

REFERENCES

American College of Gastroenterology. IBS-infographic.pdf [Internet]. North Bethesda, MD: American College of Gastroenterology; [cited 10/15/2022]. Available from: https://webfiles.gi.org/images/patients/IBS-infographic.pdf.

Bellini M, Tonarelli S, Nagy AG, Pancetti A, Costa F, Ricchiuti A, de Bortoli N, Mosca M, Marchi S, Rossi A. Low FODMAP Diet: Evidence, Doubts, and Hopes. *Nutrients*. 2020 Jan;12(1):148. doi: 10.3390/nu12010148.

Centers for Disease Control and Prevention (CDC). National Center for Health Statistics (NCHS). National Health and Nutrition Examination Survey Data. Hyattsville, MD: U.S. Department of Health and Human Services, Centers for Disease Control and Prevention; 2021. Available from: https://www.cdc.gov/obesity/data/adult.html (Accessed 10/15/2022).

Mitchell LJ, Ball LE, Ross LJ, Barnes KA, Williams LT. Effectiveness of Dietetic Consultations in Primary Health Care: A Systematic Review of Randomized Controlled Trials. *J Acad Nutr Diet*. 2017 Dec;117(12):1941–1962. doi: 10.1016/j.jand.2017.06.364.

Sastre LR, Van Horn LT. Family Medicine Physicians' Report Strong Support, Barriers and Preferences for Registered Dietitian Nutritionist Care in the Primary Care Setting. *Fam Pract*. 2021 Feb;38(1):25–31. doi: 10.1093/fampra/cmaa099.

Schiller MR, Miller M, Moore C, Davis E, Dunn A, Mulligan K, Zeller P. Patients Report Positive Nutrition Counseling Outcomes. *J Am Diet Assoc*. 1998 Sep;98(9):977–982; quiz 983-4. doi: 10.1016/S0002-8223(98)00224-7.

Xu JQ, Murphy SL, Kochanek KD, Arias E. *Mortality in the United States, 2021*. NCHS Data Brief, no 456. Hyattsville, MD: National Center for Health Statistics; 2022. doi: 10.15620/cdc:122516.

10 Type 2 Diabetes and Prediabetes

Diabetes is one of the most common reasons for referral to a dietitian from physicians (Sastre and Van Horn 2021). As of this writing, 37.3 million people in the United States have diabetes, 90%–95% of whom have type 2 diabetes (CDC 2023). Furthermore, 96 million US adults have prediabetes—that is about one in three people (CDC 2022). Therefore, it will be no surprise that many of your encounters will include nutrition counseling for diabetes or diabetes prevention.

Often, by the time a patient sees you, they have already received a lot of information about nutrition, especially about carbohydrates. From non-nutrition health professionals to well-meaning friends and family to Internet searches, people with diabetes have heard they should "avoid white carbs" or "go keto" or some other anti-carb advice.

These messages are frustrating for both patients and dietitian. For the patient, they find that "everything turns to sugar!" For dietitians who aim to promote balanced nutrition, they are challenged with refuting these misconceptions while presenting themselves as experts on nutrition. Highlighting the benefits of a variety of plant foods and asserting the importance of glucose can be particularly challenging when the patient was already told by their doctor to "cut carbs."

When I first started practicing, I also had my own misconceptions about meal planning for diabetes. I recall when a person first asked me, "How many carbohydrates do I need," I pulled up my calculator and started doing math. At 50% of calorie needs, divided by four for total grams of carbs, then divided by three meals per day, converted to carb exchanges per meal…you get the picture. Oh, the precious time I wasted, not to mention the confusion I probably caused my patient. Not only was my approach confusing for both him and myself, but by focusing on carb amount, I failed to highlight the importance of balanced meals, the effects of fat and protein, and the underlying mechanisms of impaired glucose tolerance. By omitting that information, I reinforced that diabetes was a carbohydrate issue, rather than an insulin issue.

Today, as a diabetes care and education specialist, I frequently encounter patients who say something along the lines of, "All I've been told is that I can have four or five carbs per meal." Needless to say, they are often unclear about why some meals cause higher blood sugars than others, or why their levels rise even when they have not eaten, or why even healthy carbs can still cause a spike. Conversely, for those who translate "watch your carbs" to "less is more," those who avoid carbs are unclear why their energy is low, why they are frequently hungry, or why they are experiencing more headaches. Either way, people are often primed to think carbohydrates are unhealthy.

For me, training to become certified in diabetes management helped me to develop a deeper understanding about how different foods affect blood sugar, the role of various diabetes medications and their side effects, and other factors that can cause either high or low blood sugar. With this understanding, I have become more astute at helping patients not only understand their disease but also troubleshoot the sometimes confusing patterns in their blood sugar readings.

When counseling a patient with diabetes, there are some key points that *you* will need to know, that they *want* to know, and that they *need* to know. This chapter highlights these points and prepares you for the most stated complaint, "I just need to know what to eat!"

DOI: 10.1201/9781003326038-13

WHAT YOU NEED TO KNOW

1. Their typical daily routine and eating pattern
2. Their level of physical activity
3. If they test their blood sugar, and if so, their blood sugar pattern
4. Which medications they take, if they take them as directed, and if side effects affect their eating pattern

WHAT PATIENTS *WANT* TO KNOW

1. How many carbs can I have?
2. What can I eat and what do I have to avoid?
3. Does this mean that I can never eat sweets again?
4. How can I manage this without medication?
5. How can I turn this around?

WHAT PATIENTS *NEED* TO KNOW

1. What is different in the body with prediabetes and diabetes, i.e., what is insulin resistance and how it leads to low insulin production
2. The role of glucose and insulin
3. Carbohydrate metabolism – what is supposed to happen to blood sugar after eating
4. Carbohydrate metabolism with diabetes – how insulin resistance and low insulin production affect blood sugar
5. Causes of insulin resistance and how to improve it
6. Balanced meal planning and the Diabetes Plate Method

A NOTE ABOUT TYPE 1 DIABETES AND OTHER RARE FORMS

Less than 10% of diabetes cases include the following types:
- Type 1 Diabetes
- Latent Autoimmune Diabetes in Adults (LADA)
- Mature Onset Diabetes of the Young (MODY)
- Diabetes Secondary to Underlying Conditions (e.g., pancreatic disease or lipodystrophy)
- Steroid-induced diabetes
- Post-transplant diabetes

For each of these types, the medical nutrition therapy will be similar: A personalized approach to balanced meal planning that emphasizes healthy choices, portion control, and minimal ultra-processed foods.

For those using an insulin-to-carb ratio regimen, where insulin dose is dependent on the number of grams of carbs in their meal, learning to accurately count carbs will be part of the education. However, for those on a sliding scale or set dose regimen, consistent carb portions (as represented in the Diabetes Plate Method) would be an adequate approach for those who do not want to count carbs.

For those using insulin, including those with advanced cases of type 2 diabetes, they will require medication guidance including insulin adjustments, ongoing pattern management, and for some, insulin pump training. Monitoring for hypoglycemia is critical, and an assessment of their eating pattern and physical activity in the context of their insulin regimen will indicate if they need to make nutrition changes, medication adjustments, or both. Proper treatment of hypoglycemia is also important to review, as well as the action time of insulin—both topics are commonly misunderstood and frequently underlie the wide swings in blood sugar that many people experience.

Due to the complicated nature of their treatment, these patients often receive ongoing support from certified diabetes care and education specialists. Dietitians, nurses, pharmacists, and other health professionals with these credentials can assist with MNT, medication adjustments, diabetes technology, remote patient monitoring, problem solving, patient advocacy, and overall pattern management.

More information on how to become a Certified Diabetes Care and Education Specialist (CDCES) or Board Certified in Advanced Diabetes Management (BC-ADM) is available at diabeteseducator.org.

WHAT YOU NEED TO KNOW

As with any nutrition visit, the first part of your visit will be the assessment. As there are a multitude of topics that can be covered in diabetes education, the purpose of your assessment will be to find out which topics are most relevant at that moment so you can tailor your approach, manage your time, and provide the patient with the information they need most.

As you break the ice with your patient and allow them to voice their concerns, they are likely to shed light on what they *want* to know. Once you are clear which topics they want to learn about, repeat those topics as the agenda for the visit to confirm with the patient what will be covered during their appointment. If not all topics will fit within the allotted time, ask them which topics they would like to cover now, and which they are willing to delay until the next visit. This approach allows you to manage your time effectively, include the patient in the decision-making process of their care, and sets the patient's expectations that nutrition counseling and diabetes management may require ongoing care.

Below are some clarifying questions you may need to ask to find out what else they *need* to know.

Key Assessment Questions for Diabetes Care

1. ***What does your typical day look like?*** As discussed earlier in this book, a dietary recall often reveals information about their schedules, daily responsibilities, social support, challenges, perceived barriers, and other personal values. You will also learn about their everyday eating routine. Do they prepare their own meals, or do they eat out more? Do they skip meals, or snack frequently, or eat late at night? Do they avoid certain food groups? Or are their portions excessive? Review Part 2 for other common everyday patterns.
2. ***Please describe your physical activities.*** Assess the types of activity they are able to do and how often they are able to do it.
3. ***Do you test your blood sugar?*** Clarify how often they test. This will vary per person. For those who are not on diabetes medication, their doctor may not have instructed them to test. Those on non-insulin medications may be testing once or twice a day. Those using insulin may need to test before each meal and at bedtime. Have them describe their

typical blood sugar ranges or, if available, review their blood sugar readings. Do they have concerns for recurring hyperglycemia, hypoglycemia, neither or both?

4. Confirm which diabetes medications they are taking and ask, ***"How often do you miss a dose of your medication, if at all?"*** While healthy eating is critical for managing blood sugar, even the healthiest diet will cause high blood sugar if the patient is not taking their medications properly. Also ask, ***"Have you experienced any side effects since starting this/these medications?"*** Some diabetes medications cause GI disturbances, reduced appetite, or increased risk for hypoglycemia, which should be incorporated into the nutrition education.

5. For those taking mealtime insulin, ask, ***"Do you inject before you eat, during, or after?"*** As rapid-acting insulin should be taken up to 15 minutes before eating, late doses can lead to high blood sugar, even if the meal is properly balanced.

As you listen to their story and evaluate their blood sugar pattern, consider the factors that can cause hyper- or hypoglycemia (see Table 10.1).

While listening to their story, I often ask myself, "What information is going to be most helpful for this patient today?"

Plan which information you will highlight for that visit. For example, perhaps the agenda you set with the patient focused on meal planning. However, as they described their typical day, you find out they are not taking their medication properly. You may need to highlight how their medications help them metabolize the glucose from their meals.

While the treatment of diabetes is multifaceted, nutrition is the main topic of interest for many people with type 2 diabetes. However, in order to better understand how food affects blood sugar, a detailed education about the disease itself is often warranted. Just as the dietitian's understanding of the condition improves their nutrition counseling skills, so can a patient's self-management improve once they acquire that knowledge for themselves. Therefore, sharing knowledge about how the disease works provides a better understanding of the nutrition recommendations, and subsequently a more compelling reason to follow them. The same can be said for their medications.

Therefore, the following are the most common questions that patients have about diabetes as well as the answers they did not know they needed.

WHAT PATIENTS WANT TO KNOW

How many carbs can I have? A diagnosis of diabetes can often motivate a person to start eating healthier. While there may be some misconceptions about how different foods affect blood sugar, many of the nutrition changes people initiate are beneficial. They cut out sweets or pop. They consume more vegetables. They choose lean chicken over red meat. However, some may be unnecessarily restrictive, such as avoiding all carbohydrates, or eating only salads. Such extremes can result in unsustainable changes, uncomfortable side effects, possible nutrient deficiencies, and sometimes even increased risk for complications.

To be fair, the American Diabetes Association found that there is no ideal percentage of macronutrients for people with or at risk for diabetes (Evert et al. 2019). In their review, no specific dietary pattern proved superior to another in regard to diabetes management or prevention. Reduction in A1C was observed in various eating patterns and macronutrient distributions, including the Mediterranean diet, the DASH diet, vegetarian or vegan diets, and low- and very-low-carb diets. Therefore, while some dietitians may aim to refute or promote certain popular diets, personalizing MNT to the values of the patient can be effective in glycemic management, regardless of their macronutrient distribution. Of course, incorporating other dietary concerns such as lipid management, hypertension, or other conditions must be considered, as well as risks such as

TABLE 10.1

Risk Factors for Hyperglycemia or Hypoglycemia

	Hyperglycemia	Hypoglycemia
Dietary factors		
Excessive portions of carbohydrates	✔	
Refined carbohydrates	✔	
Meals low in fiber, protein, and fat	✔	
High fat meals	✔	✔[a]
Frequent snacking between meals	✔	
Frequent snacks taken with insulin		✔
Skipped meals or prolonged fasts[b]	✔	✔
Caffeine	✔	
Physical activity[c]		
Sedentary activity	✔	
Moderate activity		✔
Vigorous activity	✔	✔
Strength training	✔	✔
Medications		
Excessive or inadequate medication regimens[d]	✔	✔
Medication non-compliance	✔	✔
Injecting mealtime insulin after eating instead of before	✔	✔
Injecting "correction" insulin between meals or too frequently (a.k.a. "stacking")		✔
Other medications or medical treatments, e.g., steroid therapy or cancer treatments	✔	
Expired insulin	✔	
Malfunction with insulin delivery devices	✔	✔
Other factors		
Poor sleep	✔	
High stress	✔	
Infection or illness[e]	✔	✔
Menstrual cycle	✔	✔
Overtreating low blood sugar with too much sugar	✔	
Overtreating high blood sugar with too much insulin		✔

[a] High fat meals can cause a delay in gastric emptying. If the patient uses rapid-acting insulin, the mismatch between insulin and food absorption can cause low blood sugar immediately after a meal. Conversely, once the fats enter the bloodstream, they can cause insulin resistance, leading to prolonged hyperglycemia.

[b] Some diabetes medications increase the risk for low blood sugar, e.g., insulin and sulfonylureas. Thus, they are at risk of low blood sugar if they go too long without eating. Conversely, prolonged fasts can result in hepatic release of glucose and can raise blood sugar, an effect often observed in fasting readings.

[c] Moderate physical activity can cause blood sugar to lower during or soon after the activity. Conversely, high intensity exercises or strength training can cause blood sugar to surge during the activity and may still be high soon after. All types of exercise increase insulin sensitivity for several hours after the exercise. Increased insulin sensitivity can improve blood sugar patterns, but depending on their medication type, may increase risk for hypoglycemia. If the patient experiences frequent low blood sugar, an adjustment to their medications may be necessary.

[d] If the patient is experiencing wide fluctuations in blood sugar regardless of medication compliance and healthy choices, refer them to their doctor for further assessment of their medication regimens. Some diabetes programs allow dietitians who are certified in diabetes care (CDCES or BC-ADM) to make medication adjustments.

[e] Infections can cause high blood sugar, but poor appetite related to illness may lead to low blood sugar.

hypoglycemia. Of note, the Mediterranean diet is the only dietary pattern that has been shown to reduce risk for major cardiovascular events, in addition to A1C reduction (Evert et al. 2019; Estruch et al. 2018), which is advantageous considering that heart disease is the leading cause of death for people with diabetes (ADA n.d.).

Some patients will ask about ***carb counting***, which can be an effective way to mindfully control carb portions. However, for some, measuring and calculating carbs may feel burdensome, overwhelming, or simply confusing. For each patient, the dietitian must assess if carb counting is an appropriate approach for them. For people using an insulin-to-carb-ratio regimen, carb counting is integral in dosing their mealtime insulin. However, the majority of people with diabetes have type 2 without intensive insulin therapy (Hodish 2018). In these cases, carb counting can be helpful, but not required.

Furthermore, focusing on carb counting may cause people to neglect the overall balance of their nutrition. When told to include 45 g of carbs per meal, people might neglect to include sufficient protein or non-starchy vegetables in their meal, subsequently resulting in rapid digestion and glycemic response. Similarly, a focus on carb amount can mislead people into thinking that refined carbs such as sugary cereals or beverages can be frequently consumed, as long as the amount is within the recommended portion. Or that non-carb foods that are high in fat can be freely consumed without regard to portion or calories, which may contribute to weight gain or hyperlipidemia. Therefore, carb counting without balanced meal planning can have some drawbacks.

The Diabetes Plate Method (ADA 2020). For most people, the Plate Method may be a more effective approach than carb counting as it is easy to understand and can be applied with little measuring or math. Furthermore, it incorporates (1) consistent carb portions, (2) the benefits of fiber, protein, and fat on glycemic response, (3) the importance of lean protein, non-starchy vegetables, and healthy fats for nutrition and satiety, and (4) overall portion control. A key message with the Plate Method is that it is an overall healthy approach to eating that provides benefits beyond glycemic control.

The Diabetes Plate Method (Figure 10.1) is slightly different than the MyPlate approach described in the Dietary Guidelines for Americans (USDA n.d.). In the diabetes version,

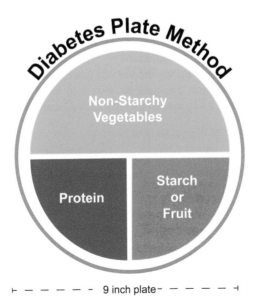

FIGURE 10.1   The diabetes plate method.

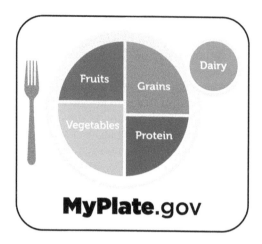

FIGURE 10.2   MyPlate is the official symbol of the five food groups in the *Dietary Guidelines for Americans 2020–2025*.

carbohydrates, such as starches and fruit, are indicated for one-quarter of the plate, non-starchy vegetables are recommended for half of the plate, and protein would make up the other quarter of the plate. This is different from the DGA's MyPlate (Figure 10.2), which has separate sections for fruit and grains, allowing almost half a plate of carbohydrates. In comparison, the Diabetes Plate Method can be described as lower in carb.

For those who are managing both diabetes and cardiovascular conditions, a Diabetes Plate shown with a glass of low-fat milk can also be used to represent the DASH diet—which is high in vegetables and fruit. The DASH diet also emphasizes the benefits of low-fat dairy.

The Diabetes Plate can also represent the Mediterranean diet, which is also high in plant foods. Plates that include fish, nuts, and/or vegetables cooked in olive oil can communicate the protective effects of healthy fats (Figure 10.3).

When showing examples without animal products, the protein portion of the plate can be used for beans, lentils, or soy foods. While legumes contain carbohydrates, the average carb count of a plant-based Plate would still be 45–60 g carbs, which is appropriate for most people. Further, the high fiber content of the meal would attenuate the glycemic response.

By emphasizing the similarities among the various eating patterns, the concern that nutrition guidelines conflict starts to subside. For patients who also have hypertension, hyperlipidemia, and/or coronary artery disease, a key message in diabetes education will be:

> "What you eat for your diabetes is good for your heart, and what you eat for your heart is good for your diabetes.

What can I eat and what do I have to avoid? In addition to being nutritionally sound, another key benefit of the Plate Method is that it communicates flexibility. Both plant and lean animal proteins can be included. Carbohydrates do not need to be avoided. A variety of non-starchy vegetables can be included, and they can be raw or cooked.

Another key message in diabetes education is that variety is important. A person with diabetes needs the same vitamins, minerals and nutrients that those without diabetes need; their brain is still reliant on glucose; their muscles still need to maintain glycogen for exercise; and polyphenols found in fruits and other plant foods can still protect their health (Pandey and Rizvi 2009). Therefore, consuming a variety of healthy foods would be advantageous compared to avoiding certain foods or food groups.

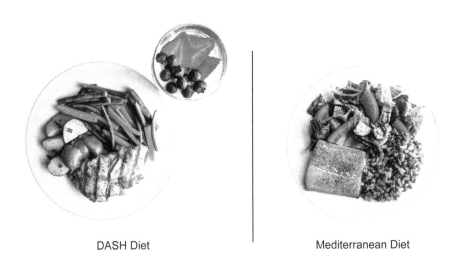

DASH Diet | Mediterranean Diet

FIGURE 10.3 The Diabetes Plate can be used when discussing the DASH Diet and the Mediterranean Diet.

Overall, focusing on the types of foods people choose (e.g., ultra-processed foods versus whole foods, or fast foods versus home-prepared meals, or high fat meats versus lean proteins), as well as their eating behaviors (e.g., grazing or night snacking), will be as important as dietary guidelines.

Does this mean that I can never eat sweets again? Dietary guidelines, on the other hand, can be vague about how to incorporate treats, which is another topic people have questions about. While the concepts of healthy eating can be clear, many fear that they can never indulge for pleasure.

In these cases, a discussion about frequency and portion may alleviate their concern. A snack in the afternoon may keep blood sugar from dropping if there is a long duration between lunch and dinner. While dietitians should encourage healthy choices, assure the patient that a mindful treat can be safely included at times as well. For those who count carbs, including a small dessert as part of the carb count for their meal can allow for occasional sweets or special occasions. Common scenarios that patients ask about are birthday parties or other social occasions. For these instances, one strategy may be to forego the carbs in the main meal to allow for the carbs in the dessert.

For patients with or without diabetes, mindful indulgences can provide pleasure and enhance quality of life, as compared to deprivation and restriction. For patients with diabetes, their A1C or their blood sugar tests can indicate whether more mindfulness is needed. Unintended weight gain, or difficulty losing weight, may also require a closer look at how much, or how often, non-nutritious foods are included.

While balance, portion control, and mindfulness can allow for most types of foods, sugary beverages like soda and juice will cause the biggest spikes in blood sugar. Unless they are being used to treat hypoglycemia, they should be substituted with sugar-free beverages, especially water. While many people with diabetes are quick to avoid sugary soda, there are some who will struggle with avoiding it. Also, those new to diabetes may be surprised to learn that juice affects blood sugar similarly to soda, or that flavored coffee drinks contain a lot of sugar. As there are some people who find water or unsweetened beverages distasteful, helping people find acceptable drink alternatives can sometimes be a challenge. Sugar-free flavor enhancers can be a safe option. If sugar alcohols are used to add sweetness, an assessment of GI issues would be required if such beverages are excessively consumed.

How can I manage this without medication? When newly diagnosed with T2DM, many people are hesitant to start medication. For some, they are leery of side effects or question how they work. Others may be medically managing other conditions and do not want to add yet another prescription to their regimen. Many are unclear about the physiological changes that cause diabetes and feel that nutritional changes are sufficient to manage blood sugar.

While diet and lifestyle are undeniably key factors in successfully managing metabolic disorders, for some, medications are necessary. The duration of disease, A1C level, and other underlying conditions are indicators as to whether or not a person can manage diabetes through lifestyle alone. For example, a patient who is newly diagnosed with an A1C of 6.6% who has a sedentary lifestyle and poor food choices may see their A1C reduced to the prediabetes range once they increase physical activity and make healthy diet changes. For a person with an A1C over 9.0%, they too may see a reduction in A1C with healthy changes. However, the higher their A1C is, the more likely their insulin production has diminished. Thus, lifestyle changes alone may not reduce their A1C sufficiently. In these cases, medication would still be necessary to manage their disease.

For those who have started taking medication, another common question is, "Can I ever get off the medication?" Often, when people do see their A1C improve, they are eager to discontinue the prescription. However, while they may have made significant lifestyle changes, some of their improvements could also be attributed to the medication. In these cases, discontinuing the therapy may diminish their improvement. On the other hand, if they are experiencing recurrent hypoglycemia, their doctor may be amenable to reducing or eliminating medication.

Therefore, the question about the need for medication can best be addressed by explaining what changes in the body with diabetes (i.e., insulin resistance and low insulin production), how it progresses over time, and a discussion about how long they have had their diabetes and the level of their A1c. With that information, along with an explanation about how their medications work, patients may better understand why they need the medication.

How can I turn this around? Addressing the question of whether diabetes is reversible requires a delicate approach. On too many occasions, I have witnessed healthcare providers quick to reply that the disease is irreversible and only gets worse over time. I was certainly guilty of this approach early in my career. However, while this information may be true, such a frank reply may demonstrate a lack of compassion, which is a key component in patient-centered care.

A diagnosis of diabetes can be quite emotional for many people. On one hand, the patient may admit that they saw it coming as their A1C had been climbing for several years. Some even feel angry with themselves for not taking action to prevent it. Others may have been taken by surprise or are in denial of the diagnosis. Many are fearful, especially if they have witnessed the effects of diabetes in people they know.

Whatever their emotional state, the provider will be most effective if they:

1. Exhibit compassion.
2. Avoid judgment.
3. Share knowledge.

A well-designed, easy-to-understand, and objectively delivered education will answer many of the patient's questions. Thus, in response to their questions, explain that "During this visit, we're going to learn about what is different in the body with diabetes, how food affects blood sugar, and what we can do to keep blood sugar levels in a safe range. A lot of this information will answer your questions today, and at the end, we'll put the puzzle pieces together to see what the right next steps are for you." Once the information is shared, the patient will better understand which actions and therapies apply to them.

WHAT PATIENTS NEED TO KNOW

Having worked in diabetes education for nearly a decade, in both individual counseling and group classes, I have found that the most common questions are answered by presenting a detailed description of the disease, what has changed in the patient's physiology, and what causes those changes. With this information, from basic metabolism to metabolism with diabetes, patients are better primed to understand the reasoning behind the nutrition recommendations.

Therefore, be sure to include the following information:

What are prediabetes and diabetes? A common misconception about diabetes is that it is caused by eating too much sugar. As such, another frequently asked question is, "But I don't even eat sweets. How could I get diabetes?"

While refined sugars can surely cause blood sugar spikes, a common misconception is that sweets alone cause diabetes or high blood sugar. This belief can be confusing for someone who does not eat a lot of sweets. For those who do, they may hope that avoiding sugar will help cure their diabetes. In either scenario, they will benefit from understanding that high blood sugar is due to a dysfunction in how their body makes or uses insulin, which is a result of several contributing factors, not just sugar.

While diet is fundamental in managing blood sugar, limiting the education to meal planning can be misleading to patients. Without a deeper understanding of what has changed in their body, they may feel that nutrition alone will manage—or reverse—their disease. Furthermore, as discussions about diabetes often focus on carbohydrates, patients often are misled into believing that carbohydrates alone affect their blood sugar levels.

Therefore, before discussing nutrition, an easy-to-understand, but detailed, explanation about the physiological changes that affect carb metabolism can help people better understand how to manage their disease, its progressive nature, related complications, and the impact of their behaviors. Often, this explanation helps to answer many of the questions they came with, including those mentioned above.

Therefore, define the type of diabetes they have, i.e., type 2 diabetes or prediabetes, and emphasize that the dysfunction is in how their body makes or uses insulin. Define relevant terms like "glucose," "insulin, and "insulin resistance." Describe how insulin resistance can lead to low insulin production. This information is critical in helping patients understand that their body is changing, which is key in helping them accept the various therapies required.

KEY POINTS: WHAT ARE PREDIABETES AND TYPE 2 DIABETES?

Diabetes is a disease that impairs how the body makes or uses insulin.

Insulin is a hormone that is produced by the pancreas. Insulin helps to lower the level of *glucose* in the blood.

In *prediabetes*, the pancreas still produces insulin, but the insulin does not work as well as it used to, which is called *insulin resistance*. This leads to higher levels of blood sugar.

Prediabetes becomes *type 2 diabetes* when the pancreas is no longer able to make enough insulin. The blood sugar level rises even higher due to the combination of insulin resistance and low insulin levels.

Basic carbohydrate metabolism. Provide a description of which foods contain carbohydrates, as well as their nutritional benefits. Highlight the importance of fiber, vitamins, minerals, and other nutrients in whole grains, starchy vegetables, fruit, legumes, milk, and yogurt. The key point here is that carbohydrates provide a variety of health benefits.

Discuss how all carbohydrates break down into glucose during digestion, then enter the bloodstream. A key point to make here is that everybody's blood sugar goes up after eating, with or without diabetes. Often, patients perceive that blood sugar levels should remain flat. This belief sometimes causes them to avoid all carbohydrates for fear of any rise in their blood sugar readings. As such, they exclude nutritious foods such as whole grains, starchy vegetables, fruit, or other plant foods.

Describe how glucose travels through the bloodstream to various cells around the body, especially the brain and muscle cells. Emphasize that the brain is dependent on glucose. Explain that glucose is the main fuel for exercise. Again, reinforce the benefits of carbohydrates and glucose. Prior to this education, many patients consider glucose as a bad thing, and therefore avoid carbohydrates. By explaining the pivotal role of glucose in brain function and energy production, they will be more amenable to balancing their meals with carbs (Figure 10.4).

A common response will be, "I thought I couldn't eat those things!" At this point, they start to feel relieved that they do not have to be as restrictive as they were initially led to believe.

Explain that the pancreas releases insulin as blood sugar starts to rise. Define insulin as a hormone that helps the glucose enter the cells and leave the bloodstream, at which point the blood sugar levels start to decline (Figure 10.5).

Carbohydrate metabolism with diabetes. Provide a description of what has changed in regard to how their body makes or uses insulin.

For patients with type 2 diabetes, prediabetes, or other conditions that cause insulin resistance (e.g., steroid therapy or PCOS), provide a simple definition of **insulin resistance**. For example, if using the key analogy, indicate that "the key doesn't fit in the lock as well as it used to, so the sugar stays in the blood longer and builds up." Many patients appreciate this analogy as they better

KEY POINTS: BASIC CARBOHYDRATE METABOLISM

1. There are many healthy carbohydrates, most of which are plant foods.
2. Glucose is the main fuel for the brain and for exercising muscle.
3. Insulin is the "key" that opens up the cells for the glucose to enter. As glucose moves into the cells, blood sugar levels decline. The glucose is used for energy in the cells.

FAQ:
But I thought carbs were bad for you?

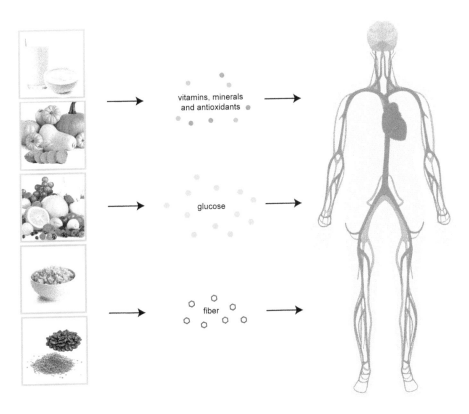

Key Message
Carbohydrates provide glucose and other important nutrients.
Glucose is the main fuel for the brain and for exercising muscle.

FIGURE 10.4   Provide a description of which foods contain carbohydrates as well as their nutritional benefits.

understand why their blood sugar levels are higher. Subsequently, people will often ask what is blocking their insulin from working, at which point a discussion about lifestyle factors would be beneficial (Figure 10.6).

Discuss that insulin resistance first develops in the prediabetes stage, when A1C is between 5.7% and 6.4%. During this stage, the pancreas detects higher blood sugar levels and produces more insulin to help move the glucose into the cells. Thus, insulin levels are typically higher with prediabetes. However, that means that the pancreas is working harder. With this point, the **progressive nature of diabetes** can be explained with another analogy:

"Over time, like anything with a lot of mileage on it, there can be some wear and tear, causing the cells on the pancreas to produce less insulin. Thus, type 2 diabetes develops when the pancreas is no longer able to produce enough insulin" (Figure 10.7).

Clarifying that diabetes is typically diagnosed when A1C is 6.5 or higher can also help them assess the progression of their disease.

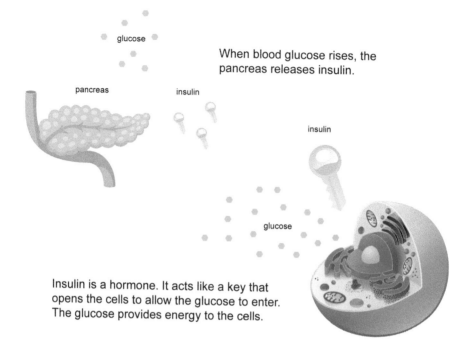

When blood glucose rises, the pancreas releases insulin.

glucose

pancreas   insulin

insulin

glucose

Insulin is a hormone. It acts like a key that opens the cells to allow the glucose to enter. The glucose provides energy to the cells.

Key Message
Glucose is an important source of energy, especially for the brain and for physical activity.

FIGURE 10.5   Comparing insulin to a key is a common analogy used to explain how insulin works.

What causes insulin resistance. For those with type 2 diabetes, once the patient understands the impact of insulin resistance, their next question will be, "What is blocking my insulin from working?"

While it is important for a patient to understand the irreversible nature of diabetes, it is equally important for them to understand that they still have the power to reduce insulin resistance through diet, physical activity, and—if applicable—moderate weight loss. To hear that diabetes cannot be reversed can be devastating. However, for people with type 2 diabetes, to learn that insulin resistance is still modifiable may be empowering. Thus, providing this information together may help minimize the blow of the diagnosis, prevent a feeling of hopelessness, and motivate the patient to take action.

KEY POINTS: CARBOHYDRATE METABOLISM WITH DIABETES

1. The body still needs glucose for energy, as well as the other vitamins, minerals, fiber, and other benefits of various carbohydrates.
2. In order to get the benefits of these foods, treatment goals are to (1) reduce the insulin resistance and/or (2) increase insulin levels with medication.

If applicable, explain how the patient's medications work. Many of them have nutritional implications such as GI side effects, risk for hypoglycemia, and weight loss or weight gain (see Table 10.2).

TABLE 10.2

Common Diabetes Medications with Nutrition-Related Side Effects

Medication Classification	Primary Action	Nutrition-Related Side Effects	Nutrition Intervention
Metformin	Improves insulin sensitivity and reduces hepatic production of glucose	GI disturbances including diarrhea, gas, or bloating May help with weight loss	Take with food Reinforce benefits of fiber
GLP-1 receptor agonists	Increases insulin production, slows gastric emptying, and lowers appetite	Prolonged feeling of satiety, sometimes accompanied by bloating, nausea, vomiting, or diarrhea Helps with weight loss	Emphasize proper portion control and small, frequent meals or snacks Caution against large and/or high fat meals Encourage soft-textured foods like cooked vegetables, fish, eggs, tofu, simmered meats, or smoothies and soups Monitor for inadequate nutrient intake.
SGLT-2 inhibitors	Excretes glucose through the urine	Increased urination and thirst May help with weight loss	Reinforce importance of hydration Of note, SGLT-2 inhibitors have been shown to increase risk for diabetic ketoacidosis (Douros 2020). Caution against the ketogenic diet with this medication.
Sulfonylureas	Stimulates insulin production	Increased risk for hypoglycemia May cause weight gain	Reinforce the importance of balanced meals that include carbohydrates Caution against skipping meals or prolonged fasting Educate on proper treatment of hypoglycemia Reinforce importance of portion control and mindful choices
Long-Acting Insulin	Raises basal insulin levels Reduces hepatic production of glucose	Increased risk for hypoglycemia May cause weight gain	Reinforce the importance of balanced meals that include consistent portions of carbohydrates Caution against skipping meals or prolonged fasting Educate on proper treatment of hypoglycemia Reinforce importance of portion control and mindful choices
Fast-acting insulin	Helps move glucose from the bloodstream into the cells and is typically injected before eating	Increased risk for hypoglycemia May cause weight gain	Reinforce the importance of balanced meals that include consistent portions of carbohydrates Caution against skipping meals or prolonged fasting Educate on proper treatment of hypoglycemia If using a carb ratio regimen, educate on proper carb counting Reinforce importance of portion control and mindful choices

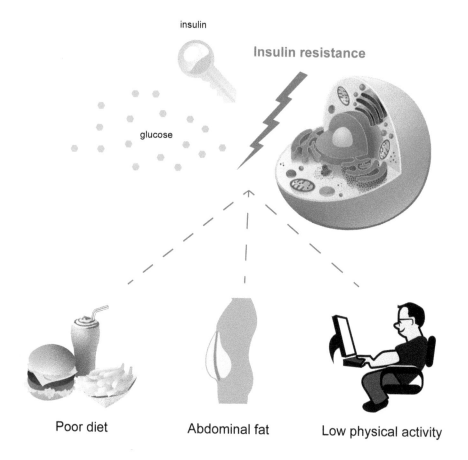

insulin

Insulin resistance

glucose

Poor diet   Abdominal fat   Low physical activity

Key Message
Poor diet, abdominal fat, and low physical activity
can lead to insulin resistance.

FIGURE 10.6   Describing what causes insulin resistance can reinforce the recommendations for what can reverse insulin resistance, i.e., healthy diet, physical activity, and if applicable, weight loss.

While type 2 diabetes is largely preventable, acknowledge their non-modifiable risk factors as well, such as family history, age, ethnicity, or other underlying conditions.

KEY POINTS: CAUSES OF INSULIN RESISTANCE

Poor diet, low physical activity, and abdominal fat can lead to insulin resistance.

Other risk factors for diabetes include family history, age, and ethnicity (i.e., African American, Hispanic or Latino, Native American, Pacific Islander, or Asian American). High stress, some medical conditions, and some medications can also cause insulin resistance.

Emphasize the factors that they can modify.

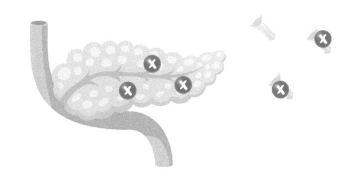

FIGURE 10.7   An explanation that type 2 diabetes is typically characterized by low insulin production helps people understand that medications are often required in addition to lifestyle changes.

Explain how ***physical activity*** affects blood sugar and insulin resistance. For this, returning to the key analogy can be helpful (Figure 10.8).

"Like insulin, physical activity is a key that opens the muscle cells. Whether you are going on a brisk walk or using a stationary bike or vacuuming, as your muscles move, they open up even without insulin. Then the sugar is able to enter your muscle cells, and your blood sugar level lowers."

Describe the *Physical Activity Guidelines for Americans* (U.S. Department of Health and Human Services 2018) along with examples of how to include activity throughout the day. Emphasize that movement of any duration and form is beneficial, with a goal of accumulating at least 150 minutes of moderate to vigorous activity per week. People often find physical activity more attainable when they learn that they can spread activity throughout the day, and that the activity does not have to be formal exercise. Walking is attainable for many people and can typically be implemented without medical clearance. For those who are unable to walk, seated upper body movements such as arm raises may be an option. Portable or table-top arm peddlers are also available in a wide range of prices and can be relatively affordable.

It is helpful to have a variety of examples ready for various barriers, including busy schedules, financial constraints, and physical limitations. These examples can include free online videos of various durations, inexpensive equipment like portable peddlers or resistance bands, and even household items like 16 oz water bottles used as hand weights.

Patients are often responsive to the information that insulin resistance is lower for several hours after the activity is over. I often refer to this as the "afterburn." This information helps reinforce the benefit of being active most days of the week. For those who test their blood sugar, they are likely to have observed these benefits.

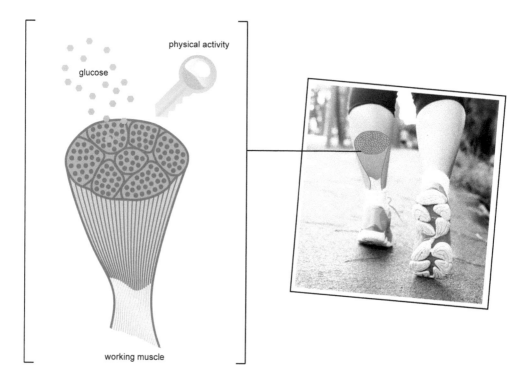

FIGURE 10.8 Physical activity facilitates glucose transport into the muscle cells. Physical activity can also increase insulin sensitivity up to 24 hours after exercise (ADA n.d.).

Some people may already be active throughout the day at their job, or taking care of their young children, or with a regular exercise routine. If they are not already including strength training, explain that resistance exercises also help to lower A1C, especially in combination with aerobic activity (Sigal et al. 2007).

In regard to *healthy eating*, it is important to understand which foods can worsen insulin resistance. As mentioned earlier, most discussions about blood sugar revolve around carbohydrates. What is not commonly discussed is the effect of fat. Specifically, foods that are excessive in *saturated fat* like fast food, some deep-fried foods, or foods laden with high fat dairy like pizza. In excess, saturated fat can directly increase insulin resistance (Riccardi et al. 2004; Luukkonen et al. 2018) (Figure 10.9).

This part of the conversation often sparks confusion, perhaps even debate. "But I heard saturated fat was not really bad," or, "but a keto diet is high in fat."

On the other hand, this information also demonstrates the overlap between a heart healthy diet and healthy eating for diabetes. As excessive intake of saturated fat can elevate LDL-cholesterol levels, a key message here is "what you do for your blood sugar is good for your heart, and what you do for your heart is good for your diabetes."

FAQ:
Can't I eat as much meat and cheese as I want since they are not carbs?

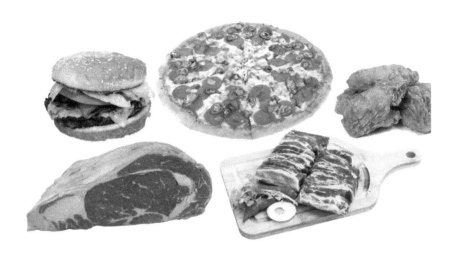

Key Message
In large amounts, foods high in saturated fat can worsen insulin resistance. Choose lean or plant proteins more often.

FIGURE 10.9   Saturated fat has been shown to worsen insulin resistance. In a typical American diet, excessive intake of saturate fat comes from high fat meat, some processed meats, fast food, some deep-fried foods, and foods heavy with high fat dairy, e.g., pizza.

The mishap occurs when saturated fats are consumed in excess, which is an important distinction to make. A slice of cheese on a turkey sandwich is typically not the culprit of high cholesterol and insulin resistance, nor is a pat of butter on toast. However, in a typical American diet, saturated fats are consumed in excess through fast food, large portions of high fat meat and dairy, and foods cooked in animal fat. Ultra-processed or packaged foods often are manufactured with palm oils, which is also high in saturated fat. These types of foods, in excess, are largely responsible for nutrition-related conditions. While saturated fat in and of itself is not harmful in light amounts, the amount that many Americans consume is the concern. For many, restaurant meals and ultra-processed foods are easily accessible—both of which are often excessive in many nutrients of concern (e.g., fat, sodium, refined carbohydrates). Furthermore, these same meals often lack fiber, vegetables, and other nutrient-dense foods, causing an overall imbalance in nutrition.

With this information, it becomes clearer to the patient that the overall diet must be addressed to manage diabetes, not just carbohydrates.

In the setting of low physical activity and poor diet, the risk of ***abdominal obesity*** increases. The portion of Americans who were overweight or obese in 2021 was 67%, an increase from 63% 10 years prior (CDC n.d.). For many, the topic of weight is a sensitive issue. In the healthcare setting, weight bias has been shown to negatively affect patient care. Providers often—consciously or unconsciously—shame patients for their weight, essentially blaming them for their conditions. Such biases undermine the patient-provider relationship, which can ultimately lead to ineffective care and negative outcomes.

In the case of diabetes, weight loss has been shown to lower insulin resistance and lower A1C. The research behind the Diabetes Prevention Program demonstrated that achieving and maintaining at least a 5% weight loss reduced the risk of type 2 diabetes by 58% (Knowler et al. 2002). In practice, it is commonly observed that weight loss helps to lower A1C and improve blood sugar readings. Therefore, it is critical to share this information with the patient. However, the educator must be mindful to present this information objectively as part of a comprehensive education, as opposed to a personal recommendation to lose weight. Again, the empowerment approach emphasizes that the role of the educator is to provide information, rather than dictate a treatment plan (Funnell and Anderson 2004).

Furthermore, while the contribution of weight to metabolic disorders is important to explain, the time spent on this specific topic can be minimized, as the lifestyle recommendations for diabetes management are beneficial for weight management as well. Nutrition education for diabetes will demonstrate balanced meal planning, portion control, healthy food choices, optimal meal timing, and overall mindfulness—all of which would be discussed for weight loss as well. In fact, I cannot tell you how many times patients return after the first visit reporting, "I've already started to lose weight," when weight loss strategies were not even part of the initial education. As such, a focus on overall healthy choices rather than weight can effectively address multiple concerns. Of note, healthy habits have also shown a reduced risk for mortality independent of weight (Matheson et al. 2012).

KEY POINTS: HOW TO IMPROVE INSULIN RESISTANCE

1. Increase physical activity.
2. Limit foods that are ultra-processed, high in saturated fat, and high in refined carbohydrates.
3. Aim to achieve and maintain at least 5% weight loss if applicable.

Meal planning for diabetes. The general components of good nutrition are similar for those with or without diabetes, including:

Food choices: Explain that carbs, fat, and protein are all important parts of the diet, but the types of food we choose matter.

Portion control: Controlling portions of carbs can help prevent high blood sugars, and portion control of all foods is important for weight management. Use the Diabetes Plate Method to demonstrate the recommended portions of each food group. Point out that a full meal can be consumed while still controlling calorie intake.

Balance: Including high fiber foods, protein, and fat helps to slow digestion, prevent hunger and cravings between meals, and minimize the rise in blood sugar after eating. Also, consuming a variety of food groups provides a variety of nutrients. The Diabetes Plate also helps to illustrate the concept of balance. Emphasize the different benefits of each food group. While carbs provide glucose for energy, protein helps to build and maintain muscle and metabolism, and the non-starchy vegetables provide vitamins, minerals, and protective compounds to help keep the body healthy.

Meal timing: Time meals to allow blood glucose to rise and fall before introducing more food. The optimal time between meals is typically around four hours. Include snacks when there will be a long gap between meals to help prevent hunger and cravings related to lower blood sugar levels, or to prevent hypoglycemia in people who use insulin, sulfonylureas, or other medication regimens that increase their risk for lows. However, caution against frequent snacking, as that can prolong and compound postprandial hyperglycemia, and/or promote weight gain through excessive calorie intake.

KEY POINTS: MEAL PLANNING FOR DIABETES

1. Use the Diabetes Plate to highlight the importance of all food groups, including non-starchy vegetables, protein, and carbohydrates, and to illustrate proper portion control.
2. Show examples of the Diabetes Plate with lean proteins, plant proteins, high fiber carbohydrates, and plenty of non-starchy vegetables. Highlight the flexibility of the Diabetes Plate, showing that a variety of foods can be included.
3. Recommend spacing meals about four hours apart, using snacks if needed. Discuss the pitfalls of skipping meals or snacking too frequently.

Regardless of the type of diabetes someone has, balanced nutrition is beneficial for all. However, food alone does not determine blood sugar patterns. Diabetes is a complicated disease that requires careful monitoring of blood sugar, food, activity, and medications. It can be an overwhelming disease to manage, as it affects every aspect of a person's life. From inexplicable high blood sugars to dangerous low blood sugars, some patients may have recurring patterns, while others have wide fluctuations that vary day to day.

For most people, a detailed explanation of what affects blood sugar can help shed light on some factors that may need addressing. Advanced training in diabetes care will be required to assist patients with medication management, problem solving, and diabetes technology like continuous glucose monitors and insulin pumps. However, food will forever be a key component in managing blood sugar, reducing risks, and preventing complications. As such, all dietitians who provide nutrition counseling can expect to treat patients with diabetes.

In most cases, the primary question you can expect to hear is, "What can I eat?" Often, the patient appears disheartened about food as they feel like they cannot eat anything. Sometimes, patients state that they were hesitant to make the appointment, as they are afraid the dietitian "will take everything good away."

Fortunately, a compassionate, well-delivered nutrition education not only provides relief to the patient, but also provides them with a sense of hope. Not only do they learn that they can still enjoy a variety of foods, but that they can take action to protect their health. All, in fact, is not lost. By the end of the visit, the burden they arrived with visibly lightens. They appear reassured, uplifted, and motivated. I recall one patient who exclaimed, "Oh thank goodness! I can eat again!"

These are the moments that dietitians strive for, the reason they entered the field.

To give people their lives back.

CLINICAL PRACTICE GUIDELINES, KEY STUDIES, MEAL PLANNING WEBSITES, AND PROFESSIONAL RESOURCES

American Diabetes Association: Standards of Medical Care in Diabetes - updated annually (ElSayed et al. 2023)

American Diabetes Association: Nutrition Therapy for Adults With Diabetes or Prediabetes: A Consensus Report (Evert et al. 2019)

Empowerment and Self-Management of Diabetes (Funnell and Anderson 2004).

The Look AHEAD study: a description of the lifestyle intervention and the evidence supporting it (Wadden et al. 2007)

Diabetes Prevention Program Research Group: Reduction in the incidence of type 2 diabetes with lifestyle intervention or metformin (Knowler et al. 2002)

National Diabetes Prevention Program, https://www.cdc.gov/diabetes/prevention/index.html

Physical Activity Guidelines for Americans, 2nd edition (USDHH 2018)

Association of Diabetes Care and Education Specialists, https://www.diabeteseducator.org/

American Diabetes Association: Diabetes Food Hub recipe website - https://www.diabetesfoodhub.org/

Platemethodpics.com – a stock photography website specializing in a variety of Plate Method examples.

Educational slides and meal planning handouts are included with this book, available online at https://resourcecentre.routledge.com/books/9781032352459

REFERENCES

American Diabetes Association. Blood Glucose and Exercise [Internet]. Arlington, VA; n.d. [cited 5/20/2023]. Available from: https://diabetes.org/healthy-living/fitness/getting-started-safely/blood-glucose-and-exercise.

American Diabetes Association. Diabetes Complications: Cardiovascular Disease [Internet]. Arlington, VA; n.d. [cited 5/14/2023]. Available from: https://diabetes.org/diabetes/cardiovascular-disease.

American Diabetes Association. What is the Diabetes Plate Method? [Internet]. Arlington, VA; February 2020 [cited 11/6/2022]. Available from: https://www.diabetesfoodhub.org/articles/what-is-the-diabetes-plate-method.html.

Centers for Disease Control and Prevention. National Diabetes Statistics Report website [Internet]; 2022 [cited 11/5/2022]. Available from: https://www.cdc.gov/diabetes/data/statistics-report/index.html.

Centers for Disease Control and Prevention. National Center for Chronic Disease Prevention and Health Promotion, Division of Nutrition, Physical Activity, and Obesity.Data, Trend and Maps [Internet]. Centers for Disease Control and Prevention. [cited May 12, 2023]. Available from: https://www.cdc.gov/nccdphp/dnpao/data-trends-maps/index.html.

Centers for Disease Control and Prevention. Type 2 Diabetes [Internet]; 2023 [cited 5/14/2023]. Available from: https://www.cdc.gov/diabetes/basics/type2.html.

Douros A, Lix LM, Fralick M, Dell'Aniello S, Shah BR, Ronksley PE, Tremblay É, Hu N, Alessi-Severini S, Fisher A, Bugden SC, Ernst P, Filion KB; Canadian Network for Observational Drug Effect Studies (CNODES) Investigators. Sodium-Glucose Cotransporter-2 Inhibitors and the Risk for Diabetic Ketoacidosis: A Multicenter Cohort Study. *Ann Intern Med.* 2020 Sep 15;173(6):417–425. doi: 10.7326/M20-0289.

ElSayed NA, Aleppo G, Aroda VR, Bannuru RR, Brown FM, Bruemmer D, Collins BS, Cusi K, Das SR, Gibbons CH, Giurini JM, Hilliard ME, Isaacs D, Johnson EL, Kahan S, Khunti K, Kosiborod M, Leon J, Lyons SK, Murdock L, Perry ML, Prahalad P, Pratley RE, Seley JJ, Stanton RC, Sun JK, Woodward CC, Young-Hyman D, Gabbay RA. On Behalf of the American Diabetes Association. Introduction and Methodology: Standards of Care in Diabetes-2023. *Diabetes Care*. 2023 Jan 1;46(Suppl 1):S1–S4. doi: 10.2337/dc23-Sint.

Estruch R, Ros E, Salas-Salvadó J, Covas MI, Corella D, Arós F, Gómez-Gracia E, Ruiz-Gutiérrez V, Fiol M, Lapetra J, Lamuela-Raventos RM, Serra-Majem L, Pintó X, Basora J, Muñoz MA, Sorlí JV, Martínez JA, Fitó M, Gea A, Hernán MA, Martínez-González MA, PREDIMED Study Investigators. Primary Prevention of Cardiovascular Disease with a Mediterranean Diet Supplemented with Extra-Virgin Olive Oil or Nuts. *N Engl J Med*. 2018 Jun;378(25):e34. doi: 10.1056/NEJMoa1800389.

Evert AB, Dennison M, Gardner CD, Garvey WT, Lau KHK, MacLeod J, Mitri J, Pereira RF, Rawlings K, Robinson S, Saslow L, Uelmen S, Urbanski PB, Yancy WS Jr. Nutrition Therapy for Adults with Diabetes or Prediabetes: A Consensus Report. *Diabetes Care*. 2019 May;42(5):731–754. doi: 10.2337/dci19-0014.

Funnell MM, Anderson RM. Empowerment and Self-Management of Diabetes. *Clin Diabetes*. 2004; 22(3):123–127.

Hodish, I. Insulin Therapy for Type 2 Diabetes - Are We There Yet? The d-Nav(r) Story. *Clin Diabetes Endocrinol*. 2018;4:8. doi: 10.1186/s40842-018-0056-5. Accessed 11/6/2022.

Knowler WC, Barrett-Connor E, Fowler SE, Hamman RF, Lachin JM, Walker EA, Nathan DM, Diabetes Prevention Program Research Group. Reduction in the Incidence of Type 2 Diabetes with Lifestyle Intervention or Metformin. *N Engl J Med*. 2002 Feb;346(6):393–403. doi: 10.1056/NEJMoa012512.

Look AHEAD Research Group, Wadden TA, West DS, Delahanty L, Jakicic J, Rejeski J, Williamson D, Berkowitz RI, Kelley DE, Tomchee C, Hill JO, Kumanyika S. The Look AHEAD Study: A Description of the Lifestyle Intervention and the Evidence Supporting It. *Obesity* (Silver Spring). 2006 May;14(5):737–752. doi: 10.1038/oby.2006.84. Erratum in: *Obesity* (Silver Spring). 2007 May;15(5):1339.

Luukkonen PK, Sädevirta S, Zhou Y, Kayser B, Ali A, Ahonen L, Lallukka S, Pelloux V, Gaggini M, Jian C, Hakkarainen A, Lundbom N, Gylling H, Salonen A, Orešič M, Hyötyläinen T, Orho-Melander M, Rissanen A, Gastaldelli A, Clément K, Hodson L, Yki-Järvinen H. Saturated Fat Is More Metabolically Harmful for the Human Liver Than Unsaturated Fat or Simple Sugars. *Diabetes Care*. 2018 Aug;41(8):1732–1739. doi: 10.2337/dc18-0071.

Matheson EM, King DE, Everett CJ. Healthy Lifestyle Habits and Mortality in Overweight and Obese Individuals. *J Am Board Fam Med*. 2012 Jan-Feb;25(1):9–15. doi: 10.3122/jabfm.2012.01.110164.

Pandey KB, Rizvi SI. Plant Polyphenols as Dietary Antioxidants in Human Health and Disease. *Oxid Med Cell Longev*. 2009 Nov-Dec;2(5):270–278. doi: 10.4161/oxim.2.5.9498.

Riccardi G, Giacco R, Rivellese AA. Dietary Fat, Insulin Sensitivity and the Metabolic Syndrome. *Clin Nutr*. 2004 Aug;23(4):447–456. doi: 10.1016/j.clnu.2004.02.006.

Sastre LR, Van Horn LT. Family Medicine Physicians' Report Strong Support, Barriers and Preferences for Registered Dietitian Nutritionist Care in the Primary Care Setting. *Fam Pract*. 2021 Feb;38(1):25–31. doi: 10.1093/fampra/cmaa099.

Sigal RJ, Kenny GP, Boulé NG, Wells GA, Prud'homme D, Fortier M, Reid RD, Tulloch H, Coyle D, Phillips P, Jennings A, Jaffey J. Effects of Aerobic Training, Resistance Training, or Both on Glycemic Control in Type 2 Diabetes: A Randomized Trial. *Ann Intern Med*. 2007 Sep;147(6):357–369. doi: 10.7326/0003-4819-147-6-200709180-00005.

US Department of Agriculture. Learn how to eat healthy with MyPlate [Internet]. Alexandria, VA. [cited 11/6/2022]. Available from: https://www.myplate.gov/.

U.S. Department of Health and Human Services. *Physical Activity Guidelines for Americans*, 2nd edition. Washington, DC: U.S. Department of Health and Human Services; 2018.

11 Heart Disease Prevention and Management

When I was working in a cardiovascular clinic, I often heard people say, "I have been following a diabetes diet, but now my doctor told me I have to follow a heart healthy diet. How can I do both?" Not surprisingly, when I moved to the diabetes clinic, I heard the exact opposite. "I was told I have to watch my cholesterol. Now I have to watch my sugar. How can I do both?"

The more complications that people develop, the more frustrated and overwhelmed they become with nutrition recommendations. And who could blame them? One day they are being told to avoid certain fats, then another day they hear they should watch their carbs. It is no surprise that a common complaint is, "I just don't know what is left to eat."

Medical nutrition therapy for the prevention or management of cardiovascular disease typically focuses on hypertension and/or dyslipidemia. Often, physicians will request that the dietitian teach specific nutrition guidelines. For example, the doctor may list "low sodium diet" and/or "DASH Diet" for patients with high blood pressure. Similarly, they may list "Mediterranean Diet" or "AHA Diet" for their patients with high LDL cholesterol, high triglycerides, or recent heart surgery.

Both the DASH and Mediterranean diets meet the nutrition recommendations from the American Heart Association/American College of Cardiology:

> Patients should consume a dietary pattern that emphasizes intake of vegetables, fruits, whole grains, legumes, healthy protein sources (low-fat dairy products, low-fat poultry (without the skin), fish/seafood, and nuts), and nontropical vegetable oils; and limits intake of sweets, sugar-sweetened beverages, and red meats.
>
> *(Grundy et al. 2019)*

In fact, the DASH Diet has been referred to as the "American Mediterranean Diet." Although DASH is lower in fat in comparison, both eating patterns emphasize vegetables, fruits, and lean proteins. Another difference is that the DASH highlights the benefit of low-fat dairy. Both eating patterns have been shown to benefit blood pressure, cholesterol levels, and blood sugar.

As stated in Chapter 10 on diabetes, both eating patterns can be represented with the Diabetes Plate Method, which demonstrates a heavy emphasis on plant foods. Therefore, a key message for patients managing both diabetes and cardiovascular conditions is that "What you do for your blood sugar is good for your heart, and what you do for your heart is good for your blood sugar."

While not all people with hypertension or hyperlipidemia have diabetes, many will have multiple metabolic concerns. About one in three adults have metabolic syndrome, which the National Heart, Lung and Blood Institute defines as having three or more of the following five criteria: central obesity, elevated blood glucose, elevated triglycerides, low levels of high-density lipoprotein cholesterol, and elevated blood pressure (Gallagher et al. 2011; NHLBI 2022). Furthermore, as stated in the diabetes chapter, cardiovascular disease is the number one cause of death for people with diabetes. Therefore, managing and preventing both heart disease and diabetes go hand in hand.

Therefore, for patients referred to you for a heart healthy diet, this chapter highlights the key points that will help you and your patient find common ground.

DOI: 10.1201/9781003326038-14

DYSLIPIDEMIA

WHAT YOU NEED TO KNOW

1. Their typical daily routine and eating pattern
2. How often they consume restaurant food and what types
3. Their main cooking fats
4. Vegetable and fruit consumption
5. Physical activity

WHAT PATIENTS *WANT* TO KNOW

1. What can I eat to lower my cholesterol?
2. Which are the bad fats and the good fats?
3. Do I need a fish oil supplement?
4. Are eggs good or bad?
5. How can I raise my good cholesterol?

WHAT PATIENTS *NEED* TO KNOW

1. What do their lab values mean?
2. What is LDL cholesterol?
3. Which foods increase LDL cholesterol?
4. What can happen when LDL cholesterol is high?
5. What are triglycerides?
6. Which foods increase triglycerides?
7. What can happen when triglycerides are high?
8. How can they improve their lipids?

WHAT YOU NEED TO KNOW

A typical American diet is often considered to be high in red meat, refined sugar, ultra-processed foods, restaurant foods, additives, and sodium; and low in fiber and plant foods. Think burgers, fries, and a soda—an iconic American meal. In other words, the exact opposite of what is recommended by the American Heart Association.

WHAT ARE ULTRA-PROCESSED FOODS?

The NOVA Classification of foods categorizes foods according to the extent of food processing. The categories include (1) unprocessed or minimally processed foods, (2) processed culinary ingredients such as salt, sugar, or oils, (3) processed foods, which are relatively simple products made by adding sugar, oil, salt, or other culinary ingredients to unprocessed foods, and (4) ultra-processed foods, which are defined below.

ULTRA-PROCESSED FOODS TYPICALLY CONTAIN:

Five or more ingredients including substances not commonly used in culinary preparations, and additives whose purpose is to imitate sensory qualities of minimally processed food, or to disguise undesirable sensory qualities of the final product (Figure 11.1).

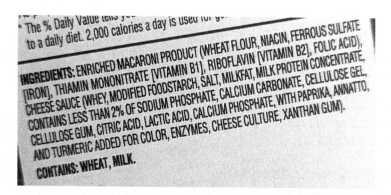

FIGURE 11.1   Ultra-processed foods have more than five ingredients, many of which are used to enhance texture or flavor, to disguise undesirable qualities, or to add or replace nutrients lost in processing.

Simply stated, ultra-processed foods are made with ingredients and manufacturing processes that cannot be used or replicated in home cooking.

Examples include carbonated drinks; sweet or savory packaged snacks; ice cream, chocolate, candies; mass-produced packaged breads and buns; margarines and spreads; cookies, pastries, cakes, breakfast cereals, and more.

Source: Monteiro et al. (2016)

Cheap packaged foods, fast food value meals, and mainstream chain restaurants with platter-sized portions are easily accessible for many people. A large pizza is often ready and waiting to go, and with a two-liter of pop and an order of breadsticks, can feed a family for under $15. Together with highly demanding work schedules, busy families, and ergo, a reduction in home cooking, these food choices help keep heart disease the leading cause of mortality in the United States.

Even home-prepared meals can be high in saturated fat, one of the key culprits in hypercholesterolemia. Higher fat meat and poultry are priced lower than their lean counterparts, making them a more accessible purchase. Fresh fish is much more expensive, therefore is less often purchased. Many feel that fresh food, overall, is priced out of their budgets, driving them to the packaged food aisles.

To be fair, people's snack and beverage *habits* are often equal contributors—if not the main contributor—to metabolic conditions. Sweets, snacks, and sugary beverages find ways of fitting into people's grocery budget. These types of foods are often overconsumed, which plays a role in elevating triglycerides, spiking insulin levels, weight gain, and related diseases.

Therefore, during the assessment portion of your visit, the key information you will need to uncover is not only what they eat but also where, why, and how much.

Key Assessment Questions for Dyslipidemia

1. ***What does your typical day look like?*** Walk your patient through a "typical day" or 24-hour dietary recall, including meals, snacks, drinks, and nutrition supplements. People often include details about their work and/or family schedules as they describe

how, and with whom, they eat throughout the day. They are likely to mention their challenges in meal planning or making healthy choices. From time constraints to budget limitations to their relationship with food, meal planning is an endeavor that requires more than nutrition knowledge or recipes.

2. *How many meals per day or week come from restaurants—whether sit-down, drive-through, or delivery? What do you typically order?* Listen for the types of foods they order as well as their dining out behaviors. Some will mention if they save part of the meal for leftovers, or if they share with their companion, or if they focus on healthier choices. Others will admit to indulging in higher fat foods, sugary or alcoholic beverages, or other splurges. If they dine out frequently, many may explain why. For example, perhaps they are empty nesters who do not want to cook for just one or two people. Or their schedules do not allow time for preparing meals at home. Or they have never developed an interest in cooking.

3. *What are your main cooking fats?* This question can provide insight into their nutrition knowledge and efforts. Those who use olive oil or avocado oil may already be mindful about healthy eating. Some who use coconut oil may demonstrate a tendency to follow diet trends. Cooking fats may also represent cultural traditions, such as the use of ghee in Indian populations, pork fat or lard in southern cooking, peanut and sesame oils in Asian cuisine, or butter in various European cuisines.

4. *How often a day or a week do you consume vegetables? Which types do you like?* As plant foods are heavily emphasized in heart healthy eating, learning which vegetables the patient likes will help personalize the education. Most people can name at least a few choices they will tolerate, even if they don't love vegetables. When you provide examples of healthy meals, you can incorporate the foods they already like, thus demonstrating that good nutrition does not have to be too different from what they are already eating. For many, they may find that they merely need to adjust the proportions of the foods in their meals—i.e., increase the vegetable portions and decrease the carb and protein portions while still including their typical foods. Again, the plate method demonstrates flexibility, where people can mix and match their favorite protein, carbs, and vegetables, while being mindful of portions.

5. *How often a day or week do you consume fruit? Which types do you like?* Similar to the previous question, the patient's fruit preferences can be incorporated into personalized meal or snack ideas. For those with a sweet tooth, a comparison of fat and/or calories between fruit and their typical treat can demonstrate the benefits of choosing fruit for snacks (Figure 11.2).

6. *How would you describe your level of physical activity?* Assess the types of activity they can do and how often they are able to do it. Be prepared to share examples that meet some barriers they may have—e.g., free or low-cost ideas, indoor activities for cold weather, or seated and low impact exercises for some physical limitations. Walking is typically considered safe to perform without medical clearance. However, for patients who are deconditioned and/or have existing cardiovascular conditions, advise them to consult with their doctor before starting any exercise program. A referral to an exercise physiologist or physical therapist will help them learn which exercises are safe for them.

From the questions above, determine their everyday eating routine, their intake of saturated fat and/or refined carbohydrates, and their intake of plant foods and fiber. Not only are you listening

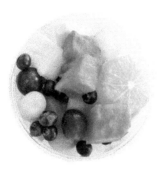

vs

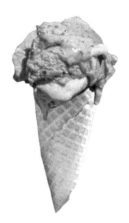

1 serving of fruit
60 calories
0g saturated fat
15g carbs
2g fiber

1 cup scoop of ice cream
253 calories
7g saturated fat
36g carbs
1g fiber

Key Message
Fruit is a healthy snack choice that is low in
calories and saturated fat.

FIGURE 11.2   For those with a sweet tooth, a comparison of fat and calories between fruit and their typical treat can demonstrate the benefits of choosing fruit for snacks.

for the foods affecting their lipids, but you are also listening for their healthy choices as well (Figure 11.3).

Most people can name some plant foods, lean proteins, or healthy fats that they would eat. Include those foods in examples of heart healthy meals. Discuss ways to include those types of foods more often in their meals. Reassure them that they do not have to overhaul their entire diet or plan unfamiliar meals. Instead, consider ways to increase the frequency and proportion of healthy choices they already enjoy while including other favorites more mindfully. Identify some healthy alternatives that the patient would be willing to try, with the goal of increasing the overlap between their food preferences and dietary guidelines.

People often feel frustrated, restricted, and even resentful when they start to make diet changes. Patients commonly report that they eat the same things every day. While they notice improvements to their lab values or how they feel, they complain that that they are getting bored. While sharing more meal ideas and recipes will be beneficial, they will also benefit from a discussion about flexibility and frequency. Many are under the impression that healthy eating

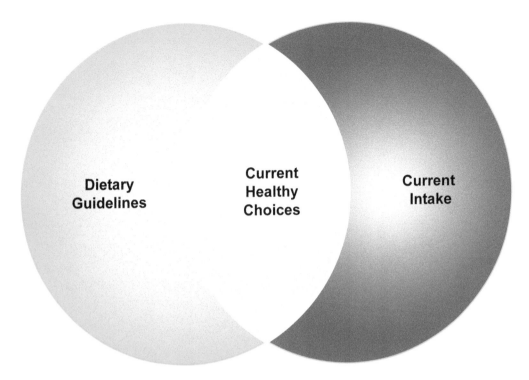

FIGURE 11.3   Identify the foods that the patient already enjoys that can fit into a heart healthy diet.

has to be "all or nothing." A kinder message to be "mostly good, most of the time" may be an easier pill to swallow (Figure 11.4).

WHAT PATIENTS WANT TO KNOW

As heart disease became the leading cause of death in the 20th century, people became more aware of the role of diet and health. While nutrition recommendations have evolved over the years, some concepts have stood the test of time. For many patients, a diagnosis of elevated cholesterol often motivates them to eat more chicken, fish, and salads. Intuitively—and for some, begrudgingly—many will start to avoid or limit red meat. Most people recognize that deep fried foods are not a healthy choice. Often, people demonstrate that knowledge during the dietary recall, stating that they bake instead of fry certain foods. Furthermore, few people would claim that fast food is healthy, or sweets are harmless.

While the key features of a healthy diet will not be new information to a patient, it is the fine details that people have questions about. In most cases, these fine details are magnified in popular diets, food marketing, and dietary supplements—and these are the concepts that frequently change and confuse people. From butter to eggs to fish oil, people are looking for an answer, an absolution, and/or both. In addition to the typical questions, "What can I eat" and "What do I have to avoid," below are other topics that people commonly ask about.

What can I eat to lower my cholesterol? While lowering foods high in saturated fat can keep LDL-C from going up, including adequate **fiber** can directly help lower cholesterol. While most people understand that fiber is generally healthy, many will not be familiar with how it binds to cholesterol (i.e., bile) in the digestive tract and takes it out of the body, thus causing the liver to take cholesterol out of the blood to make more bile—hence lowering LDL levels (Figure 11.5).

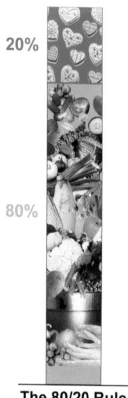

20%

80%

Key Message
A healthy diet does not have to be
all or nothing.

The occasional treat is not harmful.

However, poor food choices *in excess*
can increase risk for nutrition-related
diseases.

The 80/20 Rule

FIGURE 11.4   The 80/20 Rule is a popular concept that dietitians use to discuss healthy eating. This concept recognizes that 100% dietary compliance is impractical and difficult to maintain. On the other hand, flexibility can help prevent feelings of deprivation, thus making changes more sustainable.

Again, when people are empowered with knowledge, they may be more compelled to apply that information. Showing a sample day that includes whole grains, vegetables, fruits, legumes, and other high fiber foods demonstrates how the fiber easily adds up to the recommended 25–35 g/ day (Tables 11.1 and 11.2).

Which are the bad fats and the good fats? While the topic of **saturated fat** can spur debate among nutrition researchers and clinicians, it has been shown that excessive intake of saturated fat can directly raise LDL cholesterol (Ginsberg et al. 1998). However, the media is quick to report on nutrition controversies, pitting observational studies against landmark randomized controlled trials. Subsequently, consumers are confused about what to believe.

While dietitians are careful not to vilify any one nutrient, product manufacturers and the fad diets on which they piggyback are quick to capitalize on food trends. From palm oils to coconut oils to full fat dairy, the pendulum has completely swung from the low-fat craze of the 80s. While the concept of "healthy fat" has been adopted into the mainstream for over a decade, what is considered healthy continues to perplex people. For example, when the paleo diet was in fashion, a common statement among patients was, "But I heard that bacon was okay."

A key message that is generally better accepted is that certain types of foods *in excess* can be problematic. A pat of butter on your Saturday morning toast is not the sole cause of heart disease. A slice of cheese on a turkey sandwich is likely not going to clog arteries. A quarter-pound sirloin patty grilled at home is relatively safe. However, the third-pounder topped with bacon and cheese

FAQ:
What can I eat to lower my cholesterol?

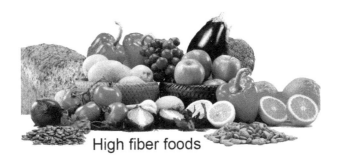

High fiber foods

○ Fiber

LDL - cholesterol

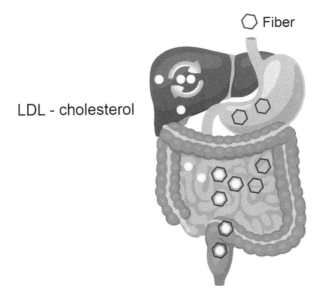

Key Message
Fiber from the diet helps to take cholesterol
out of the body, lowering LDL levels.

FIGURE 11.5 For those motivated to lower LDL-C through diet, the information that fiber lowers cholesterol by blocking it from entering the body may be novel and motivating.

for lunch, a few slices of pizza on Friday night, or a big Coney breakfast on the weekends hints at
the contribution saturated fats *in excess* make to elevated LDL-C. Focus your discussion on portion and frequency, rather than avoidance and restriction (Figure 11.5).

Reviewing your patient's everyday eating routine with them and identifying sources of excess
will be better received than a blanket warning against saturated fat. If they eat mostly at home, ask

TABLE 11.1

Sample Day with Heart Healthy Choices, Minimally Processed Foods, and Home-Prepared Meals

Meal	Calories	Saturated Fat	Sodium	Fiber
Breakfast				
Avocado toast with tomato	229	2.1	155	6
5.3 oz light vanilla greek yogurt	87	0	47	0
1/2 cup blueberries	42	0	0	2
Subtotal	359	2.5	497	9
Lunch				
Black bean and chicken wrap	353	2	569	11
2 cup side salad with cucumber and tomato	10	0	10	2
1 Tbsp oil and vinegar dressing	60	1	0	0
Subtotal	423	3	579	13
Snack				
Light string cheese	50	1.5	160	0
1 medium apple	93	0	2	4
Subtotal	143	1.5	162	4
Dinner				
Home cooked 1/4 pound sirloin burger	197	4.5	76	0
On whole grain bun	160	0	260	4
1 cup grilled zucchini/carrots/yellow squash with olive oil	67	0.7	33	1.7
2 cup side salad	10	0	10	2
1 cup low-fat milk	105	1.5	127	0
Subtotal	539	6.7	506	7.7
Snack/dessert				
Cut fruit with almonds and chocolate drizzle	148	1	2	4.6
Total	1,611	14.3	1,451	37.5

Sources: https://recipes.heart.org/en/, diabetesfoodhub.org, calorieking.com, verywellfit.com - recipe calculator.

for specifics in terms of food choices, serving sizes, and frequency. If they dine out often, show examples of common restaurant meals and their nutrient content. More often than not, a patient's personal eating pattern will reveal their eating habits of concern. Be prepared to show examples of lean options for whatever eating pattern presents—whether they are examples of heart healthy recipes, dining out tips, or healthy snack ideas.

Regarding "healthy fats," summarizing the research findings behind the Mediterranean Diet can help to demonstrate the benefit of extra virgin olive oil, walnuts, or similar types of oils, nuts, and seeds. Explaining that diets higher in fish have lower risk for cardiovascular disease can help illustrate the benefits of omega-3 fats as well (Rimm et al. 2018).

The Mediterranean Diet has been shown to lower risk for heart attack, stroke, or cardiovascular-related death by 30% (Estruch et al. 2018).

Do I need a fish oil supplement? If so, how much should I take? Omega-3 supplementation is another controversial topic that has shown various outcomes. While the American Heart Association recommends the use of prescription doses for the treatment of high triglycerides, over the counter doses for primary prevention of heart disease has not been proven effective

TABLE 11.2

Sample Day with Ultra-Processed and Restaurant Foods

Meal	Calories	Saturated Fat	Sodium	Fiber
Breakfast				
1.5 cups honey nut toasted oats	218	0	317	4
1 cup 2% milk	122	3	100	0
Subtotal	340	3	417	4
Snack				
Granola bar with chocolate chips	124	3	98	1
Lunch				
Frozen lasagna with meat sauce	377	7	832	3.6
Snacks				
Large vanilla latte	290	6	140	0
Dinner				
Fast food quarter pounder with cheese	520	12	1,140	2
Large fries	490	3	400	6
Large soda	216	0	52	0
Subtotal	1,226	15	1,592	8
Snack/dessert				
2 cups vanilla ice cream	546	18	211	2
Total	2,903	52	3,290	18.6

Source: calorieking.com.

(Skulas-Ray et al. 2019; Abdelhamid et al. 2018). On the other hand, for people who have known coronary heart disease, fish oil supplementation has been shown to lower risk for CHD mortality (Siscovick et al. 2017). Therefore, the AHA concludes that fish oil supplementation for secondary prevention is reasonable. According to the AHA advisory, the average dose used in the studies supporting this recommendation was about 1,000 mg/day. As with all supplements—which are not regulated by the Food and Drug Administration—recommending brands that have been third-party tested by organizations like the US Pharmacopeia can ensure product quality.

For patients without heart disease, while omega-3 supplements may not provide added benefits, consuming non-fried fish and seafood at least twice a week has been shown to reduce cardiovascular risks (Rimm et al. 2018).

Are eggs good or bad? Up until about a decade ago, nutrition guidelines for heart disease cautioned against egg consumption, with the primary concern being the cholesterol content. Since then, as the association between saturated fat and LDL cholesterol became more clear, the dietary guidelines around eggs and cholesterol loosened. Moreover, multiple studies have concluded that egg consumption of about 1–1.5 per day was not associated with heart disease (Darooghegi et al. 2022; Geiker et al. 2018; Krittanawong et al. 2021).

On the other hand, many studies have found that people with diabetes do have an increased risk of heart disease with egg consumption (Geiker et al. 2018). Another recent study found an increased risk for all-cause and cancer mortality with higher egg intake (Darooghegi et al. 2022). With every new study, there is a new headline, causing whiplash among patients and health professionals alike.

Therefore, erring on the side of balance and variety can be a safe way to maneuver some of these controversial and ever-changing topics. While eggs are a great source of protein and vitamins, they

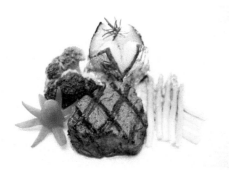
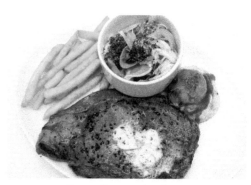

4 oz sirloin steak
207 calories
2.5g saturated fat

8 oz ribeye steak
507 calories
10.7g saturated fat

> *Key Message*
> A variety of foods can fit in a healthy diet. Consider portion,
> balance, and frequency.

FIGURE 11.6 Demonstrate that all foods can fit into a healthy diet while emphasizing portion control, leaner choices, and balance.

are not the only protein option for breakfast. Varying meal ideas throughout the week can help minimize excessive intake of any one thing. Perhaps they enjoy eggs for breakfast a couple of days per week but rotate with other proteins on other days. For example, beans, nuts and nut butter, fish, lean turkey sausage, or repurposed dinner leftovers are just some examples that can be part of the breakfast rotation. For those who desire a higher intake of eggs, swapping some of the whole eggs with egg whites or egg substitute can help keep intake in moderation (Figure 11.7).

Many people use eggs for snacks or protein supplementation. First, assess if protein supplementation is necessary. If so, offer other ideas such as low fat cheese, yogurt, or plant proteins like nuts or nut butters.

Not only can variety help ensure that people get a host of nutrients, but it helps prevent a food rut that is especially common for breakfast.

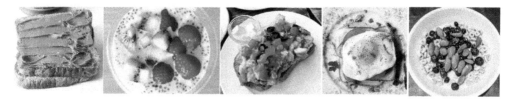

> *Key Message*
> Including a variety of foods maximizes nutrition, minimizes
> nutrients of concern, and adds enjoyment to eating.

FIGURE 11.7 A frequently asked question is, "What else can I have for breakfast?" Provide alternative protein choices to emphasize variety, maximal nutrition, and moderation.

How can I raise my good cholesterol? When faced with abnormal lab values, people have a tendency to look for a single fix—something to eat, supplement, or avoid. Low HDL values can trigger similar reactions. While some nutrients and medications have been shown to directly impact HDL levels, raising levels alone has not shown to be protective (Zakai et al. 2022; Sirtori et al. 2022). However, an overall healthy diet, especially a Mediterranean-style diet, plus physical activity will ultimately be the answer to not only raising HDL but also improving its function (Yanai and Tada 2018; Roussell and Kris-Etherton 2007; Hernáez et al. 2017). For some, other lifestyle factors may also need to be addressed, such as alcohol moderation or smoking cessation (Roussell and Kris-Etherton 2007).

What Patients Need to Know

While the general public has a basic understanding about heart healthy eating, many may not understand how foods specifically affect their lab values and disease risk. A visit to a dietitian will not be impactful if the patient only hears what they already know.

> After my heart attack, the dietitian told me not to eat too much butter or fat. I already knew that! *(cardiac rehab patient)*

On many occasions, patients are told their diagnosis without a detailed description of the condition. Worse yet, they may be given a blanket statement about how to manage the condition without explaining what, how, or why.

> I have PCOS. My doctor just told me to lose weight. *(nutrition counseling patient)*

On the other hand, a deeper education about their disease, its development, and the direct impact of food can elicit a more positive response. In the case of metabolic disorders, a brief, easy-to-understand explanation of basic metabolism helps set the stage for a discussion about the disease process. By learning what is supposed to happen in the body, followed by where the disruption occurs, patients start to see what—and how much—impact they have over the progression of their condition. As the education unfolds, details about how foods benefit—or worsen—their condition will position the patient to better understand the nutrition guidelines. With this knowledge, they may feel empowered to be proactive about their health.

> I learned something new today. I'm glad I came. *(nutrition counseling patient)*

Therefore, plan to review the following:

Their lipid values. Starting with a review of their lab values helps the patient understand their diagnoses, the reasons for referral, and when compared to the goals, may clarify the severity of their condition. Therefore, this information is helpful to include in the education. For some, the numbers alone can evoke concern and motivation. For others, the numbers may seem abstract, even meaningless, especially if medications help to lower those numbers. For many people, a detailed explanation about how those numbers translate to how their body functions helps to solidify their understanding about their disease, its severity, as well as its management.

What causes LDL to increase? While some cases of high cholesterol can be due to genetic factors, the majority of cases can be linked to poor diet quality. Saturated fat, refined sugars, low fiber, and ultra-processed foods have all been implicated in raising LDL, as well as triglycerides. In a typical American diet, high fat meat, high fat dairy, refined wheat products, sweets and sugary beverages, certain types of restaurant meals, animal fat, and generally large portions are all likely contributors to high LDL. Assess your patient's individual dietary factors to personalize the education (Figure 11.8).

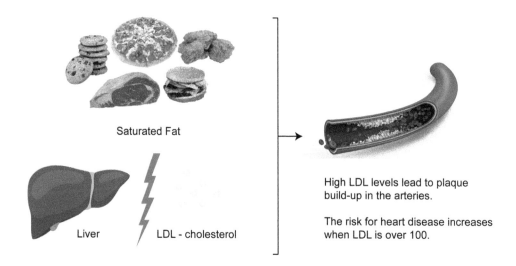

Saturated Fat

Liver   LDL - cholesterol

High LDL levels lead to plaque build-up in the arteries.

The risk for heart disease increases when LDL is over 100.

Key Message

Eating too much saturated fat stops the liver from taking cholesterol out of the blood, leading to high levels of LDL.

Extra LDL gets stuck in the blood vessels and forms plaque, which blocks blood and nutrients from flowing to the heart.

FIGURE 11.8   A brief explanation of how food that is high in saturated fat affects LDL levels may enhance the patient's understanding—and acceptance—of nutrition recommendations.

What are triglycerides? Explain that triglycerides are a compound in the blood made of fat and sugar put together. They either come directly from fats in food or they are made in the body when there is extra sugar from the diet.

What happens when triglycerides are high? When triglycerides build up in the blood, high levels can promote clot formation, which can lead to a heart attack (Olufadi and Byrne 2006). At levels over 500, the patient is at an increased risk of pancreatitis (Yuan et al. 2007) (Figure 11.9).

What causes high triglycerides? While extra triglycerides are stored in fat cells, certain conditions can prevent the triglycerides from being stored properly, such as genetic disorders, insulin resistance, uncontrolled diabetes, or obesity. Thus, they remain in the blood and build up. Excessive alcohol intake can also impair the breakdown of triglycerides (Yuan et al. 2007; Parhofer and Laufs 2019; Karanchi et al. 2022).

Plan to address the patient's individual factors affecting their lipids. Whether their elevation is related to genetics, comorbidities, or lifestyle, the fat and sugar in their diet will have a direct impact on their levels. Assess their typical intake to determine which dietary factors need to be addressed.

How can lipid values be improved? Whether your patient's goal is to lower LDL, lower triglycerides, or increase HDL, the Mediterranean Diet is the most recommended dietary pattern for heart health.

Compared to a typical American diet, the Mediterranean Diet is higher in vegetables, fruits, legumes, fish, and lean meat, as well as lower in saturated fat, red meat, and processed food. Due

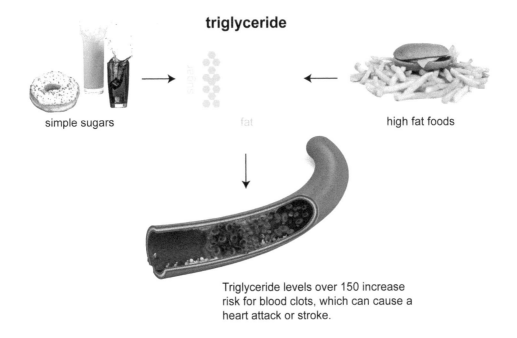

simple sugars   fat   high fat foods

Triglyceride levels over 150 increase
risk for blood clots, which can cause a
heart attack or stroke.

Key Message
Triglycerides are made of fat and sugar put together.
High triglycerides increase the risk of heart attack or stroke.

FIGURE 11.9 Explain which types of food and drinks can increase triglycerides, and that high triglycerides are also associated with an increased risk for heart disease.

to the emphasis on plant foods, it is higher in fiber. The Mediterranean Diet emphasizes the protective effects of healthy fats from nuts, extra virgin olive oil, and fatty fish. As with any nutrition guidelines, it limits sweets and sugary beverages. Those at high risk of heart disease have been shown to have a 30% lower risk of major cardiovascular events when following a Mediterranean diet with healthy fats (Estruch et al. 2018).

Overall, the beneficial effects of the Mediterranean diet may be attributed to the combined benefits of healthy fats, including improved lipid metabolism, insulin sensitivity, and anti-inflammatory effects (Calder 2015); the cholesterol-lowering benefit of the fiber; as well as the reductions in LDL-raising saturated fat and triglyceride-generating sugars. Plant foods and their phytochemical benefits are also a major component of the Mediterranean Diet and are highly recognized for being protective against heart disease (Trautwein and McKay 2020).

In addition to diet, lifestyle factors such as smoking, alcohol use, and physical activity may also need addressing. Adjustments to diet and lifestyle are likely to result in some modest weight loss, but additional weight loss strategies can be applied as needed.

MEDITERRANEAN DIET

A Mediterranean-style diet includes:

Olive oil
Tree nuts and peanuts
Fresh fruits and vegetables
Fish and seafood
Legumes
Lean poultry
Optional wine with meals

LIMIT

Sugary beverages
Sweets
Spread fats
Red and processed meat

Source: Estruch et al. (2018)

CLINICAL PRACTICE GUIDELINES, KEY STUDIES, AND MEAL PLANNING WEBSITES

Guideline on the Management of Blood Cholesterol: A Report of the American College of Cardiology/American Heart Association Task Force on Clinical Practice Guidelines (Grundy et al. 2019)

PREDIMED Study: Primary Prevention of Cardiovascular Disease with a Mediterranean Diet Supplemented with Extra Virgin Olive Oil or Nuts (Estruch et al. 2018).

American Heart Association Recipes https://recipes.heart.org/en/

Oldways Mediterranean Diet Recipes https://oldwayspt.org/traditional-diets/mediterranean-diet

Educational slides and meal planning handouts are included with this book, available online at https://resourcecentre.routledge.com/books/9781032352459

HYPERTENSION

Nearly half of U.S. adults have hypertension (CDC 2021). Lifestyle factors are one of the key determinants of primary hypertension, which makes up most hypertension cases (Whelton et al. 2018). Therefore, nutrition and lifestyle counseling continue to be critical components of therapy.

Regarding diet, while many comparisons can be made between the Mediterranean Diet and the DASH diet, the latter is highlighted in the clinical practice guidelines developed by the American College of Cardiology and American Heart Association (Whelton et al. 2018).

As high blood pressure is a common condition, many people are already aware of some recommendations, such as lowering sodium intake and generally eating healthier. Other factors may also need addressing, i.e., weight loss and physical activity. Alcohol intake may require interventions beyond the dietitian's scope of practice. For many, making healthy changes can feel challenging.

Therefore, as with all assessments, identifying what the patient already knows, wants to know, and needs to know provides for a personalized and more effective patient experience.

WHAT *YOU* NEED TO KNOW

1. Their typical daily routine and eating pattern
2. How often they consume restaurant food and what types
3. Their vegetable and fruit intake
4. Their dairy intake
5. Their level of physical activity

WHAT PATIENTS *WANT* TO KNOW

1. I don't like a lot of vegetables. Is there a supplement I can take?
2. Produce is expensive. How can I eat healthy on a budget?
3. I don't drink milk. How can I get more dairy?
4. I have diabetes. Doesn't fruit have too much sugar?
5. I eat out a lot because I'm always on the go. What are some quick recipes I can make at home?
6. Do I have to give up coffee?

WHAT PATIENTS *NEED* TO KNOW

1. What is hypertension?
2. Why it matters?
3. How sodium affects blood pressure?
4. The DASH Diet and other ways to lower blood pressure

WHAT YOU NEED TO KNOW

Treatment guidelines recognize lifestyle modification as the first line of treatment for high blood pressure, with strong evidence supporting the benefit of medical nutrition therapy from a registered dietitian nutritionist (Unger et al. 2020; Lennon et al. 2017). The key points of education will include the low-sodium DASH diet, as well as the effects of potassium, weight, physical activity, and alcohol on blood pressure (Lennon et al. 2017; NIH NHLBI 2021).

Therefore, when assessing the patient, look for ways their diet and lifestyle can align with the DASH diet and hypertension guidelines.

DASH DIET

The DASH diet is high in vegetables and fruit with moderate amounts of lean protein. DASH also highlights the benefit of low-fat dairy.

A typical 2,000 calories/day DASH diet includes[a]:

4–5 servings of vegetables (one serving = 1 cup raw or ½ cup cooked)
4–5 servings of fruit (one serving = 1 average-size piece of fruit or 1 cup cut fruit or berries)
6–8 servings of whole grains (one serving = 1/3 cup grains or 1 slice whole grain bread)
Less than 6 ounces of lean animal protein

2–3 servings of low-fat dairy (one serving = 1 cup milk or 3/4 cup plain yogurt)
2–3 teaspoons of fats and oils
1 serving of beans, nuts, or seeds (one serving = ½ cup beans or 2 tbsp nuts or seeds)

Sources: National Heart, Lung, and Blood Institute 2021; American Dietetic Association Exchange Lists (as cited by NHLBI).
[a]Calorie needs vary per person. Adjust number of servings accordingly.

Key Assessment Questions for Hypertension

1. *What does your typical day look like?* Walk your patient through a "typical day" dietary recall, including meals, snacks, drinks, and nutrition supplements. Listen for sources of excess sodium like packaged foods, salty snacks, sports drinks, and restaurant foods. Also note if their caffeine or alcohol consumption may need addressing.

2. *How many meals per day or week come from restaurants—whether sit-down, drive-through, or delivery? What do you typically order?* Many will be unfamiliar with the typical amount of sodium found in restaurant foods. Be prepared to give examples, especially from restaurants they frequent.

3. *How often a day or a week do you consume vegetables? Which types do you like?* As the DASH Diet recommends four to five servings per day, assess how closely their current intake meets those recommendations. Look for opportunities to increase intake if needed.

4. *How often a day or week do you consume fruit? Which types do you like?* Similar to the previous question, see how closely they already meet the recommendation of four to five servings for a standard 2,000 calorie diet. As fruit has more calories than non-starchy vegetables, adjust the recommendation per the patient's personal energy needs. Also, due to the carb content, be prepared to demonstrate how to incorporate fruit into a consistent carb diet for people with diabetes.

5. *How often in a day or week do you consume low-fat milk, yogurt, or dairy alternatives?* Again, most people do not meet the therapeutic level of two to three servings per day. Clarify which types of dairy they prefer, then be prepared to include them in a sample meal plan.

6. *What types of physical activity are you able to do, and how often do you do them?* Both moderate-intensity physical activity and strength training are beneficial for those with hypertension. However, caution against heavy resistance training which can increase blood pressure and cause vascular damage (Biagioli 2019). If the patient is not currently following an exercise routine, advise them to consult with their doctor before starting a new program. Otherwise, be prepared to share examples that meet any barriers they may have—e.g., free or low-cost ideas, indoor activities for cold weather, or seated or low impact exercises for some physical limitations. Clarify that physical activity is not limited to formal exercise, and provide examples of how to increase activity throughout the day, e.g., taking the stairs, parking at the back of the lot, walking breaks, etc. Emphasize that any bout of duration is beneficial with a cumulative goal of at least 150 minutes per week. Many respond positively upon hearing that three bouts of 10-minute activity is as beneficial as one 30-minute session.

WHAT PATIENTS WANT TO KNOW?

I don't like a lot of vegetables. Is there a supplement I can take? While there are plenty of vegetable extractions and powders on the market, they are not listed among proven treatments. They may not capture the additive effects of the various nutrients and phytochemicals in whole foods. Also, the ultra-processing may diminish the therapeutic benefits. As supplements can be costly, they may not be worth the expense.

Find out which vegetables they do enjoy. Most people can name at least a few, including salads. Some may be more amenable to vegetables in soups or stews. Vegetable and fruit smoothies may also be an option they are willing to try. Show plenty of variety as people often find themselves in a vegetable rut. Many people struggle with including vegetables in breakfast or find that preparing vegetables is a time-consuming task. Be prepared to show quick and easy examples of how to include vegetables throughout the day (Figure 11.10).

Produce is expensive. How can I eat healthy on a budget? The cost of fresh food can be a barrier for many people, especially when there is a risk of spoilage and food waste. A common complaint is that people forget to use the vegetables or cannot find the time to prepare them before they go bad. Further, many people assume that frozen or canned vegetables are not as healthy as their fresh counterparts, or they do not like how they taste.

Reassure people that frozen or canned vegetables and fruit are healthy and economical choices. Be prepared to guide them in label reading to select low sodium options and products with no added sugar. Encourage them to stock up on sale items (Figure 11.11).

For fresh vegetables, guide them in planning meals prior to shopping so they do not purchase more than they need. Provide quick and easy recipes for using up vegetables on the brink of going bad—such as soups, stews, casseroles, and baked goods. Encourage them to set aside time to cut and portion vegetables so they are easy to grab and go as a snack.

Have a list ready of nearby food pantries, farmers' markets, or community-supported agriculture (CSA) programs. Provide guidance on how to preserve vegetables by freezing, jarring, or canning.

FAQ:
I'm tired of salads. How else can I eat more vegetables?

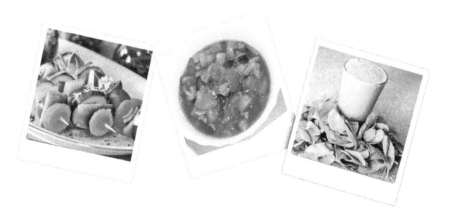

Key Message
Whether raw, cooked, fresh, or frozen, vegetables provide fiber, potassium, calcium, and other vitamins, minerals, and nutrients that protect the heart.

FIGURE 11.10   To prevent a food rut, provide ideas and recipes for a variety of vegetable preparations.

FAQ:
Doesn't healthy food cost more?

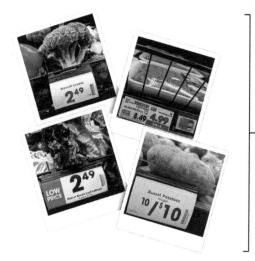

Sirloin burgers, potatoes, and fresh vegetables:

4 servings
$3.75* per serving

Compare to a
fast food combo
meal: $8* per meal

*Estimated prices at the
time of this writing.

Key Message
Meals prepared at home are often less expensive than fast food and can be much healthier.

For more savings, stock up on discounted items and plan meals around sales.

FIGURE 11.11   When purchasing simple ingredients and sale items, cooking at home can be more affordable and much healthier than other seemingly "cheap" options.

Also be prepared with information about government nutrition assistance programs for those who may qualify. Some healthcare systems have even implemented prescription programs for healthy foods.

I don't drink milk. How can I get more dairy? If the patient is intolerant to lactose or allergic to milk, discuss dairy alternatives that are fortified with calcium, such as soy or almond drinks. If they do not enjoy milk as a beverage, yogurt may be more acceptable for them. Adding milk or yogurt to recipes like oatmeal, low-fat cream soups, sugar free puddings, smoothies, or berry parfaits may help.

Some may ask if a calcium supplement will suffice. Again, the therapeutic effects of dairy can be attributed to both calcium and potassium, so a calcium supplement may not be sufficient to replicate the blood pressure benefit.

I have diabetes. Doesn't fruit have too much sugar? Reinforce the importance of glucose, the benefits of fiber, and the antioxidant benefits of various fruits. Demonstrate how to include fruit in the total carb portions that are appropriate for the patient—either as part of a meal or as snacks. Berries are a lower sugar choice. Emphasize that fruit is low in calories compared to sweets.

I eat out a lot because I'm always on the go. What are some quick recipes I can make at home? Discuss time-saving tips such as large-batch cooking, cutting and chopping vegetables

FAQ:
I have a busy schedule. How can I find more time to cook?

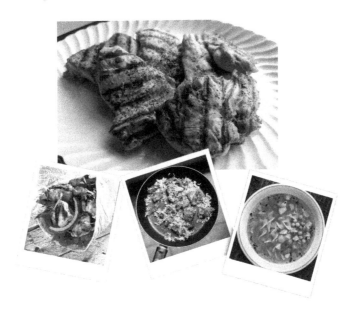

Key Message
Batch cook, prep ahead, and stock up on staples to
cut cooking time later in the week.

FIGURE 11.12 Provide quick and easy meal ideas that use time-saving tips like batch cooking, pre-prepping ingredients, and staple ingredients.

ahead of time, using a slow cooker or pressure cooker, or leftover makeovers (Figure 11.12). Suggest some convenience products like salad kits, pre-cut vegetables, frozen vegetables, or lower sodium frozen meals. Demonstrate how to incorporate prepared foods into balanced meals, such as serving rotisserie chicken with fresh or frozen vegetables and a microwave-baked potato.

Do I have to give up coffee? For mild to moderate cases, limiting caffeine to less than 300 mg/day is recommended (Whelton et al. 2018). The average cup of coffee can range from 80 to 100 mg (USFDA 2018). Be sure to counsel on other sources of caffeine that may be present in the patient's diet, such as soda, tea, or energy drinks. Even decaf coffee can have up to 15 mg per cup (USFDA 2018). Avoidance of caffeine is warranted for uncontrolled cases (Whelton et al. 2018).

WHAT PATIENTS NEED TO KNOW?

Patients are often advised on what to do, without a detailed education on why to do it. Dietitians, on the other hand, are afforded the time to provide more information, for which the patients and referring providers often appreciate.

Most people have a general understanding that high blood pressure can burden their heart. However, beyond "it makes the heart work harder," they may not be clear on the extent to which blood pressure affects their overall cardiovascular health, as well as other risks such as eye damage, kidney disease, and stroke.

First, an explanation about what hypertension is can help reinforce the importance of managing blood pressure.

What is hypertension? In plain language, hypertension is also known as "high blood pressure." With this condition, the blood is putting too much pressure on the arteries and other blood vessels.

The extra pressure could be due to various factors: (1) The blood vessels are not opening up enough to allow the blood to flow freely, (2) the amount of water in the blood is too much, increasing the volume of fluid flowing through the blood vessels, or (3) there are blockages in the arteries slowing the flow of blood, which builds up pressure where the blood is backed up (Figure 11.13 and Table 11.3).

Why it matters? Damaged blood vessels, including the coronary arteries, are susceptible to cholesterol build up, leading to the formation of plaques. As those plaques increase in size, blood flow is restricted and backed up, further building up pressure. This strains the heart as it must work harder to pump blood throughout the body. Reduced blood flow would also slow delivery of oxygen and nutrients to the heart, further damaging heart tissue and causing heart disease.

With the increased pressure, some plaques in the arterial walls could be loosened and flushed through the blood vessel, and later get lodged further down where the blood vessel is more narrow. Or, at the point where the plaque was initially dislodged, a blood clot could form. In both cases, the flow of blood to the heart could be blocked and thus cause a heart attack.

The wear and tear that high blood pressure can cause is especially hard on smaller blood vessels. As blood flows through the kidneys, increased pressure can progressively damage the organ, impair its function, and increase risk for **chronic kidney disease**. In advanced cases of CKD,

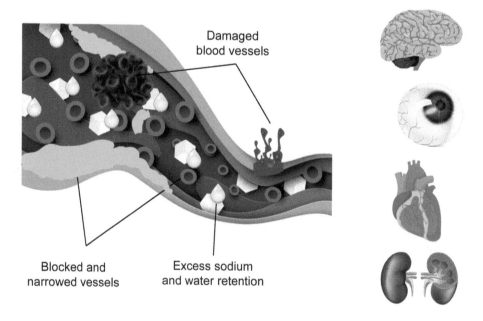

Key Message

High blood pressure can damage blood vessels, increasing risk for stroke, vision loss, heart disease, and kidney disease. Risks increase for blood pressure higher than 120/80.

FIGURE 11.13   Relate blood pressure levels to the risk for complications.

TABLE 11.3

Blood Pressure Categories (Whelton et al. 2018)

Category	Systolic Blood Pressure/Diastolic Blood Pressure (mmHg/mmHg)
Normal	Less than 120/less than 80
Elevated	120–129/less than 80
Hypertension	
Stage 1	130–139/80–89
Stage 2	Greater or equal to 140/greater or equal to 90

heart disease is the leading cause of death as kidneys help regulate various factors that affect the heart, including blood vessel function and electrolyte balance (Jankowski et al. 2021). Electrolytes are nutrients that keep the heart pumping properly. When those nutrients are out of balance, the heart can beat irregularly, which is a risk for sudden cardiac death.

In the brain, high blood pressure can promote damage to blood vessels and/or plaque formation. Thus, the blood vessels in the brain are susceptible to blockage or bleeding, which can cause a **stroke**.

Similarly, increased blood pressure in the eyes can damage the vessels and lead to **vision loss**.

How does sodium affect blood pressure? One of the first things that patients hear when they are diagnosed with hypertension is to lower their **sodium** intake. However, not all have been educated on how sodium affects blood pressure, nor which types of foods contain too much. Thus, many people stop using the salt shaker, unaware that their intake may still be too high. They may also be reading labels looking for the lowest sodium products, only to feel frustrated if they feel their choices are limited.

First, sodium plays an important role in the body. Therefore, the goal is not to avoid it completely. With the help of sodium, the kidneys maintain a level amount of fluid in the body, keeping or excreting water as needed. As blood flows through the kidneys, any extra water in the blood will be taken out in the urine. Or, if fluid levels are lower, the sodium helps the kidneys retain some water to prevent dehydration. Sodium works like a key that locks the floodgates, keeping the water in if needed.

When the diet is high in sodium, the extra sodium can cause the kidneys to retain even more water. The water retention increases the blood volume, which increases pressure on the blood vessels. Thus, reducing sodium intake can help reduce blood pressure by reducing fluid retention and blood volume.

The typical American diet that is high in processed and/or restaurant foods takes in about 3,600 mg of sodium per day (Mattes and Donnelly 1991). Of that 3,600 mg, about 77% of the sodium came from salt added in processed and restaurant foods. The salt shaker contributes a minimal amount of only about 11%, even less than the 12% that is naturally occurring in foods. Therefore, for those who state that they have stopped adding salt, clarifying where excess sodium is typically found will be key (Table 11.4).

The DASH-Sodium trials showed that sodium reduction to about 1,500 mg/day combined with a DASH diet reduces blood pressure (Sacks et al. 2001).

What is the DASH diet? Some patients are given a handout about the DASH diet when they are diagnosed with hypertension. However, until they speak to a dietitian, many need more information about why the DASH diet works, as well as how to effectively implement it.

The research showed that the reduction in blood pressure was twice as much with the DASH diet compared to simply increasing fruit and vegetables alone, with even further reductions when sodium was reduced to 1,500 mg/day (Sacks et al. 2001; Appel et al. 1997). Since then, the DASH diet continues to be rated as one of the top overall diets for heart health (US News 2023). This approach has also shown benefits in treating the factors of metabolic syndrome, as well as weight

TABLE 11.4

Relative Contributions of Dietary Sodium Sources (Mattes and Donnelly 1991)

Typical American Diet	~3,600 mg/day
Processed and restaurant foods	77%
Naturally occurring sodium in food	12%
Salt shaker	11%

management and diabetes (Challa et al. 2022)—all key factors in preventing and managing heart disease. For patients with congestive heart failure, the low-sodium DASH approach may also be beneficial (Wickman et al. 2021).

The DASH diet provides therapeutic benefits from the following nutrients:

Potassium helps the kidneys to rid the body of excess fluid and sodium, hence lowering fluid retention and blood pressure. Adequate intakes of potassium for adult males and females are 3,400 and 2,600 mg respectively (NIH 2022b). Of note, there may be potassium restrictions for people with hyperkalemia related to kidney disease or some blood pressure medications.

Among healthy individuals, Americans typically consume less potassium than needed (NIH 2022b). In fact, the Dietary Guidelines for Americans lists potassium as a "nutrient of concern," likely because the typical American diet tends to be lower in plant foods and/or higher in processed foods (Snetselaar et al. 2021). For example, beans, lentils, dark leafy greens, potatoes, squash, and various fruits are high in potassium. However, foods that are ultra-processed lose potassium. For example, white rice has two-thirds less potassium than brown rice (NIH 2022b). Milk and yogurt are also good sources of potassium, but as reported by the Dietary Guidelines Advisory Committee (2020), the National Health and Nutrition Survey indicates that 88% of Americans do not consume enough dairy.

Calcium, another nutrient found in abundance in dairy, further helps the kidneys to excrete sodium and fluid. Furthermore, low calcium intake promotes hormonal activity that causes constriction, or narrowing, of blood vessels (Villa-Etchegoyen et al. 2019). The DASH trials showed that including three servings a day of low-fat dairy lowers blood pressure twice as much as the same dietary pattern with a lower dairy intake (Appel et al. 1997).

Magnesium, which is highly available in nuts, seeds, dark leafy greens, legumes and whole grains, helps with dilating, or widening, blood vessels, thus reducing blood pressure (NIH 2022a; Houston 2011). Nearly half of Americans do not meet the estimated average requirement for magnesium (USDA 2019).

While potassium, calcium, and magnesium each play an individual role in blood pressure, supplementation of these minerals has not proven to be effective in treating hypertension. However, the result of these nutrients working together from a diet rich in fruits, vegetables, and low-fat dairy foods, with reduced fat and sodium, does lower blood pressure (Appel et al. 1997). Due to the heavy emphasis on plant foods, phytochemical compounds may also contribute to the therapeutic effects of DASH (Most 2004) (Figure 11.14).

Lifestyle changes. In addition to diet, many patients will hear advice on weight, physical activity, and other lifestyle factors. For some, these are lectures that they have heard before, perhaps for other conditions. Most people recognize that healthy choices are beneficial. However, for some, more quantifiable details may help bolster the point and motivate them to take action. Table 11.5 shows the average impact of various diet and lifestyle factors on blood pressure.

Further, many of the factors above also play a role in lipid and glucose metabolism. Therefore, treatment of hypertension will benefit other comorbidities. For patients with diabetes, managing blood pressure further protects against diabetes-related complications such as kidney disease, eye damage, or stroke.

FAQ:
What can I eat to lower my blood pressure?

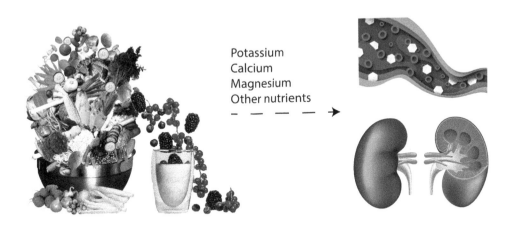

Potassium
Calcium
Magnesium
Other nutrients

Key Message
The nutrients in vegetables, fruit, and low-fat dairy help to
open blood vessels and remove extra water and sodium
through the kidneys.

FIGURE 11.14   Explain that the nutrients that are abundant in a DASH diet help to dilate blood vessels, reduce water retention, remove extra sodium through the kidneys, and overall protect the heart.

TABLE 11.5
The Best Proven Diet and Lifestyle Interventions for Treating Hypertension (Whelton et al. 2018)

Treatment	Effect on Systolic Blood Pressure (mm Hg)
Weight loss	−5
Healthy diet (DASH diet)	−11
Reduced intake of sodium to <1,500 mg/day	−5 to −6
Enhanced intake of potassium (DASH diet/high in vegetables and fruit)	−4 to −5
Physical Activity	
Aerobic 90–150 min/week	−5 to −8
Resistance 90–150 min/week	−4 to −5
Moderation in alcohol intake (2 or less drinks per day for men; 1 or less for women)	−4

PRACTICE TIP: MINIMIZE THE MATH

After reading hundreds of food logs from tracking apps, I noticed that when people made general efforts at healthy food choices and portion control, the numbers we tend to count tend to fall within the recommended ranges. Whether it's calories, sodium, fiber, or saturated fats, counting becomes unnecessary when people mindfully include healthy foods, practice portion control, eat at home more often, and limit packaged or ultra-processed foods.

It is common for nutrition departments to hand out food lists that include nutrient content. However, for somebody who does not want to measure, count, and track, those lists can seem overwhelming, incomprehensible, or impractical.

On the other hand, a comparison of eating patterns may drive the point home more easily—see Tables 11.1 and 11.2.

For many patients, seeing the examples in Tables 11.1 and 11.2 may be their first look at the nutrient content in various foods. The information can be quite surprising. When comparing the two eating patterns, key points of interest will be that healthier choices result in:

1. More food
2. Less calories
3. Less saturated fat
4. Less sodium
5. More fiber

For those who previously found "dieting" to be restrictive and unsatisfying, these examples demonstrate that healthy eating allows for filling meals, variety, and treats. With the right recipes, tips, and troubleshooting, a heart healthy diet can be both attainable and sustainable, thus relieving pressure both inside and out.

CLINICAL PRACTICE GUIDELINES, KEY STUDIES, AND MEAL PLANNING WEBSITES

Guideline for the Prevention, Detection, Evaluation, and Management of High Blood Pressure in Adults (Whelton et al. 2018)

Effects on Blood Pressure of Reduced Dietary Sodium and the Dietary Approaches to Stop Hypertension (DASH) diet (Sacks et al. 2001)

Relative Contributions of Dietary Sodium Sources (Mattes and Donnelly 1991)

National Heart, Lung, and Blood Institute DASH-Friendly recipes https://healthyeating.nhlbi.nih.gov/

Dash Diet https://dashdiet.org/dash-diet-recipes.html

American Heart Association Recipes https://recipes.heart.org/en/

Physical Activity Guidelines for Americans, 2nd edition (USDHH 2018)

Educational slides and meal planning handouts are included with this book, available online at https://resourcecentre.routledge.com/books/9781032352459

REFERENCES

Abdelhamid AS, Brown TJ, Brainard JS, Biswas P, Thorpe GC, Moore HJ, Deane KH, AlAbdulghafoor FK, Summerbell CD, Worthington HV, Song F, Hooper L. Omega-3 Fatty Acids for the Primary and Secondary Prevention of Cardiovascular Disease. *Cochrane Database Syst Rev.* 2018 Jul;7(7):CD003177. doi: 10.1002/14651858.CD003177.pub3. Update in: *Cochrane Database Syst Rev.* 2018 Nov 30;11:CD003177.

Appel LJ, Moore TJ, Obarzanek E, Vollmer WM, Svetkey LP, Sacks FM, Bray GA, Vogt TM, Cutler JA, Windhauser MM, Lin PH, Karanja N. A Clinical Trial of the Effects of Dietary Patterns on Blood Pressure. *N Engl J Med.* 1997 Apr;336(16):1117–1124. doi: 10.1056/NEJM199704173361601.

Biagioli B. *Advanced Concepts of Personal Training.* 2nd edition. Coral Gables, FL: National Council on Strength & Fitness; 2019 [English].

Calder PC. Functional Roles of Fatty Acids and Their Effects on Human Health. *JPEN J Parenter Enteral Nutr.* 2015 Sep;39(1 Suppl):18S–32S. doi: 10.1177/0148607115595980.

Centers for Disease Control and Prevention (CDC). *Hypertension Cascade: Hypertension Prevalence, Treatment and Control Estimates among US Adults Aged 18 Years and Older Applying the Criteria from the American College of Cardiology and American Heart Association's 2017 Hypertension Guideline-NHANES 2015–2018.* Atlanta, GA: US Department of Health and Human Services; 2021. Accessed 11/30/2022.

Karanchi H, Muppidi V, Wyne K. *Hypertriglyceridemia* [Internet]. Treasure Island, FL: StatPearls Publishing; 2022 [updated 2022 Aug 22, cited 5/31/2023]. Available from: https://www.ncbi.nlm.nih.gov/books/NBK459368/.

Challa HJ, Ameer MA, Uppaluri KR. *DASH Diet to Stop Hypertension.* Treasure Island, FL: StatPearls Publishing; 2022 [updated 2022 May 15]. Available from: https://www.ncbi.nlm.nih.gov/books/NBK482514/.

Darooghegi Mofrad M, Naghshi S, Lotfi K, Beyene J, Hypponen E, Pirouzi A, Sadeghi O. Egg and Dietary Cholesterol Intake and Risk of All-Cause, Cardiovascular, and Cancer Mortality: A Systematic Review and Dose-Response Meta-Analysis of Prospective Cohort Studies. *Front. Nutr.* 2022;9:878979. doi: 10.3389/fnut.2022.878979.

Dietary Guidelines Advisory Committee. *Scientific Report of the 2020 Dietary Guidelines Advisory Committee: Advisory Report to the Secretary of Agriculture and the Secretary of Health and Human Services.* Washington, DC: U.S. Department of Agriculture, Agricultural Research Service; 2020.

Estruch R, Ros E, Salas-Salvadó J, Covas MI, Corella D, Arós F, Gómez-Gracia E, Ruiz-Gutiérrez V, Fiol M, Lapetra J, Lamuela-Raventos RM, Serra-Majem L, Pintó X, Basora J, Muñoz MA, Sorlí JV, Martínez JA, Fitó M, Gea A, Hernán MA, Martínez-González MA, PREDIMED Study Investigators. Primary Prevention of Cardiovascular Disease with a Mediterranean Diet Supplemented with Extra-Virgin Olive Oil or Nuts. *N Engl J Med.* 2018 Jun;378(25):e34. doi: 10.1056/NEJMoa1800389.

Gallagher EJ, Leroith D, Karnieli E. The Metabolic Syndrome--From Insulin Resistance to Obesity and Diabetes. *Med Clin North Am.* 2011 Sep;95(5):855–873. doi: 10.1016/j.mcna.2011.06.001.

Geiker NRW, Larsen ML, Dyerberg J, Stender S, Astrup A. Egg Consumption, Cardiovascular Diseases and Type 2 Diabetes. *Eur J Clin Nutr.* 2018 Jan;72(1):44–56. doi: 10.1038/ejcn.2017.153.

Ginsberg HN, Kris-Etherton P, Dennis B, Elmer PJ, Ershow A, Lefevre M, Pearson T, Roheim P, Ramakrishnan R, Reed R, Stewart K, Stewart P, Phillips K, Anderson N. Effects of Reducing Dietary Saturated Fatty Acids on Plasma Lipids and Lipoproteins in Healthy Subjects: The DELTA Study, Protocol 1. *Arterioscler Thromb Vasc Biol.* 1998 Mar;18(3):441–449. doi: 10.1161/01.atv.18.3.441.

Grundy SM, Stone NJ, Bailey AL, Beam C, Birtcher KK, Blumenthal RS, Braun LT, de Ferranti S, Faiella-Tommasino J, Forman DE, Goldberg R, Heidenreich PA, Hlatky MA, Jones DW, Lloyd-Jones D, Lopez-Pajares N, Ndumele CE, Orringer CE, Peralta CA, Saseen JJ, Smith SC Jr, Sperling L, Virani SS, Yeboah J. 2018 AHA/ACC/AACVPR/AAPA/ABC/ACPM/ADA/AGS/APhA/ASPC/NLA/PCNA Guideline on the Management of Blood Cholesterol: A Report of the American College of Cardiology/American Heart Association Task Force on Clinical Practice Guidelines. *Circulation.* 2019 Jun;139(25):e1082–e1143. doi: 10.1161/CIR.0000000000000625.

Hernáez Á, Castañer O, Elosua R, Pintó X, Estruch R, Salas-Salvadó J, Corella D, Arós F, Serra-Majem L, Fiol M, Ortega-Calvo M, Ros E, Martínez-González MÁ, de la Torre R, López-Sabater MC, Fitó M. Mediterranean Diet Improves High-Density Lipoprotein Function in High-Cardiovascular-Risk Individuals: A Randomized Controlled Trial. *Circulation.* 2017 Feb;135(7):633–643. doi: 10.1161/CIRCULATIONAHA.116.023712.

Houston M. The Role of Magnesium in Hypertension and Cardiovascular Disease. *J Clin Hypertens (Greenwich)*. 2011 Nov;13(11):843–847. doi: 10.1111/j.1751-7176.2011.00538.x.

Jankowski J, Floege J, Fliser D, Böhm M, Marx N. Cardiovascular Disease in Chronic Kidney Disease: Pathophysiological Insights and Therapeutic Options. *Circulation*. 2021 Mar;143(11):1157–1172. doi: 10.1161/CIRCULATIONAHA.120.050686.

Karanchi H, Muppidi V, Wyne K. *Hypertriglyceridemia* [Internet]. Treasure Island, FL: StatPearls Publishing; 2022 [updated 2022 Aug 22, cited 5/31/2023]. Available from: https://www.ncbi.nlm.nih.gov/books/NBK459368/.

Krittanawong C, Narasimhan B, Wang Z, Virk HUH, Farrell AM, Zhang H, Tang WHW. Association between Egg Consumption and Risk of Cardiovascular Outcomes: A Systematic Review and Meta-Analysis. *Am J Med*. 2021 Jan;134(1):76–83.e2. doi: 10.1016/j.amjmed.2020.05.046.

Lennon SL, DellaValle DM, Rodder SG, Prest M, Sinley RC, Hoy MK, Papoutsakis C. 2015 Evidence Analysis Library Evidence-Based Nutrition Practice Guideline for the Management of Hypertension in Adults. *J Acad Nutr Diet*. 2017 Sep;117(9):1445–1458.e17. doi: 10.1016/j.jand.2017.04.008.

Mattes RD, Donnelly D. Relative Contributions of Dietary Sodium Sources. *J Am Coll Nutr*. 1991 Aug;10(4):383–393. doi: 10.1080/07315724.1991.10718167. Accessed 10/21/2022.

Monteiro CA, Cannon G, Levy RB, Moubarac J-C, Jaime P, Martins AP, Canella D, Louzada ML, Parra D; with Ricardo C, Calixto G, Machado P, Martins C, Martinez E, Baraldi L, Garzillo J, Sattamini I. NOVA. The Star Shines Bright. [Food Classification. Public Health]. *World Nutrition*. 2016;7:1–3, 28–38. Contributions to World Nutrition are owned by their authors.

Most MM. Estimated Phytochemical Content of the Dietary Approaches to Stop Hypertension (DASH) Diet Is Higher Than in the Control Study Diet. *J Am Diet Assoc*. 2004 Nov;104(11):1725–1727. doi: 10.1016/j.jada.2004.08.001.

National Institutes of Health Office of Dietary Supplements. *Magnesium: Fact Sheet for Health Professionals* [Internet]. Bethesda, MD: National Institutes of Health; 2022a, June 2 [cited 2023, February 5]. Available from: https://ods.od.nih.gov/factsheets/Magnesium-HealthProfessional/.

National Institutes of Health Office of Dietary Supplements. *Potassium: Fact Sheet for Health Professionals* [Internet]. Bethesda, MD: National Institutes of Health; 2022b, June 2 [cited 2023, February 5]. Available from: https://ods.od.nih.gov/factsheets/Potassium-HealthProfessional/#en26.

National Institutes of Health, National Heart, Lung, and Blood Institute. *Dash Eating Plan* [Internet]. Bethesda, MD: National Institutes of Health; 2021, December 29 [cited 2023, February 5]. Available from: https://www.nhlbi.nih.gov/education/dash-eating-plan.

National Institutes of Health, National Heart, Lung, and Blood Institute. *What Is Metabolic Syndrome?* [Internet]. Bethesda, MD: National Institutes of Health; 2022, May 18 [cited 2023, February 5]. Available from: https://www.nhlbi.nih.gov/health/metabolic-syndrome.

Olufadi R, Byrne CD. Effects of VLDL and Remnant Particles on Platelets. *Pathophysiol Haemost Thromb*. 2006;35(3–4):281–291. doi: 10.1159/000093221.

Parhofer KG, Laufs U. The Diagnosis and Treatment of Hypertriglyceridemia. *Dtsch Arztebl Int*. 2019 Dec;116(49):825–832. doi: 10.3238/arztebl.2019.0825.

Rimm EB, Appel LJ, Chiuve SE, Djoussé L, Engler MB, Kris-Etherton PM, Mozaffarian D, Siscovick DS, Lichtenstein AH, American Heart Association Nutrition Committee of the Council on Lifestyle and Cardiometabolic Health, Council on Epidemiology and Prevention, Council on Cardiovascular Disease in the Young; Council on Cardiovascular and Stroke Nursing; and Council on Clinical Cardiology. Seafood Long-Chain n-3 Polyunsaturated Fatty Acids and Cardiovascular Disease: A Science Advisory from the American Heart Association. *Circulation*. 2018 Jul;138(1):e35–e47. doi: 10.1161/CIR.0000000000000574.

Roussell MA, Kris-Etherton P. Effects of Lifestyle Interventions on High-Density Lipoprotein Cholesterol Levels. *J Clin Lipidol*. 2007 Mar;1(1):65–73. doi: 10.1016/j.jacl.2007.02.005.

Sacks FM, Svetkey LP, Vollmer WM, Appel LJ, Bray GA, Harsha D, Obarzanek E, Conlin PR, Miller ER 3rd, Simons-Morton DG, Karanja N, Lin PH, DASH-Sodium Collaborative Research Group. Effects on Blood Pressure of Reduced Dietary Sodium and the Dietary Approaches to Stop Hypertension (DASH) Diet. *N Engl J Med*. 2001 Jan;344(1):3–10. doi: 10.1056/NEJM200101043440101. Accessed 10/21/2022.

Sirtori CR, Corsini A, Ruscica M. The Role of High-Density Lipoprotein Cholesterol in 2022. *Curr Atheroscler Rep*. 2022 May;24(5):365–377. doi: 10.1007/s11883-022-01012-y.

Siscovick DS, Barringer TA, Fretts AM, Wu JH, Lichtenstein AH, Costello RB, Kris-Etherton PM, Jacobson TA, Engler MB, Alger HM, Appel LJ, Mozaffarian D, American Heart Association Nutrition Committee of the Council on Lifestyle and Cardiometabolic Health, Council on Epidemiology and Prevention, Council on Cardiovascular Disease in the Young, Council on Cardiovascular and Stroke Nursing; and Council on Clinical Cardiology. Omega-3 Polyunsaturated Fatty Acid (Fish Oil) Supplementation and the Prevention of Clinical Cardiovascular Disease: A Science Advisory From the American Heart Association. *Circulation.* 2017 Apr;135(15):e867–e884. doi: 10.1161/CIR.0000000000000482.

Skulas-Ray AC, Wilson PWF, Harris WS, Brinton EA, Kris-Etherton PM, Richter CK, Jacobson TA, Engler MB, Miller M, Robinson JG, Blum CB, Rodriguez-Leyva D, de Ferranti SD, Welty FK, American Heart Association Council on Arteriosclerosis, Thrombosis and Vascular Biology; Council on Lifestyle and Cardiometabolic Health, Council on Cardiovascular Disease in the Young, Council on Cardiovascular and Stroke Nursing, Council on Clinical Cardiology. Omega-3 Fatty Acids for the Management of Hypertriglyceridemia: A Science Advisory from the American Heart Association. *Circulation.* 2019 Sep;140(12):e673–e691. doi: 10.1161/CIR.0000000000000709.

Snetselaar LG, de Jesus JM, DeSilva DM, Stoody EE. Dietary Guidelines for Americans, 2020-2025: Understanding the Scientific Process, Guidelines, and Key Recommendations. *Nutr Today.* 2021 Nov-Dec;56(6):287–295. doi: 10.1097/NT.0000000000000512.

Trautwein EA, McKay S. The Role of Specific Components of a Plant-Based Diet in Management of Dyslipidemia and the Impact on Cardiovascular Risk. *Nutrients.* 2020 Sep;12(9):2671. doi: 10.3390/nu12092671.

U.S. Department of Agriculture, Agricultural Research Service. *Usual Nutrient Intake from Food and Beverages, by Gender and Age, What We Eat in America, NHANES* 2013-2016 [Internet]. Beltsville, MD: USDA; 2019 [cited 2023, February 5]. Available from: www.ars.usda.gov/nea/bhnrc/fsrg.

U.S. Department of Health and Human Services. *Physical Activity Guidelines for Americans*, 2nd edition. Washington, DC: U.S. Department of Health and Human Services; 2018.

U.S. Food and Drug Administration. *Spilling the Beans: How Much Caffeine is too Much?* [Internet]. Silver Spring, MD: FDA; 2018 [cited 5/31/2023]. Available from: https://www.fda.gov/consumers/consumer-updates/spilling-beans-how-much-caffeine-too-much.

U.S. News and World Report. *Best Heart-Healthy Diets* 2023 [Internet]. 2023, January 3 [cited 2023, February 5]. Available from: https://health.usnews.com/best-diet/best-heart-healthy-diets.

Unger T, Borghi C, Charchar F, Khan NA, Poulter NR, Prabhakaran D, Ramirez A, Schlaich M, Stergiou GS, Tomaszewski M, Wainford RD, Williams B, Schutte AE. 2020 International Society of Hypertension Global Hypertension Practice Guidelines. *Hypertension.* 2020 Jun;75(6):1334–1357. doi: 10.1161/HYPERTENSIONAHA.120.15026. Accessed 10/21/2022.

Villa-Etchegoyen C, Lombarte M, Matamoros N, Belizán JM, Cormick G. Mechanisms Involved in the Relationship between Low Calcium Intake and High Blood Pressure. *Nutrients.* 2019 May;11(5):1112. doi: 10.3390/nu11051112.

Whelton PK, Carey RM, Aronow WS, Casey DE Jr, Collins KJ, Dennison Himmelfarb C, DePalma SM, Gidding S, Jamerson KA, Jones DW, MacLaughlin EJ, Muntner P, Ovbiagele B, Smith SC Jr, Spencer CC, Stafford RS, Taler SJ, Thomas RJ, Williams KA Sr, Williamson JD, Wright JT Jr. 2017 ACC/AHA/AAPA/ABC/ACPM/AGS/APhA/ASH/ASPC/NMA/PCNA Guideline for the Prevention, Detection, Evaluation, and Management of High Blood Pressure in Adults: A Report of the American College of Cardiology/American Heart Association Task Force on Clinical Practice Guidelines. *Hypertension.* 2018 Jun;71(6):e13–e115. doi: 10.1161/HYP.0000000000000065.

Wickman BE, Enkhmaa B, Ridberg R, Romero E, Cadeiras M, Meyers F, Steinberg F. Dietary Management of Heart Failure: DASH Diet and Precision Nutrition Perspectives. *Nutrients.* 2021 Dec;13(12):4424. doi: 10.3390/nu13124424.

Yanai H, Tada N. Which Nutritional Factors Are Good for HDL? *J Clin Med Res.* 2018 Dec;10(12):936–939. doi: 10.14740/jocmr3646.

Yuan G, Al-Shali KZ, Hegele RA. Hypertriglyceridemia: Its Etiology, Effects and Treatment. *CMAJ.* 2007 Apr;176(8):1113–1120. doi: 10.1503/cmaj.060963.

Zakai N, Minnier J, Safford M, et al. Race-Dependent Association of High-Density Lipoprotein Cholesterol Levels with Incident Coronary Artery Disease. *J Am Coll Cardiol.* 2022 Nov;80(22):2104–2115. doi:10.1016/j.jacc.2022.09.027.

12 Chronic Kidney Disease

When I started practicing ten years ago, counseling for chronic kidney disease seemed to run counter to the basic tenets of healthy eating. Guidelines cautioned against whole grains and legumes due to their phosphorus content. Several vegetables and fruits were limited due to potassium. As is the case with many patient education materials, foods are often categorized as "allowed" or "not allowed." Patients with CKD and other comorbidities complained that the foods they were allowed were bad for their diabetes or their heart. As the dietitian, I dutifully recommended the appropriate guidelines, but I was intuitively uncomfortable advising against the very foods that generally protect health.

Fast forward to today. Guidelines have started to shift. Nutrition research is focusing more on dietary patterns rather than individual nutrient restrictions. Naturally occurring potassium and phosphorus from plant foods are recognized as less bioavailable than inorganic additives, thus implicating ultra-processed foods as the larger concern for these nutrients (Picard 2019; Naismith and Braschi 2008; D'Alessandro et al. 2015). Currently, the Mediterranean Diet and diets high in vegetables and fruit are included in the guidelines (Ikizler et al. 2020; Kelly et al. 2017; Pérez-Torres et al. 2022). Higher fiber diets promote glycemic control, which is imperative for renal protection, as well as lipid management for cardiovascular protection. High vegetable and fruit intake helps to lower inflammation, reduce oxidative stress, and manage blood pressure—all critical for cardiometabolic health. And plant-based proteins like legumes and nuts have been shown to be safe and beneficial for patients with CKD (Joshi et al. 2019).

Once again, healthy eating prevails. What you do for your diabetes is good for your kidneys, protecting your kidneys protects your heart, and what is heart healthy is healthy overall. One almost wonders why there was ever any doubt (Figure 12.1).

But doubt there is. While research is evolving, the word can be slow to get out. Experienced practitioners are sometimes set in their ways. They may either be resistant to change or unaware that change is happening. As such, some clinicians are still recommending refined over whole grains, advising against beans, and handing out lists of vegetables and fruits to avoid. In turn, when patients hear the newest guidelines, they express their own hesitancy, saying, "but the dietitian at my dialysis center said…" or "my doctor told me never to eat…."

While more research is needed to define recommended dietary patterns for various stages of CKD, the registered dietitian can help guide patients in achieving a varied diet within the parameters of their individual nutrient concerns. Instead of describing foods as allowable, dietitians can demonstrate how proper portions and healthy choices can help them meet—and not exceed—their needs. As in all nutrition counseling, recommendations must be tailored to the individual needs and lab values of the patient.

The following are the key points that you need to know to help bring your patients—and other clinicians—up to date on healthy eating for kidney disease.

DOI: 10.1201/9781003326038-15

FAQ:
I have heart disease, diabetes, and kidney disease.
How do I combine all the different diets?

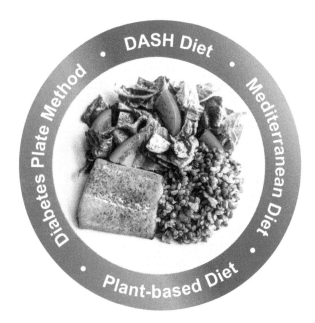

Key Message
What you do for your diabetes is good for your kidneys,
protecting your kidneys protects your heart, and
what is heart healthy is healthy overall.

FIGURE 12.1   Recent guidelines recognize that diets high in plant foods such as the Mediterranean Diet, DASH Diet, and plant-based diets are protective of the kidneys.

WHAT YOU NEED TO KNOW
1. Your patient's stage of kidney disease.
2. Their dialysis status and/or transplant status.
3. Which comorbidities are present.
4. Electrolyte status.
5. Current dietary intake.
6. Their appetite.

WHAT PATIENTS *WANT* TO KNOW
1. What foods can I eat? What do I need to avoid?
2. I have [diabetes and/or heart disease] too. How do I combine all the different diets?
3. How can I improve my kidneys, or keep them from getting worse?

WHAT PATIENTS *NEED* TO KNOW

1. The role of the kidneys.
2. The meaning of eGFR.
3. How kidney disease, heart health, and diabetes are related.
4. That the latest nutrition guidelines for kidney disease, heart health, and diabetes are similar.
5. The risks of high potassium or high phosphorus levels.

WHAT YOU NEED TO KNOW

KEY CONSIDERATIONS FOR CKD

The recommendations below are included in the *KDOQI Clinical Practice Guidelines for Nutrition in CKD: 2020 Update* unless otherwise noted.

What stage of kidney disease is your patient? While nutrition guidelines evolve, various stages of CKD may affect whether or not certain nutrients need restriction or supplementation (Table 12.1).

For patients with **CKD stages 1–5 *without* dialysis or electrolyte abnormalities,** a Mediterranean-style diet that provides the recommended dietary allowance for all vitamins and minerals can be beneficial for lipid management.

For patients with **CKD stages 3–5 *without* dialysis**, there is an increased risk for electrolyte abnormalities such as potassium and phosphorus. If lab values are elevated, phosphorus or potassium binders can be used. Dietary adjustment may be required. Assess the patient's typical intake to identify which foods or beverages may need limiting. A protein restriction is also recommended to prevent progression to end-stage renal disease. Current guidelines recommend limiting protein to 0.6 g/kg/day for those without diabetes or 0.8 g/kg/day with diabetes. The higher protein limit for patients with diabetes recognizes the mitigating effect of protein on post-prandial excursions.

For **patients on dialysis**, protein needs will increase to 1.0–1.2 g/kg/day, and electrolytes will require continued monitoring. Specially trained renal dietitians are typically on staff at dialysis centers to monitor lab values and guide the patients.

Post-kidney transplant patients also may benefit from a Mediterranean-style diet, although intake may need to be adjusted for electrolyte imbalances.

For all patients, they should be monitored for adequate intake. Supplementation may be needed for those who are at risk for malnutrition, protein energy wasting, or micronutrient deficiencies.

TABLE 12.1

Stages of Kidney Disease, eGFR, and Kidney Function (NKF 2022)

Stage of CKD	eGFR	Kidney Function
Stage 1	90 or above, with other signs of kidney damage, such as protein in the urine	90%–100% function
Stage 2	60–89	60%–89% function
Stage 3a	45–59	45%–59% function
Stage 3b	30–44	30%–44% function
Stage 4	15–29	15%–29% function
Stage 5	<15	Less than 15% function - dialysis will be required and kidney transplant may be considered

If on dialysis, are they on hemodialysis or peritoneal dialysis? For all patients on dialysis, protein needs increase to 1.0–1.2 g/kg/day. Monitor for adequate dietary intake and assess risk for protein energy wasting.

For those receiving peritoneal dialysis, dextrose-based solutions increase calorie intake and can result in weight gain. Therefore, dietary recommendations should include guidance on energy intake to prevent unwanted weight gain. For those with diabetes, the dextrose can increase blood sugar levels. The dialysis team will determine if amino acid-based solutions should be used instead. Blood sugar should be monitored for diet and/or medication adjustment.

Fluid restrictions for dialysis patients are generally required and will vary depending on urine output.

Patients on dialysis should be followed regularly by specially trained renal dietitians. However, patients are often referred to other outpatient dietitians for other comorbidities, in which case all dietitians must be aware of dialysis-specific guidelines.

What comorbidities are present? Patients with CKD often have other cardiometabolic abnormalities including diabetes, hypertension, dyslipidemia, and heart disease. Some are at risk of malnutrition due to reduced appetite and/or nutrient losses from dialysis. Therefore, medical nutrition therapy must be personalized to the metabolic needs of the patient.

What are they currently consuming that may be affecting their lab values? A 3-day food record or 24-hour recall can be used to assess dietary intake.

For **elevated potassium or phosphorus** levels, Pérez-Torres et al. (2022) outlines the following steps:

Monitor for other possible causes that can elevate levels (Table 12.2). Some medications can increase potassium levels, as can uncontrolled diabetes. Inquire if the patient has been using phosphate or potassium binders to help lower absorption of these nutrients. Constipation can also increase phosphorus levels.

Listen for ultra-processed foods or beverages, as additives are more readily absorbed than the naturally occurring nutrients in plant foods.

Also monitor for portion sizes of foods high in potassium or phosphorus. Proper portion control can help keep nutrient amounts within recommended intakes.

Advise on cooking techniques that can help lower the potassium content in foods. As potassium is water soluble, soaking and simmering foods—and discarding the liquid—can help lower ⁀ount in the food.

⁀*heir appetite affecting their intake?* Renal decline is often associated with reduced ⁀009), thus increasing risk for malnutrition. For those on dialysis, renal dietitians ⁀ry intake, dry body weight changes, anthropometric measures, and bio- ⁀d protein catabolic rate, albumin, and prealbumin to monitor nutri-

⁀e seeing a dialysis patient for other conditions, the 7-point ⁀ls recommended in the KDOQI Clinical Practice ⁀alize nutrition recommendations accordingly ⁀ micronutrient supplementation are available intake. Consulting with their dialysis dietitian ⁀ efforts.

(Continued)

to avoid? Unfortunately, patients continue to rec⁀ ⁀KD. While recent guidelines are recognizing the⁀ ⁀ are still quick to recommend against legumes an⁀ ⁀s and potassium content.

TABLE 12.2

Possible Causes for High Potassium or Phosphorus Levels (Pérez-Torres et al. 2022; NKF 2017)

Possible Cause	Recommendation
Medications Examples: angiotensin-converting enzyme (ACE) inhibitors, angiotensin receptor blockers (ARBs), or immunosuppressants can increase potassium	Discuss with doctor
Diet	
Ultra-processed foods or beverages with additives	Reduce or discontinue
Nutritional drinks, powders, or multivitamins	Recommend renal-friendly products
Salt substitutes (i.e., potassium chloride)	Discontinue use
High potassium or high phosphorus foods	Discuss portion control and wet-cooking methods
	Recommend increasing plant proteins and reducing animal proteins
	If applicable, recommend alternatives (e.g., rice milk instead of cow's milk, or apple juice instead of orange juice)
	Recommend phosphate or potassium blockers
	As poor appetite is common in patients with CKD, take caution with food restrictions
Herbal supplements or remedies	Discontinue use
Physiological Causes	
Constipation can increase phosphorus	If fiber intake is low, recommend increasing high fiber foods
	Refer to doctor for medication recommendations
	Take caution in regard to fluid intake as some patients have a fluid restriction
Uncontrolled diabetes due to insufficient insulin can increase potassium	Refer to diabetes specialists for medication assessment

TABLE 12.3

The 7-Point Subjective Global Assessment (Churchill et al. 1996; Lim et al. 2016)

Assessment	Points					
Weight change in the past 6 months	7	6	5	4	3	2
7 – 0%						
6 – <3%						
5 – 3%–<5%						
4 – 5%–<7%						
3 – 7%–<10%						
2 – 10%–15%						
1 – ≥15%						
If ↑ weight trend, add 1 point, if ↓ weight trend within 1 month, minus 1 point						
Dietary intake (past 2 weeks)	7	6	5	4		
Full share of usual meals						
⬤ full share of usual meals						
¾ of usual meal, but increasing						

TABLE 12.3 (*Continued*)

The 7-Point Subjective Global Assessment (Churchill et al. 1996; Lim et al. 2016)

Assessment	Points						
4 – ½ to ¾ of usual meal, no change or decreasing							
3 – less than ½ of usual meal, but increasing							
2 – less than ½ of usual meal, no change or decreasing							
1 – less than ¼ of usual meal							
GI symptoms	7	6	5	4	3	2	1
❏ nausea ❏ vomiting ❏ diarrhea							
7 – no symptoms							
6 – few and intermittent symptoms							
5 – 2–3 times per day, but improving							
4 – 2–3 times per day, no change							
3 – 2–3 times per day, and worsening							
1 or 2 – some or all symptoms, >3 times per day							
Functional status	7	6	5	4	3	2	1
6 to 7 – Full functional capacity							
3 to 5 – Mild to moderate loss of stamina							
1 to 2 – Severe loss of functional ability (bedridden)							
Disease state affecting nutritional requirements	7	6	5	4	3	2	1
6 to 7 – No or low metabolic stress							
3 to 5 – Mild to moderate increase in metabolic stress							
1 to 2 – High metabolic stress							
Muscle waste in at least 3 areas	7	6	5	4	3	2	1
6 to 7 – No depletion							
3 to 5 – Mild to moderate depletion							
1 to 2 – Severe depletion							
Fat stores	7	6	5	4	3	2	1
6 to 7 – No depletion							
3 to 5 – Mild to moderate depletion							
1 to 2 – Severe depletion							
Edema (nutrition related)	7	6	5	4	3	2	1
6 to 7 – None							
3 to 5 – Mild to moderate							
1 to 2 – Severe							
Sum of total points = _____							
Nutritional status	7	6	5	4	3	2	1
Overall SGA rating = Sum of total points ÷ 8							
6 to 7 – Well nourished							
3 to 5 – Mildly to moderately malnourished							
1 to 3 – Severely malnourished							

First, as discussed earlier, the bioavailability of these nutrients from plant foods is lower than the phosphorus or potassium compounds added in processing, which are highly absorbed. Therefore, patient education should focus on identifying additives on food labels and using minimally processed foods (Table 12.4). Regardless of electrolyte status, limiting ultra-processed foods is advisable for the preservation of kidney function and overall health.

Second, restrictions are indicated only if labs are indicative of hyperkalemia or hyperphosphatemia. While current guidelines do not specify an allowable amount of potassium

TABLE 12.4

Examples of Food Additives Used in Food Manufacturing (NKF 2019; Sherman and Mehta 2009)

Phosphorus Additives	Potassium Additives
Dicalcium phosphate	Potassium chloride
Disodium phosphate	Potassium tripolyphosphate
Monosodium phosphate	Tetrapotassium phosphate
Phosphoric acid	Dipotassium phosphate
Sodium hexameta-phosphate	Dipotassium monohydrogen orthophosphate
Trisodium phosphate	Potassium phosphate dibasic
Sodium tripolyphosphate	
Tetrasodium pyrophosphate	
Potassium tripolyphosphate	
Tetrapotassium phosphate	
Dipotassium phosphate	
Dipotassium monohydrogen orthophosphate Potassium phosphate dibasic	

or phosphorus, a careful review of the individual's dietary intake will help identify which foods may need restricting. If indeed abnormalities are present, then wet-cooking methods in which the liquid is discarded can help further lower the phosphorus and potassium content of foods.

Of note, potassium is generally considered a nutrient of concern as most Americans do not achieve recommended intakes, likely due to lower consumption of vegetables and fruits (Snetselaar et al. 2021). In U.S. adults, the main sources of potassium are milk, coffee, tea, or other non-alcoholic beverages, and potatoes (O'Neil et al. 2012). The potassium in liquids will be more readily absorbed than that in whole foods, plus the content will be higher relative to the amount of beverage consumed. Cola drinks typically have potassium or phosophorus additives as well. Thus, a careful investigation of the patient's drink preferences is important. For potatoes, soaking them followed by boiling them and discarding the liquid can help further reduce the potassium.

In the case of phosphorus, protein is one of the main dietary sources. For patients not on dialysis, the protein restriction will help to minimize phosphorus. However, for those on dialysis who require more protein, phosphorus restriction should not be at the expense of protein intake. Compared to animal protein, plant proteins such as soy foods and legumes are good sources of protein with lower phosphorus bioavailability. Thus, someone who consumes large meat portions will fare better reducing portions and including more meatless meals with legumes.

For many people, vegetable and fruit intake is already low. Thus, a discussion about food and beverage choices and portion control may be more beneficial than providing lists of "high potassium" or "high phosphorus" foods, which often include healthful plant foods. Careful assessment is needed as intake varies per person, and global restrictions on certain vegetables and fruits may not apply or be beneficial (Figure 12.2).

How can I improve my kidneys, or keep them from getting worse? While nutrition recommendations will vary depending on the patient's stage of kidney disease, dialysis status, nutrient needs, and metabolic concerns, opting for more plant-based meals has shown to protect and sometimes improve kidney function (Moe et al. 2011; Tyson et al. 2016). Managing

Percent of potassium or phosphorus absorbed from different types of food.

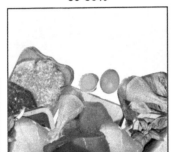
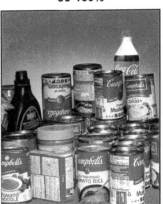

90-100%

60-80%

40-60%

Plant foods   Animal foods   Additives

Key Message
Vegetables, fruit, and other plant foods do not significantly increase potassium and phosphorus levels compared to ultra-processed foods and beverages.

FIGURE 12.2   Due to differences in bioavailability, dietary counseling should focus more on food choices and portions rather than foods "high" in potassium or phosphorus.

blood pressure and blood sugar are also critical for preventing further microvascular damage (Figure 12.3). Physical activity and weight management are also recommended for improved outcomes (de Boer et al. 2022).

WHAT PATIENTS NEED TO KNOW

The role of the kidneys. One of the key functions of the kidneys is to filter out waste, excess water, and excess electrolytes (e.g., potassium and phosphorus) from the blood. The excess is excreted through the urine. Explain that the **eGFR** (estimated glomeruler filtration rate) is an indication of how well their kidneys are filtering. Their eGFR value determines their stage of kidney disease, and the value can be translated to the kidney's percentage of function (see Table 12.1). When kidneys do not work properly, waste, water, and electrolytes build up in the blood.

Another function of the kidneys is to regulate the widening (dilation) and narrowing (constriction) of blood vessels to manage blood pressure. Thus, poor kidney function can result in high blood pressure due to impaired dilation of the blood vessels together with fluid retention.

The kidneys also play a key role in red blood cell production. Thus, declining kidney function can result in anemia, or low blood count.

How kidney disease, diabetes, and heart health are related A common complaint from patients is that managing multiple diseases is not only overwhelming, but often seems contradictory.

FAQ:
How can I keep my kidneys from getting worse?

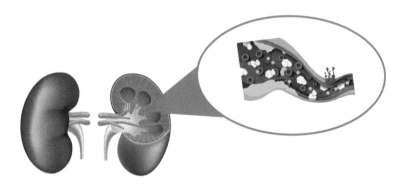

High blood glucose and high blood pressure
damage blood vessels in the kidneys.

Key Message
Managing blood pressure and blood sugar protects the kidneys.

FIGURE 12.3   Diabetes and hypertension are the leading causes of kidney damage and disease.

It may be helpful to clarify that the conditions are often intertwined, rather than distinct and separate disorders.

Diabetes and hypertension are the leading risk factors for kidney disease (NKF 2023). The combination of uncontrolled blood sugar and high blood pressure is especially damaging to the vasculature of the kidneys. Therefore, proper management of both conditions is critical in protecting the kidney.

The complications of kidney disease can be exacerbated by comorbidities as well. For example, in the case of diabetes, low insulin production and/or insulin resistance increases the risk for hyperkalemia, as insulin is involved with cellular uptake of potassium (Sousa et al. 2016). Thus, correcting insufficient insulin and reducing insulin resistance are important for both glucose and potassium regulation (Figure 12.4).

Similarly, hypertension is a leading cause of heart disease, which in turn is the number one cause of death for patients with CKD, as well as those with diabetes (National Institute of Diabetes and Digestive and Kidney Disease 2016). The effect of kidney disease is equally reciprocal to the management of blood pressure and diabetes, as its role in regulating sodium, potassium, blood volume, vascular function, glucose, and insulin is compromised (Figure 12.5).

For patients with diabetes, their A1C values may be inaccurate. As A1C measures the amount of glycated hemoglobin—or the amount of sugar attached to red blood cells—the value is related to red blood cell production. As the kidneys play a role in the production of red blood cells, impaired kidney function can lead to anemia. Thus, low levels of red blood cells may result in low A1C levels, even if blood glucose is elevated. Therefore, many patients misinterpret a lower A1C

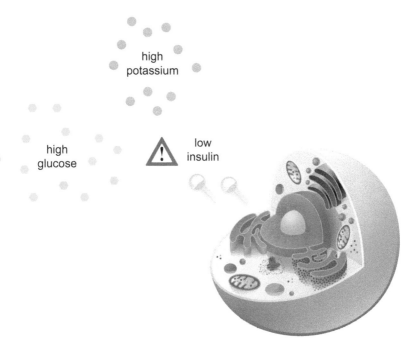

Key Message

Insulin helps lower potassium.
Uncontrolled diabetes due to low insulin
can cause high potassium.

FIGURE 12.4   High potassium levels can be a result of inadequate insulin related to diabetes. Thus, correcting insulin doses or other diabetes medications can help manage potassium.

as improved glucose control and decide to stop testing blood sugar. Thus, an important message to patients with diabetes is that they should continue to test their blood sugar regularly, even if A1C appears to have improved (Figure 12.6).

To further complicate matters, the kidneys are also responsible for the clearance of insulin. Thus, when kidney function declines, the half-life of insulin increases. Higher levels of insulin can indeed improve glucose control, but may also increase risk of hypoglycemia. In this case, continued blood sugar testing is important to inform medication doses and assess risk for lows.

Nutritional management for cardiovascular health, diabetes, and kidney disease is also intertwined. In stages 1 and 2 of CKD, and in the absence of metabolic abnormalities such as hyperkalemia or hyperphosphatemia, a well-balanced diet that includes vegetables, fruits, whole grains, and lean proteins is beneficial for glucose management, blood pressure, and overall heart health.

In stage 3 or later, a well-balanced diet is still recommended, although with a modest protein restriction to lighten the burden on the kidneys. While some additional diet modifications may be

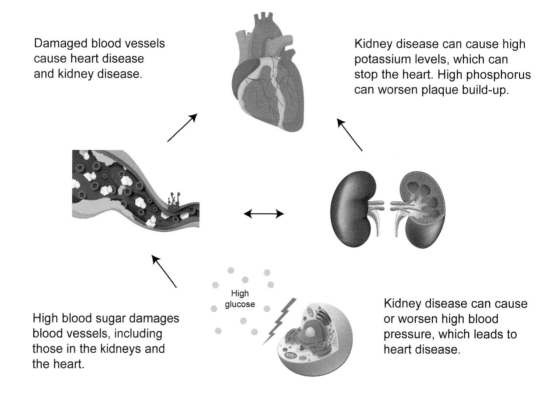

Damaged blood vessels cause heart disease and kidney disease.

Kidney disease can cause high potassium levels, which can stop the heart. High phosphorus can worsen plaque build-up.

High glucose

High blood sugar damages blood vessels, including those in the kidneys and the heart.

Kidney disease can cause or worsen high blood pressure, which leads to heart disease.

Key Message
Kidney disease, diabetes, and heart disease are related.

FIGURE 12.5 Kidney disease, diabetes, and heart disease are closely related, which is why nutrition guidelines are more similar than different.

necessary as discussed earlier in this chapter, a variety of healthy foods can still be included in a kidney friendly diet. When proper portion control, healthy food choices, and certain cooking methods are applied, nutrients of concern such as potassium, phosphorus, and sodium can be consumed without exceeding recommended intakes. Tables 12.5 and 12.6 demonstrate that a variety of foods can be included in a well-balanced diet.

The risks of high potassium or phosphorus levels. A major concern of hyperkalemia is its effect on the heart. As potassium is an electrolyte that regulates heart rhythm, high levels can cause arrythmias. Severe cases can lead to life-threatening cardiac events (Viera and Wouk 2015). Simply stated, high potassium levels can stop the heart.

In the case of phosphorus, high levels pull calcium out of the bones and can weaken them (IOM 1997). The extra calcium in the blood can be deposited in the kidneys, thus worsening renal function (IOM 1997). Calcium deposits can also occur in vascular tissue, increasing risk of heart disease (Zhou et al. 2021).

A key message for patients will be that kidney disease impacts, and is impacted by, blood pressure, blood sugar, and overall cardiovascular health. The conditions are related, thus nutritional management for each condition will be more similar than different. For many

FAQ:
My A1c went down. Does that mean that my diabetes went away?

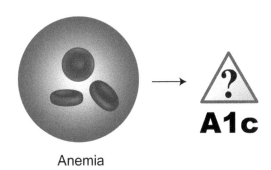

Anemia

Key Message
Kidney disease can cause anemia, which can make A1c values
falsely low. People with diabetes and kidney disease should
continue testing with fingersticks to monitor blood sugar.

FIGURE 12.6   Due to inaccurate A1C values, some people with kidney disease believe their diabetes improved. Continued monitoring through fingersticks is important to prevent further damage from uncontrolled diabetes.

TABLE 12.5

Example Meals and Their Nutrient Content – Sample Day 1

Food	Kcal	Pro	Na	K+	PO₄
Breakfast					
2 eggs cooked in 1 tsp oil	194	12	124	126	172
1 slice whole wheat toast with 1 tsp marjarine	97	3	109	60	60
1 sliced tomato	22	1	6	292	30
1 cup coffee	2	0	5	116	7
Lunch					
Tuna sandwich					
2 oz tuna	66	15	192	135	178
2 slices whole wheat bread	138	6	218	120	120
2 tsp mayo	263	0	59	0	1
1 celery stalk, sliced	6	0	32	104	15
1 cup almond milk, unsweetened	19	1	59	49	19
Snack					
1 Tbsp unsalted peanut butter	98	4	3	104	55
1 medium apple	93	0	0	192	10
Dinner					
2 oz roasted turkey breast	77	17	29	166	123

(Continued)

TABLE 12.5 (*Continued*)

Example Meals and Their Nutrient Content – Sample Day 1

Food	Kcal	Pro	Na	K+	PO$_4$
1/2 cup asparagus roasted with 1 tsp oil	53	1	1	135	32
1/2 medium sweet potato, boiled	57	1	20	174	24
1 tsp margarine-like oil spread	28	0	0	0	0
Snack					
Unsalted tortilla chips (10 chips)	91	1	3	39	36
1/4 cup salsa	19	1	462	179	22
Total	1,323	63	1,322	1,991	903

TABLE 12.6

Example Meals and Their Nutrient Content – Sample Day 2

Food	Kcal	Pro	Na	K+	PO$_4$
Breakfast					
1 packet plain instant oatmeal made with water plus:	120	4	87	108	136
11 roasted almonds, no salt	85	3	0	101	67
¼ cup blueberries	21	0	0	29	5
1 cup almond milk	40	1	118	98	38
Lunch					
Salad made with:					
1 cup romaine lettuce, shredded	8	1	4	116	14
5 grape tomatoes	15	0	3	129	14
1/2 cup cucumber slices	8	0	1	76	13
½ cup chick peas, low sodium	88	5	132	144	80
2 tbsp crumbled feta cheese	75	4	323	18	96
2 Tbsp Italian dressing	70	0	292	24	4
6.5" whole wheat pita	165	6	322	72	58
1 medium apple	95	0	2	195	20
Snack					
3 cups oil popped popcorn, no salt added	120	2.16	0.72	54	60
Dinner					
3 oz grilled salmon	175	19	52	326	214
1 cup brown rice	248	6	8	174	208
1 cup steamed, frozen green beans	37	2	3	263	47
Total	1,370	53	1,348	1,927	1,074

patients, this information may help to ease some of the frustration they felt in meal planning. However, if the patient continues to receive mixed messages, they will continue to feel conflicted and discouraged. Therefore, while a thorough yet comprehensible education will be important for the patient, ensuring communication among care team members will further enhance their care.

CLINICAL PRACTICE GUIDELINES, PROFESSIONAL AND PATIENT RESOURCES, NUTRIENT DATA, AND MEAL PLANNING WEBSITES

KDOQI Clinical Practice Guideline for Nutrition in CKD: 2020 Update (Ikizler et al. 2020)

National Kidney Foundation https://www.kidney.org/

National Institutes of Health Office of Dietary Supplements: Fact Sheets for Health Professionals (e.g., potassium, phosphorus) - https://ods.od.nih.gov/factsheets/list-all/#P

US Department of Agriculture: FoodData Central https://fdc.nal.usda.gov/

National Kidney Foundation recipes - https://www.kidney.org/nutrition

DaVita Kidney Care recipes - https://www.davita.com/diet-nutrition/recipe-search

Educational slides and meal planning handouts are included with this book, available online at https://resourcecentre.routledge.com/books/9781032352459

REFERENCES

Chazot C. Why Are Chronic Kidney Disease Patients Anorexic and What Can Be Done about It? *Semin Nephrol*. 2009 Jan;29(1):15–23. doi: 10.1016/j.semnephrol.2008.10.003.

Churchill DN, et al. Adequacy of Dialysis and Nutrition in Continuous Peritoneal Dialysis: Association with Clinical Outcomes. Canada-USA (CANUSA) Peritoneal Dialysis Study Group. *J Am Soc Nephrol*. 1996 Feb;7(2):198–207. doi: 10.1681/ASN.V72198.

D'Alessandro C, Piccoli GB, Cupisti A. The "Phosphorus Pyramid": A Visual Tool for Dietary Phosphate Management in Dialysis and CKD Patients. *BMC Nephrol*. 2015 Jan;16:9. doi: 10.1186/1471-2369-16-9.

de Boer IH, Khunti K, Sadusky T, Tuttle KR, Neumiller JJ, Rhee CM, Rosas SE, Rossing P, Bakris G. Diabetes Management in Chronic Kidney Disease: A Consensus Report by the American Diabetes Association (ADA) and Kidney Disease: Improving Global Outcomes (KDIGO). *Diabetes Care*. 2022 Dec;45(12):3075–3090. doi: 10.2337/dci22-0027.

Ikizler TA, Burrowes JD, Byham-Gray LD, Campbell KL, Carrero JJ, Chan W, Fouque D, Friedman AN, Ghaddar S, Goldstein-Fuchs DJ, Kaysen GA, Kopple JD, Teta D, Yee-Moon Wang A, Cuppari L. KDOQI Clinical Practice Guideline for Nutrition in CKD: 2020 Update. *Am J Kidney Dis*. 2020 Sep;76(3 Suppl 1):S1–S107. doi: 10.1053/j.ajkd.2020.05.006.

Institute of Medicine (US) Standing Committee on the Scientific Evaluation of Dietary Reference Intakes. *Dietary Reference Intakes for Calcium, Phosphorus, Magnesium, Vitamin D, and Fluoride*. Washington, DC: National Academies Press (US); 1997.

Joshi S, Shah S, Kalantar-Zadeh K. Adequacy of Plant-Based Proteins in Chronic Kidney Disease. *J Ren Nutr*. 2019 Mar;29(2):112–117. doi: 10.1053/j.jrn.2018.06.006.

Kelly JT, Palmer SC, Wai SN, Ruospo M, Carrero JJ, Campbell KL, Strippoli GF. Healthy Dietary Patterns and Risk of Mortality and ESRD in CKD: A Meta-Analysis of Cohort Studies. *Clin J Am Soc Nephrol*. 2017 Feb;12(2):272–279. doi: 10.2215/CJN.06190616.

Lim SL, Lin XH, Daniels L. Seven-Point Subjective Global Assessment Is More Time Sensitive Than Conventional Subjective Global Assessment in Detecting Nutrition Changes. *JPEN J Parenter Enteral Nutr*. 2016 Sep;40(7):966–972. doi: 10.1177/0148607115579938.

Moe SM, Zidehsarai MP, Chambers MA, Jackman LA, Radcliffe JS, Trevino LL, Donahue SE, Asplin JR. Vegetarian Compared with Meat Dietary Protein Source and Phosphorus Homeostasis in Chronic Kidney Disease. *Clin J Am Soc Nephrol*. 2011 Feb;6(2):257–264. doi: 10.2215/CJN.05040610.

Naismith DJ, Braschi A. An Investigation into the Bioaccessibility of Potassium in Unprocessed Fruits and Vegetables. *Int J Food Sci Nutr*. 2008;59:438–450.

National Institute of Diabetes and Digestive and Kidney Disease. *Heart Disease and Kidney* Disease [Internet]. Bethesda, MD: National Institutes of Health; 2016 [cited 2023 June 6]. Available from: https://www.niddk.nih.gov/health-information/kidney-disease/heart-disease.

National Kidney Foundation. *Your Kidneys and High Potassium (Hyperkalemia). Are You at Risk?* [Internet]. New York: National Kidney Foundation; 2017 [cited 2023 June 6]. Available from: https://www. kidney.org/sites/default/files/01-10-7269_ABG_PatBro_Hyperkalemiap7.pdf.

National Kidney Foundation. *Phosphorus and Your Diet* [Internet]. New York: National Kidney Foundation, Inc.; 2019 [cited 2023 June 9]. Available from: https://www.kidney.org/atoz/content/phosphorus.

National Kidney Foundation. *Estimated Glomerular Filtration Rate (eGFR)* [Internet]. New York: National Kidney Foundation, Inc.; 2022 [cited 2023 June 9]. Available from: https://www.kidney.org/sites/default/files/01-10-8374_2212_patflyer_egfr.pdf.

National Kidney Foundation. *Kidney Disease: The Basics* [Internet]. New York: National Kidney Foundation; 2023 [cited 2023 June 6]. Available from: https://www.kidney.org/news/newsroom/fsindex#what-causes-kidney-disease.

O'Neil CE, Keast DR, Fulgoni VL, Nicklas TA. *Food Sources of Energy and Nutrients among Adults in the US: NHANES 2003-2006. Nutrients.* 2012 Dec;4(12):2097–2120. doi: 10.3390/nu4122097.

Pérez-Torres A, Caverni-Muñoz A, González García E. Mediterranean Diet and Chronic Kidney Disease (CKD): A Practical Approach. *Nutrients.* 2022 Dec;15(1):97. doi: 10.3390/nu15010097.

Picard K. Potassium Additives and Bioavailability: Are We Missing Something in Hyperkalemia Management? *J Ren Nutr.* 2019 Jul;29(4):350–353. doi: 10.1053/j.jrn.2018.10.003.

Sherman RA, Mehta O. Potassium in Food Additives: Something Else to Consider. *J Ren Nutr.* 2009 Nov;19(6):441–442. doi: 10.1053/j.jrn.2009.08.010.

Snetselaar LG, de Jesus JM, DeSilva DM, Stoody EE. Dietary Guidelines for Americans, 2020-2025: Understanding the Scientific Process, Guidelines, and Key Recommendations. *Nutr Today.* 2021 Nov-Dec;56(6):287–295. doi: 10.1097/NT.0000000000000512.

Sousa AG, Cabral JV, El-Feghaly WB, de Sousa LS, Nunes AB. Hyporeninemic Hypoaldosteronism and Diabetes Mellitus: Pathophysiology Assumptions, Clinical Aspects and Implications for Management. *World J Diabetes.* 2016 Mar;7(5):101–111. doi: 10.4239/wjd.v7.i5.101.

Tyson CC, Lin P, Corsino L, et al. Short-term Effects of the DASH Diet in Adults with Moderate Chronic Kidney Disease: A Pilot Feeding Study. *Clin Kidney J.* 2016;9:592–598.

Viera AJ, Wouk N. Potassium Disorders: Hypokalemia and Hyperkalemia. *Am Fam Physician.* 2015 Sep;92(6):487–495.

Zhou C, Shi Z, Ouyang N, Ruan X. Hyperphosphatemia and Cardiovascular Disease. *Front Cell Dev Biol.* 2021 Mar;9:644363. doi: 10.3389/fcell.2021.644363.

13 IBS and the Low FODMAP Diet

My youngest son said to me recently, "You're lucky. You can just walk around and eat anything and not worry about it."

Since he started school, he has been trained to be cautious of certain foods due to his peanut allergy. As he got older, it also became clear that he inherited my husband's "sensitive stomach." From lactose to onions to some beans, or foods too hot or too fatty, the triggers are not always obvious. He explained that whenever a food is too "something" it does not sit well with him.

He has found that lactase supplements are helpful enough. His symptoms are irritating but not intolerable or debilitating. Like any teenager, he's willing to sacrifice a little discomfort for a pizza. But if he has an exam to sit through, he is more mindful about what he eats before that—all behaviors I have observed in his father throughout the years.

At home, we have learned what foods work well and what do not. In cooking, I will withhold certain ingredients or find substitutions as needed. As a mother and dietitian, I am driven to ensure that my family gets enough balance and variety. Even for me, there is a learning curve as we observe reactions and try to pick up on patterns.

The bigger challenges are traveling, socializing, or dining out. Like everybody, we sometimes need a break from cooking. However, because of my family's food allergies and intolerances, there is not a lot of variety in our choices.

For some, such food restrictions can significantly reduce their quality of life. People with food intolerances may feel anxious or isolated during social events, which often center around food. They find themselves either unable to fully participate in the meal, or subject to symptom flares when they do. For those with severe symptoms, avoiding unfamiliar foods is non-negotiable, to the point that some may choose to limit socialization overall. Even with their own families, they may feel like a burden as they require special accommodations.

Unfortunately, people with gastrointestinal symptoms are not commonly referred to a registered dietitian. They may be provided with generalized advice by their doctor, along with lists of foods to eat or avoid (Trott et al. 2019). But without the guidance of a dietitian, they have difficulty applying the information to their everyday meal planning. Without proper guidance, many are unable to find true relief from their symptoms and may be lacking certain nutrients.

In some cases, people may have self-diagnosed themselves and initiated dietary changes on their own. A common misconception among people with GI issues is that gluten is the cause of their symptoms. As such, they put themselves on a gluten-free diet without confirming a diagnosis with their doctor. While they may observe some improvement to their symptoms, the true trigger may actually be fructans, an oligosaccharide present in wheat. Without proper identification of their triggers, they may have symptom flares when they consume other foods with fructans. Another risk with a gluten-free diet is that it can be lower in fiber without proper guidance.

While there are various conditions that can cause gastrointestinal symptoms, the American College of Gastroenterology estimates that about 1 in 20 Americans suffer from IBS (ACG n.d.). While referrals to dietitians specifically for IBS are low, RDNs sometimes encounter patients with diagnosed IBS who were referred for other reasons. In these cases, the nutrition assessment often

DOI: 10.1201/9781003326038-16

reveals that the patient suffers recurring symptoms and limited food variety. While people have identified which foods cause them trouble, they sometimes become fearful of entire food groups or categories and may avoid some foods unnecessarily, hence increasing their risk of nutrient deficiencies.

In cases where IBS has been confirmed by their doctor, the low FODMAP diet is increasingly recommended for identifying food triggers and treating symptoms. The low FODMAP diet was initially designed by a group of researchers at Monash University in Australia and has been further tested and championed by experts around the world (Gibson 2017). While this three-phase elimination trial can be rigorous and lengthy, several studies have found this approach to be safe and effective, especially with the guidance of a registered dietitian (Bellini et al. 2020; Trott et al. 2019).

While registered dietitians are generally competent to assist with proper meal planning, in-depth training is important to prepare the dietitian to effectively guide their patient through this challenging and tedious trial. Furthermore, advanced training can help the dietitian (1) screen for other conditions that may be causing symptoms, (2) modify the approach to meet the needs of the patient, (3) provide reliable tools and resources, and (4) discuss alternative or supplemental treatments. Monash University offers the "Online FODMAP and IBS Training for Dietitians," a 10-module course approved by the Commission on Dietetic Registration for continuing professional education (Monash University 2019a). Online education and resources are also available from the GI Institute, a collaborative developed by the University of Michigan and FODMAP Friendly (GI Institute 2021).

Along with proper training, the information provided in the following pages will prepare you for the questions and challenges patients commonly have about the low FODMAP diet.

WHAT YOU NEED TO KNOW

1. Whether or not their doctor assessed and diagnosed IBS.
2. Their symptoms and severity.
3. Do they struggle more with constipation, diarrhea, or both?
4. How their symptoms affect their life.
5. Their diet and lifestyle.
6. Their level of stress.
7. If they have a history of eating disorders.

WHAT PATIENTS *WANT* TO KNOW

1. What is a FODMAP?
2. What foods have FODMAPs?
3. Do I have a gluten intolerance?
4. What can I eat?

WHAT PATIENTS *NEED* TO KNOW

1. The Low FODMAP Diet is a temporary, three-phase trial.
2. The challenge phase is worth completing.
3. Nutrients of concern on a low FODMAP diet.
4. Which supplements may help.
5. Which natural laxatives to choose.
6. Dining out tips.

7. Which ingredients to watch out for in packaged foods.
8. Portions matter.
9. The benefits of physical activity.
10. Pharmacological therapy.

WHAT YOU NEED TO KNOW

Patients who suffer GI symptoms in response to certain foods are likely to allude to this during a nutrition assessment, even if those symptoms were not the reason for referral. For example, as you guide them through a dietary recall, they may clarify that they choose gluten-free products or lactose free milk. Or as you provide nutrition education and describe various food groups, they may point out foods that they "can't have." On several occasions, I have heard patients say, "A lot of the foods that are supposed to be healthy I can't eat." Worse yet, they may have been given a list of high FODMAP foods in the past and blanketly avoid them all. Consequently, they describe a bland diet with limited variety, sometimes deficient in certain nutrients.

If IBS is their primary reason for referral, the three-phase low FODMAP trial may be an option. If they were referred for another reason, you may need to determine when, or if, another session focusing on their GI symptoms would be appropriate. In some cases, their symptoms may be so severe that they are unable to apply the nutrition recommendations related to their initial referral. On the other hand, those with milder symptoms may have successfully identified healthy alternatives and are able to achieve a balanced diet with the foods they can tolerate. For some, the lifestyle changes required for their original referral may be challenging enough, that trying to tackle a stringent elimination diet at the same time may be too overwhelming. As with any counseling session, the dietitian should engage the patient in a shared approach to their nutrition therapy to determine how to prioritize and balance the patient's concerns.

If your patient expresses trouble managing IBS, listen for the high FODMAP foods they are currently consuming. Ask clarifying questions regarding portions and frequency. In addition, the following questions will be necessary in determining what options should be explored.

KEY ASSESSMENT QUESTIONS FOR IRRITABLE BOWEL SYNDROME

1. *Has the patient been diagnosed with IBS by their doctor?* As the symptoms of IBS are similar to other diseases, it is critical that their doctor has already ruled out other causes. As a low FODMAP trial can take several months, initiating the trial first may delay appropriate, and sometimes urgent, treatment. Examples of other conditions that can cause GI issues include, but are not limited to, Celiac Disease, inflammatory bowel diseases, colon cancer, and endometriosis.

   Also, for the patient, the effort of the trial can be burdensome. It will change how they plan meals at home, for work, or for their families. Some may find it costly to purchase different foods or specialty items. Social occasions may be challenging and uncomfortable. A low FODMAP approach is a lot to ask if it is not justified. For example, if it turns out that they actually have Celiac Disease, avoiding gluten alone may have been sufficient without avoiding other high FODMAP foods.

   If the patient has not yet been diagnosed with IBS, refer them back to their doctor for assessment.

2. *What are their symptoms, and for how long have they experienced them?* The symptoms of IBS include:

Abdominal pain

Diarrhea or constipation or both

Gas

Bloating and abdominal distension

If their symptoms developed more recently, determine if there have been any changes in their diet or medications, or if there are other significant changes that would affect bowel habits or abdominal pain. Also assess for other symptoms or scenarios that may indicate the presence of other possible disease.

SYMPTOMS AND SCENARIOS SUGGESTING OTHER POSSIBLE CAUSES OF GI ISSUES

Unintended weight loss
Family history of IBD, Celiac Disease, or colon cancer
Over age 50
Rectal bleeding
Nocturnal bowel movements
Daily diarrhea
Recurrent vomiting
Fever
Progressive worsening of symptoms
Painful menstruation
Pain during sex

Before the appropriate nutrition therapy can be determined, refer the patient back to their primary care physician to verify the cause of their symptoms.

ROME IV DIAGNOSTIC CRITERIA FOR IBS (MEARIN ET AL. 2016)

1. Abdominal pain at least one day a week over the last three months
2. Plus two or more of the following:
   Pain is related to defecation.
   Change in frequency of bowel movements.
   Change in form of stool.
   Symptoms started at least six months ago.
      Their IBS can be classified as predominantly diarrhea (IBS-D), constipation (IBS-C), or mixed (IBS-M). Some cases may be considered unclassified (IBS-U).

3. ***Do they struggle more with constipation, diarrhea, or both?*** If the patient has been diagnosed with IBS, the low FODMAP trial may be beneficial regardless of their predominant type. However, additional therapies may also be beneficial.

   For example, someone who struggles more with constipation may also benefit from an insoluble fiber supplement or certain laxatives. Ensuring adequate hydration and physical activity are also important. For someone who suffers more from diarrhea, soluble fiber supplements and probiotics may be additionally beneficial.

4. ***How severe are their symptoms, and to what extent does it affect their quality of life?*** The severity of their symptoms can determine whether a full elimination trial is needed, or if a modified, gentler approach is possible. Those with severe symptoms would benefit from the full elimination trial, which may bring relief sooner. On the other hand, those with milder symptoms may choose to eliminate high FODMAP foods only, but still include FODMAPs in moderate amounts. The severity of the patient's symptoms may also affect their motivation to agree, or adhere, to the trial. Compliance will be critical in determining the efficacy of the diet.

5. ***What current foods or lifestyle habits may be exacerbating symptoms?*** During the dietary recall, listen for which types of high FODMAP foods they consume, how frequently, and in what portion sizes. For those with mild or moderate symptoms, they may need only slight adjustments to their current diet. For example, somebody who drinks a lot of juice may find relief by eliminating the beverage and choosing water more often. Or someone who consumes one or two large meals per day may find improvement by having smaller, more frequent meals. If they struggle more with constipation, assess if their fiber and fluid intake are adequate. Caffeine and alcohol intake can also trigger symptoms in some people. If they are sedentary, physical activity may also help with constipation.

6. ***What is their stress level?*** For patients with IBS, stress and anxiety can exacerbate symptoms. There is much research about the gut-brain connection, in which stress can affect intestinal permeability, gut motility, microbiota, and other factors that can cause IBS symptoms (Konturek et al. 2011). Furthermore, the cause of their stress may affect their ability to implement dietary changes. For example, their food purchases may be limited by financial constraints. Or their hectic schedule may prohibit proper meal planning and preparation. Or emotional stress may impair their motivation to commit to an elimination trial. In some cases, a referral to a therapist or social worker may be required as an adjunct or alternative therapy.

7. ***Do they have a history of eating disorders, or exhibit signs of an eating disorder?*** A focus on food restriction would not be suitable for somebody with a history of disordered eating. In these cases, coordinate care with their doctor for medication options. A referral to a mental health professional can also be made if the patient is not already receiving therapy. See "A Note About Eating Disorders" in Chapter 8 of this book for information about proper screening and treatment of eating disorders.

As with any nutrition assessment, the goal of the dietitian is to determine which diet therapies would be appropriate and acceptable to the patient. While a strict low FODMAP trial would be most effective at identifying triggers sooner, it may not be the right approach for everybody. But for those who may benefit, a detailed education about how FODMAPs cause their symptoms can help them decide if they are willing to commit to the trial. Many feel relieved to hear that there is an explanation for their symptoms, and that there is hope to improve them.

WHAT PATIENTS WANT TO KNOW

What is a FODMAP? Unfortunately, neither the acronym nor the words it stands for are informative for the general public: Fermentable Oligo-, Di-, Monosaccharides, and Polyols. Furthermore, they do not represent the FODMAP categories: fructose, lactose, fructans, galacto-oligosaccharides, mannitol, and sorbitol. What a health literacy nightmare!

Another term nutrition experts may use is "short chain carbohydrates," which is not much easier to understand. If anything, the term probably causes further vilification of carbohydrates in general.

Define complicated terminology with plain language and simple terminology whenever possible (Figure 13.1).

The following key points may help patients better understand what FODMAPs are:

- FODMAPs include different types of sugars that are naturally found in various foods. An example that many people are familiar with is lactose in milk. Provide a list of different FODMAP categories and lists of foods within each category.
- Explain that FODMAPs also include "sugar free" sweeteners like sorbitol and mannitol (also called sugar alcohols). Show them how to locate these sweeteners in the ingredient list on product packages.
- People with IBS are unable to digest and absorb large amounts of some of these types of sugars or sweeteners. Small amounts may be tolerable.

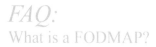

FAQ:
What is a FODMAP?

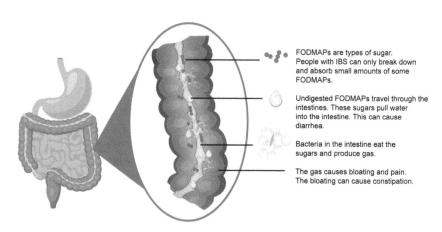

FODMAPs are types of sugar. People with IBS can only break down and absorb small amounts of some FODMAPs.

Undigested FODMAPs travel through the intestines. These sugars pull water into the intestine. This can cause diarrhea.

Bacteria in the intestine eat the sugars and produce gas.

The gas causes bloating and pain. The bloating can cause constipation.

Key Message
FODMAPs are different types of sugar. People with IBS can only digest small amounts of some FODMAPs. The sugars stay in the intestine and can cause diarrhea, gas, bloating, pain, or constipation.

FIGURE 13.1   Use plain language and simple imagery to explain how FODMAPs cause symptoms.

- Undigested FODMAPs move down the digestive tract where the sugars can attract water, which causes diarrhea.
- *F* stands for "fermentable," which means that the bacteria in the intestines feed on FODMAPs. After feeding, they produce gas which builds up and contributes to bloating and constipation.
- For patients with IBS, the bloating expands the intestines, causing abdominal pain.
- Monash University's online video "IBS Symptoms, the Low FODMAP Diet and the Monash App That Can Help" provides a nice animation of how FODMAPs cause bloating, gas, and/or constipation and diarrhea. The video is available on YouTube (Monash University, Department of Gastroenterology, Central Clinical School, 2015).

Which foods have FODMAPs? Once a patient learns about FODMAPs, a common misconception is that they need to avoid them completely. Binary lists that categorize FODMAPs as "low" or "high" mislead people into thinking that foods on the "high" list must be completely avoided. This leads to frustration as people feel they are unable to enjoy a variety of foods.

For many foods, a smaller serving size of a "high FODMAP food" may be included in a low FODMAP diet. The low FODMAP app from Monash University is a helpful tool for people to determine how to enjoy a variety of foods, rather than simply avoiding all high FODMAP foods (Monash University 2019b). For example, a ripe, medium-sized banana is high in fructans. However, the app shows that one-third of a medium banana is considered a low FODMAP serving size. Therefore, a small amount of banana that is part of a meal or snack may be tolerated by most people with IBS, as long as the other foods or ingredients are also low in FODMAPs. For example, almond milk yogurt topped with some blueberries, almonds, and one-third of a medium banana would be a low FODMAP snack (Figure 13.2).

Do I have a gluten intolerance? In recent years, gluten, a protein found in wheat, became a frequent scapegoat for GI symptoms. While Celiac Disease is well established as an autoimmune response to gluten, Non-Celiac Gluten Sensitivity (NCGS) is an alternative—albeit controversial—diagnosis. Due to a rise in gluten awareness and gluten-free products, some people suffering from GI symptoms self-initiate a gluten-free diet. While they may find relief by avoiding gluten, there is a possibility that the true trigger of their symptoms are fructans, a fermentable oligosaccharide that is also found in wheat. However, fructans are also found in other foods, such as garlic and onions. Thus, if they continue to have symptom flares even while avoiding gluten, the dietary trigger may be fructans rather than gluten. Once their doctor has ruled out Celiac Disease and other possible conditions, then a low FODMAP approach may be beneficial in identifying the true culprit of their GI issues.

What can I eat? Once the patient understands what FODMAPS are and how they cause their symptoms, the following information will guide them through a low FODMAP trial:

- A description of balanced meal planning using either The Plate Method or the MyPlate approach from the Dietary Guidelines for Americans.
- A list of foods categorized by food group, i.e., protein, starchy vegetables, grains, fruits, legumes, non-starchy vegetables, dairy, and condiments/ingredients.
- For each food, include the high FODMAP serving, medium FODMAP serving, and low FODMAP serving. Like in the previous example, 1 whole banana is high, but 1/3 of a banana is low.
- Meal ideas, snack ideas, and recipe resources.
- An education about food labels and ingredient lists.

High FODMAP	Low FODMAP
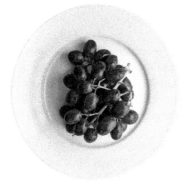	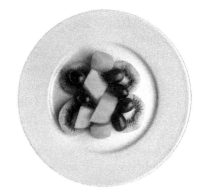
15 or more grapes	*6 or less grapes* *served with other* *low FODMAP foods*
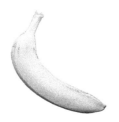	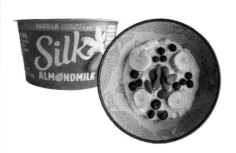
1 medium-sized ripe banana	*1/3 medium banana* *served with other* *low FODMAP foods*

Key Message

Some high FODMAP foods can be enjoyed in smaller portions with other low FODMAP foods.

FIGURE 13.2   Provide several meal and snack ideas showing how to enjoy a variety of foods.

- Low FODMAP products and meal delivery services.
- As discussed above, The Monash Low FODMAP app has an expansive list of foods with their FODMAP content, as well as recipe ideas, products, and services that support a low FODMAP diet. FODMAP Friendly is another program that certifies low FODMAP products and services as well as offers online recipes and a meal planning app.

WHAT PATIENTS NEED TO KNOW

The low FODMAP diet is a temporary, 3-phase trial. Time and again, people are misled to believe that they need to remove all high FODMAP foods from their diet permanently. They are handed lists of high and low FODMAP foods and told they can only choose from the low FODMAP foods. Consequently, patients feel overwhelmed, restricted, and fearful of many foods.

Explain that an elimination diet is a short-term trial consisting of three phases. While the trial takes some time, reassure them that most people discover that they only need to limit certain types of FODMAPs, not all of them. Throughout the trial, they will learn how to safely expand their diet. Also reinforce the importance of a varied diet for balanced nutrition (Figure 13.3).

During **Phase 1**, the diet includes low FODMAP foods, as well as small servings of some moderate and high FODMAP foods—thus, there is the possibility of more variety than people realize. The elimination phase typically lasts from 2 to 6 weeks, providing time for the body to wash out the excess FODMAPs previously consumed and recover from symptoms.

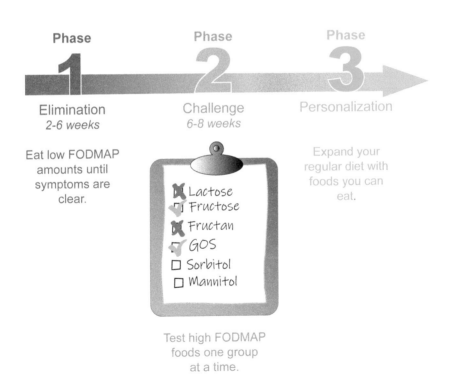

FAQ:
What is the Low FODMAP Diet?

Phase 1 — Elimination — *2-6 weeks* — Eat low FODMAP amounts until symptoms are clear.

Phase 2 — Challenge — *6-8 weeks* — Test high FODMAP foods one group at a time.

- ☒ Lactose
- ☑ Fructose
- ☒ Fructan
- ☑ GOS
- ☐ Sorbitol
- ☐ Mannitol

Phase 3 — Personalization — Expand your regular diet with foods you can eat.

Key Message
The Low FODMAP diet is a short-term trial designed to identify the FODMAP groups that cause symptoms. Most people only need to limit or avoid some groups.

FIGURE 13.3 Provide the patient with a description of each phase and an estimated timeline.

If the patient experiences a reduction in symptoms during this phase, then it would be appropriate to proceed with the next phase. If no improvement is observed, then the dietitian must determine if either (a) the patient followed the diet appropriately or (b) if there is possibility of other conditions or diseases, in which case a referral back to their doctor is required.

Phase 2 is the challenge phase, in which people systematically challenge foods from each FODMAP group. Each challenge would last three days. On the first day, a moderate amount of the test food is consumed, followed by a larger portion on the second day, and if still tolerated, a second serving of a large portion on the third day (see Figure 13.4). The result of each test determines if and how much of each FODMAP can be included in Phase 3.

After each challenge, a three-day return to a low FODMAP intake is recommended before challenging a new food from a different FODMAP group, allowing any residual impact from the

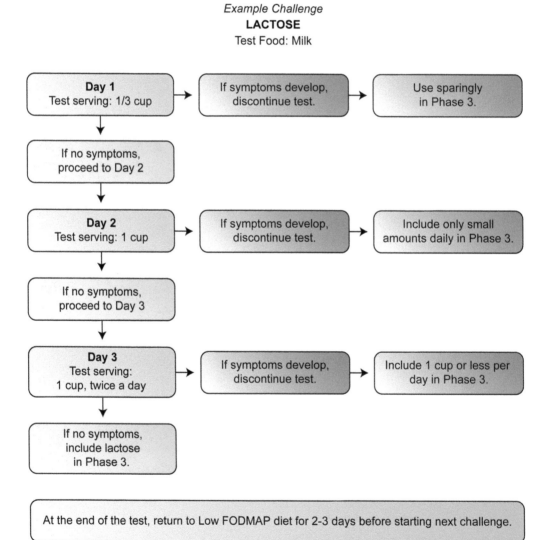

Example Challenge
LACTOSE
Test Food: Milk

| Day 1 Test serving: 1/3 cup | If symptoms develop, discontinue test. | Use sparingly in Phase 3. |

If no symptoms, proceed to Day 2

| Day 2 Test serving: 1 cup | If symptoms develop, discontinue test. | Include only small amounts daily in Phase 3. |

If no symptoms, proceed to Day 3

| Day 3 Test serving: 1 cup, twice a day | If symptoms develop, discontinue test. | Include 1 cup or less per day in Phase 3. |

If no symptoms, include lactose in Phase 3.

At the end of the test, return to Low FODMAP diet for 2-3 days before starting next challenge.

FIGURE 13.4 Each FODMAP challenge will last one to three days. Allow a two- to three-day washout period between each challenge.

previous challenge food to wash out. Each category must be challenged in isolation of the other categories. A food and symptom diary is recommended to track each challenge result.

The order of the tests may vary. If there are certain foods that the patient has been missing most, they may decide to start with those categories. However, if a patient suffers predominantly from constipation, they may benefit from testing categories that could promote laxation, such as fructose and polyols.

Upon completion of Phase 2, the trigger FODMAPs may have been identified, and the long-term diet plan can be established. Thus, in **Phase 3**, the patient implements a personalized plan that restricts the triggers yet expands their diet with the foods that do not trouble them.

Of note, tolerance has been shown to change over time. Foods that triggered symptoms in the past may be less troublesome later. Thus, it is worthwhile to periodically re-challenge foods to further expand the diet as much as possible.

The challenge phase is worth completing. Some people will feel so much better when they stop eating high FODMAP foods that they may be reluctant to advance to the challenge phase. For those with severe symptoms, they may be quite amenable to limiting their diet indefinitely for fear of their symptoms returning. However, it is likely that their symptoms were caused by only certain FODMAPs, not necessarily all of them. Thus, they may end up avoiding some foods unnecessarily. Consequently, the burden of severely restricting their diet may negatively impact their quality of life. Furthermore, their diet may end up lacking certain nutrients.

For these patients, a slower transition through the challenge phase may be more acceptable. They may choose to try only small amounts of test foods or challenge every other day instead of three days in a row. Reassure the patient that they have options, and that the results would be worthwhile knowing in the long run.

Nutrients of concern on a low FODMAP diet. Without proper guidance from a dietitian, those restricting their diet may become deficient in fiber, calcium, or iron. A low fiber diet may impair the proliferation of beneficial gut microbes that contribute to intestinal health, disease prevention, and possible other health benefits (Wong et al. 2006). By limiting lactose, some may become deficient in calcium if they do not include suitable dairy alternatives and other high-calcium foods. For people who are vegetarian or vegan, some of their typical sources of iron become restricted, such as whole grains and some legumes, so they will need to be advised on adequate iron intake and monitored for iron deficiency.

Supplements that may help. Fiber supplements may be helpful for patients with IBS, but it's important to understand the different types of fiber supplements on the market. Monash University provides the following guidance (McNamara and Iacovou 2017):

Fiber supplements made with **psyllium husk** are high in soluble fiber, which helps absorb water. This can help reduce diarrhea or add bulk to stool to improve constipation. However, some of the fiber in psyllium husk is fermentable, so may not be tolerated by some people with IBS.

Fiber supplements made with **methylcellulose** are known for their laxative effects and can be beneficial for constipation, but can be an alternative fiber supplement for diarrhea if psyllium husk is not tolerated. This type of fiber is not fermentable, so it should be appropriate for many people with IBS.

Watch out for fiber supplements made with FODMAPs such as inulin, fructooligosaccharides, or galactooligosaccharides. Other supplements may be made with other fiber types that have been found ineffective or lack scientific evidence of efficacy.

Of note, if the patient is already consuming adequate fiber from their food, additional fiber supplementation may not be beneficial and may even worsen symptoms.

The evidence and recommendations regarding **probiotics** is mixed, but may be worth trying, especially for those with mild symptoms. The risk of adverse events or safety issues is low. However, the cost of supplementation must also be considered. Probiotic preparations include capsules, powders, or products like yogurt or probiotic drinks. Monash University's FODMAP app includes a variety of products that are low in FODMAPs. The effects of probiotics may take 4–8 weeks before their benefits are realized. If no benefit is observed in that time frame, then the supplement can be discontinued as it may be an unnecessary expense.

Vitamin and mineral supplements may be needed for those who are unable to meet their needs through diet. While a variety of foods and food groups are available on a low FODMAP diet, certain food preferences may inhibit somebody from planning a balanced diet. For example, somebody who does not like milk alternatives may struggle with meeting their calcium needs. Be sure to monitor nutrient intake, advise on appropriate substitutions, assess for symptoms of nutrient deficiencies, and recommend mineral or vitamin supplements as needed. Supplement only the amounts needed to meet the recommended daily allowance. The Monash app contains a "dietary supplement" category listing products that are low FODMAP certified.

As with all supplements, patients need to know that they are not regulated by the FDA. Without oversight, products may lack therapeutic qualities required for positive results, may be subject to harmful manufacturing practices, or may contain potentially harmful compounds. Educate patients in identifying products that have been tested for quality by independent organizations such as the U.S. Pharmacopoeia, Consumerlab, or NSF.

Be selective about natural laxatives. Some patients might try foods and beverages that are known for their laxative effect. However, some may be high in FODMAPs. For example, prunes and prune juice are high in sorbitol, so should be avoided during the first phase of the low FODMAP diet. Caffeine is also known for promoting laxation. However, for some people, caffeine can trigger GI symptoms. Two kiwi, on the other hand, is a low FODMAP serving that has been shown to be effective in treating IBS-C (Lee 2021).

Dining out tips. As with other dietary guidelines, dining out can be challenging. In the case of FODMAPs, ingredients such as dairy, garlic, onion, and high fructose corn syrup may be present in sauces and dips. Many meals contain bread and/or pasta. In general, large portions at American restaurants can exacerbate IBS symptoms. However, there are healthy choices that can still be appropriate on a low FODMAP diet, such as lean proteins, potato, rice or rice noodles, salads, and vegetables. Gluten-free meals may be available. Dips and sauces can be requested on the side and used sparingly. Avoid foods made with stocks like stews and soups as they often contain garlic and onions. If menus are available online, review options ahead of time.

Read ingredient lists on packaged foods. Educate patients in identifying high FODMAP ingredients in packaged foods. Fructose, fruit, fruit juices, various types of sugar alcohols, garlic, onion, wheat, and fiber additives like chicory root extract (also listed as inulin) are commonly included in packaged foods.

Portions matter. Just as small portions of some high FODMAP foods can be safely consumed, large portions of low FODMAP foods may trigger symptoms. For most people, overeating at any one meal can cause GI discomfort in the form of bloating and indigestion, but for those with IBS, those symptoms can be even more debilitating. As with any dietary approach, mindful eating should be applied.

Benefits of physical activity. While there are numerous health benefits of physical activity, research suggests a therapeutic effect for patients with IBS. While the mechanisms are unclear, improvements have been found in GI symptoms, as well as depression, stress, and anxiety—each of which can influence GI function (Zhou et al. 2019). Aerobic exercise has been specifically shown to improve constipation (Gao et al. 2019).

Pharmacological therapy. In addition to the low FODMAP approach, patients should consult with their doctor to discuss if medications are also needed. According to the International Foundation for Gastrointestinal Disorders (2023), various drug therapies are used in IBS, from over-the-counter laxatives and antidiarrheals to prescription antispasmodics, antibiotics, antidepressants, secretagogues, or serotonin receptor agonists/antagonists.

While more research is needed in evaluating the long-term effects of the low FODMAP approach, the American College of Gastroenterology Clinical Guidelines includes the three-phase trial in their treatment recommendations for IBS. Furthermore, the guideline reinforces the importance of using a GI trained registered dietitian in leading the dietary intervention. The Monash University online course "Online FODMAP and IBS Training for Dietitians" provides 30 hours of continuing education credits and an in-depth training in screening for red flags, implementing the diet, addressing emotional and psychological barriers, and protecting against nutrient deficiencies. As the total duration of an elimination diet can take upwards of three months for a patient, a few days of training for the dietitian is a small ask.

CLINICAL PRACTICE GUIDELINES, PROFESSIONAL AND PATIENT RESOURCES, AND MEAL PLANNING WEBSITES

The American College of Gastroenterology Clinical Guideline: Management of Irritable Bowel Syndrome (Lacy et al. 2021)

Monash University. Online FODMAP and IBS Training for Dietitians - https://www.monashfodmap.com/online-training/dietitian-course/

GI Institute: FODMAP Institute (education and resources for health professionals) - https://giinstitute.com/

Monash University: IBS Central (app, resources, recipes, products) - http://www.monashfodmap.com/

FODMAP Friendly (app, resources, recipes, products) - https://fodmapfriendly.com/

Educational slides and meal planning handouts are included with this book, available online at https://resourcecentre.routledge.com/books/9781032352459

REFERENCES

American College of Gastroenterology. *About Irritable Bowel Syndrome* [Internet]. North Bethesda, MD: American College of Gastroenterology; n.d. [cited 2022 October 15]. Available from: https://webfiles.gi.org/images/patients/IBS-infographic.pdf.

Bellini M, Tonarelli S, Nagy AG, Pancetti A, Costa F, Ricchiuti A, de Bortoli N, Mosca M, Marchi S, Rossi A. Low FODMAP Diet: Evidence, Doubts, and Hopes. *Nutrients*. 2020 Jan;12(1):148. doi: 10.3390/nu12010148.

Gao R, Tao Y, Zhou C, Li J, Wang X, Chen L, Li F, Guo L. Exercise Therapy in Patients with Constipation: A Systematic Review and Meta-analysis of Randomized Controlled Trials. *Scand J Gastroenterol*. 2019 Feb;54(2):169–177. doi: 10.1080/00365521.2019.1568544.

Gibson PR. History of the Low FODMAP Diet. *J Gastroenterol Hepatol*. 2017 Mar;32(Suppl 1):5–7. doi: 10.1111/jgh.13685.

GI Institute. *FODMAP Institute* [Internet]. Ringwood, VIC: GI Institute; 2021 [cited 2023 June 16]. Available from: https://giinstitute.com/fodmap-home/.

International Foundation for Gastrointestinal Disorders. *Medications for IBS* [Internet]. Mount Pleasant, SC: IFFD; 2023 [cited 2023 June 15]. Available from: https://aboutibs.org/treatment/medications-for-ibs/.

Konturek PC, Brzozowski T, Konturek SJ. Stress and the Gut: Pathophysiology, Clinical Consequences, Diagnostic Approach and Treatment Options. *J Physiol Pharmacol*. 2011 Dec;62(6):591–599.

Lacy BE, Pimentel M, Brenner DM, Chey WD, Keefer LA, Long MD, Moshiree B. ACG Clinical Guideline: Management of Irritable Bowel Syndrome. *Am J Gastroenterol.* 2021 Jan;116(1):17–44. doi: 10.14309/ ajg.0000000000001036.

Lee, J. *Research Update: Kiwifruit, Psyllium and Prunes, Which One Is Better for Constipation?* [Internet]. Monash University. 2021 [cited 2023 June 15]. Available from: https://www.monashfodmap.com/blog/ research-update-kiwifruit-psyllium-and-prunes-which-one-better-constipation/.

McNamara L, Iacovou M. *Fibre Supplements & IBS* [Internet]. Monash University. 2017 [cited 2023 June 15]. Available from: https://www.monashfodmap.com/blog/fibre-supplements-ibs/.

Mearin F, Lacy BE, Chang L, Chey WD, Lembo AJ, Simren M, Spiller R. Bowel Disorders. *Gastroenterology.* 2016 Feb:S0016-5085(16)00222-5. doi: 10.1053/j.gastro.2016.02.031.

Monash University. *Online FODMAP and IBS Training for Dietitians* [Internet]. 2019a [cited 2022 December 12]. Available from: https://www.monashfodmap.com/online-training/dietitian-course/.

Monash University. *Get the APP* [Internet]. 2019b [cited 2022 December 12]. Available from: https://www. monashfodmap.com/ibs-central/i-have-ibs/get-the-app/

Monash University, Department of Gastroenterology, Central Clinical School. *IBS Symptoms, the Low FODMAP Diet and the Monash App That Can Help* [Internet]. 2015 [cited 15 June 2023]. Available from: https://www.youtube.com/watch?v=Z_1Hzl9o5ic

Trott N, Aziz I, Rej A, Surendran Sanders D. How Patients with IBS Use Low FODMAP Dietary Information Provided by General Practitioners and Gastroenterologists: A Qualitative Study. *Nutrients.* 2019 Jun;11(6):1313. doi: 10.3390/nu11061313.

Wong JM, de Souza R, Kendall CW, Emam A, Jenkins DJ. Colonic Health: Fermentation and Short Chain Fatty Acids. *J Clin Gastroenterol.* 2006 Mar;40(3):235–243. doi: 10.1097/00004836-200603000-00015.

Zhou C, Zhao E, Li Y, Jia Y, Li F. Exercise Therapy of Patients with Irritable Bowel Syndrome: A Systematic Review of Randomized Controlled Trials. *Neurogastroenterol Motil.* 2019 Feb;31(2):e13461. doi: 10.1111/nmo.13461.

14 Weight Counseling

Let's face it. The topic of weight is fraught with challenges. Historically, the healthcare industry has treated people with obesity with discrimination, insensitivity, and bias, both implicit and explicit (Phelan et al. 2015). While some providers may have good intentions to treat or prevent weight-related conditions, others can be shameless in their victim blaming. I once heard one patient complain:

> "No matter what my appointment is for, they always comment on my weight. I could go in for a skin tag and they'll tell me to lose weight."

Dietitians are not off the hook on this matter, either. As mentioned earlier in this book, research suggests that over 60% of dietitians demonstrate implicit weight bias (Wijayatunga et al. 2021). As nutrition and lifestyle are key components of weight management, outpatient dietitians are integral members of the healthcare team. Therefore, developing and conveying compassion will be critical for dietitians to effectively support the patient.

Supporting the patient, however, may mean different things. While their doctor may have referred them for weight loss, the patient may have different needs or goals. While BMI may be positively associated with poor health outcomes (CDC 2022), studies suggest that societal weight stigma, as well as self-internalized weight bias, may contribute to those outcomes (Wu and Berry 2018; Hilbert et al. 2014). In other words, the psychological impact of weight bias may negatively impact health behaviors, thus increasing the risk for poor health.

Moreover, research shows that the more healthy habits someone adopts, the lower their risk for mortality, regardless of BMI (Matheson et al. 2012). Those healthy habits include eating five or more fruits and vegetables daily, regular exercise, alcohol moderation, and not smoking.

To be fair, weight loss also results in health improvements, including reductions in blood pressure, triglycerides, LDL-cholesterol, and blood glucose levels (NIH 1998). Whether through intensive lifestyle change programs, weight loss medications, meal replacement plans, or bariatric surgery, improvements to cardiometabolic profiles are generally reported.

But let's not forget the *obesity paradox*, where increased BMI has been shown to be protective in patients with cardiovascular disease (Antonopoulos and Tousoulis 2017; Gruberg et al. 2002). The Association for Size Diversity and Health also cites studies showing that intentional weight loss may actually worsen outcomes and increase the risk of death (Ingram and Mussolino 2010 as cited by ASDAH 2020).

The relationship between weight and health proves to be complex. For the healthcare provider, mediating factors further complicate the treatment. Genetics, environment, access to healthy food and healthcare, and life stressors cannot be treated with prescriptions or meal plans.

However, not all people seek, want, or feel the need for treatment. The Health at Every Size® principles convey that the pursuit of health "is neither a moral imperative nor an individual obligation," and healthcare should be provided equitably and without judgment in regard to the person's individual goals and priorities.

The body positivity movement that originated during the 1960s aimed to fight discrimination against people with obesity, including in healthcare (Frazier and Mehdi 2021). As discussed earlier in this book, discrimination and bias negatively impact the type or amount

DOI: 10.1201/9781003326038-17

of care physicians provide. Furthermore, such negative treatment may prohibit people from seeking care when they need it (ASDAH 2020; Phelan et al. 2015). Both cases contribute to poor health outcomes. One of the goals of the movement was to establish laws and policies that protect people with obesity.

Since then, policy change has gained traction, especially since obesity was classified as a disease (American Medical Association 1995–2023). While the definition or criteria for "disease" is unclear, the benefits of this label informed this decision: increased healthcare coverage for obesity treatment; increased funding for research; improved training for medical professionals; increased protections against workplace discrimination or consumer fraud (i.e., weight loss supplements); and increased public awareness about the various causes of obesity (Kyle et al. 2016).

On the other hand, some argue that labeling obesity as a disease increases fat stigma (Hansen 2014).

Today, the body positivity movement has evolved to include self-acceptance and self-love of *all* body types, in addition to social acceptance (Frazier and Mehdi 2021; Ospina 2016). To be clear, many argue that the current dialogue dilutes the movement's original fight for fat acceptance, fair treatment, and legal protections (Frazier and Mehdi 2021; Ospina 2016). However, in regard to health outcomes, research has shown an association between positive body image, health behaviors, and health-related indicators, regardless of weight (Gillen 2015). Therefore, while obesity is considered a disease in the medical field, people with higher weights do not conclusively have poor health. Thus, "weight management" in the name of health, but in the absence of poor health, may actually signify and perpetuate fat stigmatization.

While the public debate wages on about weight management versus body positivity, the personal goals of the patient will set the agenda in nutrition counseling. Inevitably, there will be patients who are seeking assistance for weight loss, with or without comorbidities. The National Health and Nutrition Examination Survey from 2017 to March 2020 (Stierman et al. 2021) showed that the prevalence of obesity in the US was 41.9%, up from 30.5% in the 1999–2000 survey (CDC 2022). Therefore, dietitians must be prepared to discuss strategies for weight loss if that is what the patient requests.

BEYOND CALORIES

A common misconception about weight counseling is that the dietitian simply prescribes calorie-specific meal plans. Referring providers expect that the patient will learn how to count calories and eat accordingly. Patients expect—and often request—specific foods to eat. Some say, "I just want to be told what to eat."

If only it were that easy. Indeed, people certainly have achieved weight loss by consuming certain foods prescribed by a nutritionist or weight loss program. Perhaps they stocked up on chicken, fish, and vegetables and established a specific eating schedule. They may have even purchased protein powders, meal replacement products, or prepared meals to include in the plan. Likely, the meal plan and supplements were nutritionally balanced and calorie-controlled. Also likely, they did not allow for excess sweets, treats, or other extras. Motivated and committed, those following such plans often do see results. Having adopted a healthy mindset, they might also increase other health behaviors, like physical activity, alcohol moderation, or stress management. With these changes, those with health concerns may see improvements to lab values, biomarkers, or symptoms.

Even without a specific meal program, some people have observed weight changes when their life situation changes. For example, one patient reported that she had lost weight while studying abroad. She noted that portion sizes were smaller in the country she was visiting, and the main mode of transportation was walking. Thus, she was eating less and moving more. Upon returning to the States, she found herself regaining the weight she had lost. While she could identify the causes of her weight loss abroad (i.e., reduced intake and increased physical activity), she struggled with adopting those strategies in her usual environment.

Weight loss stories are often similar. Commercial programs, popular diets, weight loss products, apps, and websites have all been shown to be effective. However, equally similar are the stories about what happened after the programs were discontinued: "...and then the weight came back."

The concept of yo-yo dieting is familiar to most people. What is less intuitive, however, are the causes. Often, people blame themselves. "I just don't have the willpower," they might say. Or, "I hit a plateau, got frustrated, and stopped." Or they recognized that their approach "was just unsustainable," but did not know how to modify it to something more livable.

Needless to say, for many patients who desire weight loss, their visit to the dietitian will not be their first attempt. Many will be quite versed in the concepts of calorie counting and portion control. They may already be ordering their salad dressing on the side and comparing their chicken to a deck of cards. For them and for most others, detailed meals and shopping lists did not provide the long-term answer in the past, so they likely will not be the answer moving forward.

Nor is there just one answer. Like other conditions, the causes of obesity are multifactorial, many of which are non-modifiable. Genetics, age, environment, race, and ethnicity can be determinants of weight, body composition, and body shape. Health, on the other hand, can be mediated by lifestyle—nutrition, physical activity, stress management, and overall healthy choices. Lifestyle, in turn, is impacted by cultural traditions and values, access to education, nutritious foods, safe spaces for physical activity, healthcare, medications, and social and psychological support. Underlying all of this will be the patient's experiences and relationship with food, as well as their motivation to maintain or improve health.

In public health, the role of the dietitian must be part of a greater socio-ecological intervention. However, for the individual patient, the dietitian will be their personal guide to information. Upon identifying the patient's needs, the dietitian provides not only knowledge about food and health but also about available resources for various barriers. For example, the dietitian might inform those with financial constraints about nutrition assistance programs and local food pantries. Or for those who exhibit emotional eating behaviors, the dietitian can screen for eating disorders and refer them to a mental health professional for further evaluation if needed. Or for those who are inexperienced in cooking, the dietitian can educate the patient on cooking basics, and/or direct them to community cooking classes.

The complexity of weight counseling will require more training than can be covered in this chapter.

Certification programs are available from various organizations including the Commission on Dietetic Registration. Continuing education on the latest treatments for obesity including medications, bariatric surgery, and medically supervised weight loss programs is critical as nutrition therapy will be adjunctive to these treatments. And deeper insight into the psychological impact— or causes—of obesity is necessary to develop the compassion needed for patient-centered care. To get started, this book covers the most frequently asked questions and reported challenges in weight counseling and how to address them.

WHAT YOU NEED TO KNOW.

1. Does the patient have underlying conditions that affect their weight?
2. Are they taking medications or supplements that cause weight gain?
3. Are they currently taking medication for weight loss?
4. Do they have a family history of obesity?
5. What was their lowest adult weight?
6. What previous weight loss strategies have they tried?
7. Are emotional or mental health issues contributing to their eating pattern?
8. What are their socioeconomic barriers, if any?

WHAT PATIENTS *WANT* TO KNOW.

1. What is the best way to lose weight?
2. How many calories can I have?
3. How much protein do I need?
4. How do I manage my cravings for sugar?
5. What snacks can I have?
6. What is the best exercise for weight loss?
7. Is there a menu I can follow?

WHAT PATIENTS *NEED* TO KNOW.

1. Basic metabolism.
2. Macronutrients.
3. Glucose metabolism and insulin.
4. Timing of meals.
5. Strategies for successful, long-term weight loss.
6. Strategies for handling the weight loss plateau.

WHAT YOU NEED TO KNOW

As unwanted weight gain can be multifactorial, a careful assessment must be conducted to determine which factors are most pertinent to—and modifiable by—the individual. While the effects of healthy eating, calorie reduction, and physical activity for weight loss have been repeatedly demonstrated, other factors determine the sustainability of lifestyle change.

Key Considerations for Weight Counseling

1. *Are there underlying conditions contributing to unintended weight gain?* In preparation for the visit, review the patient's medical history and lab results. Some common conditions that affect weight include hypothyroidism, polycystic ovarian syndrome, or prediabetes. Also look for conditions that can cause fluid retention, such as heart failure or kidney disease, to differentiate between weight gain and fluid overload.

    If underlying conditions are present, incorporating the appropriate medical nutrition therapy will be key to mitigating its impact on weight.

    Other factors that can cause unintentional weight gain include stress, age, and age-related conditions like menopause. Some people may believe that weight gain is inevitable in these cases. However, a thorough assessment may reveal modifiable factors that can help them maintain or achieve a healthier weight.

While a host of factors may be involved, reinforcing the benefits of a healthy lifestyle will be applicable to all. Moreover, many people find that when they make changes for their health, they inadvertently achieve some weight loss as well.

2. *Are they taking medications or supplements that can cause weight gain?* Corticosteroids, some diabetes medications including insulin and sulfonylureas, and some mental health medications like some antidepressants can cause weight gain. Identifying other modifiable factors like food choices or physical activity can help mitigate the effects of these medications.

Common misconceptions about nutrition can also result in weight gain through excessive calorie intake. For example, many people unnecessarily add protein powders, shakes, or bars to their diet, only to exceed their calorie needs. Or they may overconsume juice products to address certain conditions, such as cranberry juice for urinary tract infections, cherry juice for gout, or prune juice for constipation. Whatever their nutrition goals, provide a more comprehensive education about those conditions to clarify what works, what doesn't, and how to properly meet those goals.

3. *Have they been prescribed weight loss medications?* FDA-approved weight loss medications include phentermine and topiramate capsules, lorcaserin HCl, and the injectable medication semaglutide, a GLP-1 receptor agonist (USFDA 2015, 2021). Some diabetes medications have been used off-label to treat obesity, such as other GLP-1 agonists or Metformin. Become familiar with these medications, their mechanisms of action, as well as their side effects. Some side effects can affect the patient's ability to achieve balanced meal planning or physical activity. For example, GLP-1 agonists can cause some nausea, sometimes vomiting, and can reduce appetite to the point that people are unable to consume enough nutrients. In these cases, the patient will benefit from an education on how the drugs work and how to plan meals to combat those side effects.

Unfortunately, weight loss is big business for the supplement industry. The FDA lists hundreds of tainted weight loss products, many containing hidden drug ingredients (USFDA 2023), and these are just the ones who got caught. Due to the lack of federal regulation of the supplement industry, the risk of drug–drug interactions, food–drug interactions, and other dangerous side effects are high. Be sure to screen for supplements during your assessment and educate the patient about these risks if necessary.

4. *Do they have a family history of obesity?* While genetics are a non-modifiable factor, the CDC has found that genetic disorders are not the sole cause of obesity for most people (CDC 2013). Obesity is largely multifactorial, and for some gene variants, studies have shown that physical activity can attenuate their impact on obesity (Kilpeläinen et al. 2011).

While genetics and epigenetics contribute to the predisposition for obesity, other factors likely compound the risk. A family history of obesity, itself, may implicate not only genetics but also nutrition knowledge, food choices, meal planning skills, family and cultural traditions, and psychosocial factors around food.

In the case of nutrition counseling, family history may or may not come up in discussion. If it does, the topic may be more focused on food preferences, lifelong habits, and maybe their relationship with food.

5. *What was their lowest adult weight?* A discussion about the person's weight history can help shed light on which factors contributed to their weight gain, and which strategies would be most applicable to them. Often, a person can pinpoint when they started to gain weight in the first place. Some commonly reported experiences include:

I used to play a lot of sports, but then I hurt my [knee/shoulder/other], and then I stopped exercising.

I started to gain weight after I got married. My spouse is such a good cook!

I had trouble losing weight after each pregnancy.

Once I retired, I wasn't as active at home as I was at work.

After our kids moved out, we started eating out more.

I was able to get my weight down by exercising and really watching what I was eating.

My weight started increasing once I started this medication.

As patients reflect on their experiences, they begin to identify some strategies that are most pertinent to them, and the barriers they need to overcome. Some examples include:

I need to start planning ahead so I can prepare more meals at home.

I have a stationary bike in my basement. I could move it upstairs in front of the TV.

I do better when I'm writing down my food. I need to start that again.

To be fair, the answer is not always straightforward. Some barriers are harder to overcome than others. Underlying conditions—physical or emotional—may need to be addressed. Misconceptions about diet or physical activity may need to be cleared up. Logistical barriers like time, finances, or available resources must be recognized. Some medications do not have alternatives. However, exploring a person's weight history with them can help the dietitian and patient work together in developing a personalized action plan that goes beyond calorie counting.

6. ***What previous weight loss strategies have they tried? What worked? What did not?*** Some people will have cycled through the whole gamut of weight loss strategies, from commercial programs to popular diets to cleanses to supplements. Some may have even worked with a different dietitian in the past. Likely, they even saw results. In most cases, they will be coming to you because they subsequently regained the weight.

A recall of past efforts will reinforce for the patient what actions can help with weight loss, which usually will include diet changes and physical activity. It will also remind them of the planning and effort that were required. Even more so, it may boost their self-efficacy in making changes as they remember what they were able to achieve before.

Just as importantly, however, is to clarify why they discontinued those strategies. Some frequently reported reasons include:

The program was too expensive.

I stopped losing weight and I got frustrated.

I just got really busy with work.

It was too hard cooking different meals for myself and for my family.

It was just unsustainable.

I just crave sweets too much.

Understanding the person's viewpoint will guide the education and action planning. Perhaps their barriers are more logistical (e.g., time or budget), in which case you might initiate the problem solving process and have them brainstorm solutions. They might exhibit some emotional behaviors (e.g., negative self-talk, all-or-nothing tendencies, or stress eating), for which a discussion about mindful eating practices may be helpful. For those with a history of fad dieting, they may find an education about metabolism enlightening, clarifying that a more flexible approach can be both effective and more sustainable.

7. ***Are there underlying emotional or mental health issues contributing to their eating pattern? Do they have a history of disordered eating?*** Individuals with eating disorders should be referred to ED specialists. However, on occasion, you may encounter patients with a history of ED who have received treatment in the past and are often willing to talk

openly about their disorder. Some may be in remission but will acknowledge that restrictive eating approaches are not appropriate for them.

First, clarify if they currently see a therapist. Be sure to ask if they specifically address their eating disorder with their therapist, as they may be in therapy for other issues such as anxiety, depression, or other mental health concerns. You may need to reach out to their therapist to coordinate a care plan to monitor for and prevent relapse.

Secondly, ask the patient to specify their goals for nutrition counseling. If they are trying to lose weight, you and they will be better served by referring them to a dietitian or program that specializes in ED. However, some may be seeking nutrition therapy for other concerns. For example, perhaps they were recently diagnosed with prediabetes. In such a case, an education that focuses on how food affects blood sugar, insulin resistance, and health—without emphasis on weight management—would be appropriate. Again, in follow up, monitor for signs of ED behaviors and coordinate care as needed (see Table 8.3 for screening eating disorders).

8. ***What are their socioeconomic barriers, if any?*** During the nutrition assessment, as people describe their typical day, some may share that they are on a limited income, or that they receive nutrition assistance benefits, or explicitly state that they cannot afford healthy foods. On the other hand, some may not offer that information outright out of pride or embarrassment. However, the prevalence of obesity in adults with food insecurity is 35.1%, and adults with food insecurity have a 32% increased odds of being obese compared to food secure adults (Pan et al. 2012).

If they have not explicitly reported that they struggle with food costs, but you suspect it may be an issue, the following two questions have proven effective in quickly screening for food insecurity (Hager et al. 2010):

1. Within the past 12 months, how often have you worried that food would run out before you got money to buy more: often, sometimes or never?

2. Within the past 12 months, how often has the food you bought run out and you didn't have money to get more: often, sometimes, or never?

   If they answer "often" or "sometimes" to the above two questions, provide them with information about nutrition assistance programs in their area.

NUTRITION ASSISTANCE PROGRAMS, DIRECTORIES, AND RESOURCES

The USDA Supplemental Nutrition Assistance Program (SNAP). Visit www.fns.usda.gov/snap/state-directory for your local SNAP office

Feeding America. Search for local food pantries, senior programs, child feeding programs, and more at https://www.feedingamerica.org/

***Good and Cheap: Eat Well on $4/Day* by Leanne Brown**, a free downloadable cookbook available at www.leannebrown.com/cookbooks/

Refer them to a social worker who can provide them with more resources for financial assistance. Also encourage them to contact their health insurance to inquire about nutrition and transportation benefits. For more guidance on how to counsel patients with food insecurity, check out the "Food Insecurity Screening Toolkit" developed by Feeding America and Humana, available online at https://hungerandhealth.feedingamerica.org/resource/food-insecurity-screening-toolkit/.

During your assessment, as you listen to their dietary recall, you will get a sense of the types of foods to which they already have access. As with any nutrition counseling, incorporate their current foods into a healthful meal plan. Be prepared to discuss meal planning on a budget. Leanne Brown's *Good and Cheap: Eat Well on $4/Day* is a beautiful cookbook available as a free PDF at www.leannebrown.com/cookbooks/.

What Patients Want to Know

1. ***What is the best way to lose weight?*** And this is it. Perhaps the most common question asked of dietitians. If dietitians had a dime for every time they hear this question, the salary disparity for this Masters-requiring profession would be rectified. But I digress.

   From low fat to low carb to fasting, the most *popular* diets are ironically the most restrictive. It is no wonder they tend to be the most unsustainable.

   To be fair, some popular diets do induce faster *initial* weight loss than the traditional, reduced-calorie approaches. In ketogenic diets, the initial water loss in the first week alone can show changes on the scale (Rabast et al. 1981). However, time and again, studies show evidence of weight loss in various eating patterns—regardless of macronutrient composition—without one proving to be more superior to others (Sacks et al. 2009; Evert et al. 2019; Nield et al. 2007; Johnston et al. 2014).

   These findings are typically observed by the patients themselves. A common experience is, "I've tried everything. Weight Watchers, Keto, Atkins. They all worked, but once I stop, the weight just comes back."

   Hence the bigger challenge: weight loss *maintenance*. Again, research continues to show little difference when comparing various dietary patterns for long-term weight loss (Jabbour et al. 2022). While many comparisons suggest a slight advantage with low carb diets, the definition of "low carb" can vary from study to study, with some including carbs up to 45% of total calorie intake (Jabbour et al. 2022).

   Therefore, when fielding the "best diet for weight loss" question, the patient themselves will hold the answer. The key will be finding the strategies and changes that they can adopt for the long term. Assure them that a variety of approaches can work; that flexibility is not only allowed, but recommended; that maintaining overall health is part of the goal; and that lifestyle change, rather than *dieting*, will be the ultimate key to success.

   Overall, dietary changes should be planned based on the following:
   1. What strategies will the patient find most preferable and sustainable?
   2. What health conditions or lab values must be considered?
   3. What is the patient's ultimate goal for their health and/or weight? In other words, why is it important to them?

2. ***How many calories can I have?*** Counting calories as a strategy for weight loss is controversial. While the concept of "a calorie is a calorie" can spur all sorts of debate, most dietitians can agree that 1,400 calories of a balanced diet and 1,400 calories of jellybeans will not produce the same long-term results. The latter could result in protein malnourishment, muscle wasting, reduction in metabolic rate, insulin spikes, reactive hypoglycemia, frequent hunger, fatigue and reduced physical activity. The body composition decline alone would increase risk for regression. Lack of nutritional balance is a likely contributor to the common complaint, "Once I stopped, I gained back all of the weight and more!" (Figure 14.1)

   Similarly, 1,400 calories consumed in balanced meals spread throughout one's waking hours will be metabolized differently than 1,400 mostly consumed before bed. In the second scenario, diurnal metabolic changes, sedentary activity, and an elevated insulin response may promote more fat storage than the first.

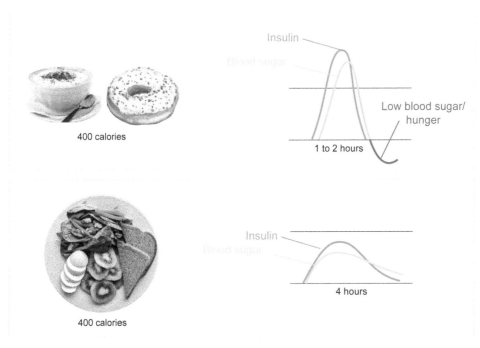

FIGURE 14.1   An explanation about how different types of food affect blood sugar, insulin, and hunger reinforces the importance of balanced nutrition.

Hence, calorie restriction, alone, may not be effective (Figures 14.2 and 14.3).

That is not to say, however, that calculating somebody's estimated energy requirement for weight loss is not worthwhile. Whether you use a Mifflin-St. Jeor calculator or some other BMR equation, estimating somebody's energy needs provides a reference to compare to their current calorie intake. This information will provide a starting point for troubleshooting what dietary factors may be contributing to their current weight. Clinical guidelines indicate that 1,200–1,500 calories per day are effective for women for weight loss, and 1,600–1,800 calories for men; alternatively, a 500–750 calorie reduction to their average intake may be effective (Jenson et al. 2014).

With an EER to compare to, a short-term calorie tracking plan can help the patient identify if their average calorie intake exceeds their needs. Often, the act of tracking alone leads to more mindful eating, in which a person is able to identify some habits they may not have noticed before.

FAQ:
How can I manage my hunger and cravings?

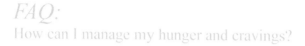

Example Day*

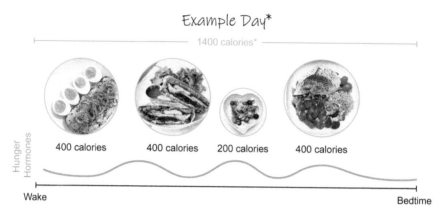

FIGURE 14.2   A brief explanation about the existence of hunger hormones helps explain why balanced meal planning helps prevent hunger and cravings.

Calorie counting as a long-term strategy, however, may not be practical. It can be time-consuming, inconvenient, and for some, emotionally burdensome. Again, for those who have attempted weight loss in the past, they have likely counted calories before, only to find it an unsustainable task. Some, in fact, may dread the idea of resuming the practice.

Nonetheless, calorie reduction continues to be the common denominator among weight loss strategies, thus should be part of the discussion. How the patient reduces calories, however, can be accomplished in a variety of ways.

1. ***Identify the source(s) of excess calories.*** A carefully conducted diet recall can often reveal which foods, beverages, portions, or dietary patterns are contributing unnecessary calories. For example, someone may report a grazing pattern of eating that includes some snacks and sweets. For them, establishing more balanced meals may help reduce cravings for snacks. Another may dine out frequently, where portions, ingredients, and cooking methods typically result in very high calorie meals. Preparing more meals at home will likely reduce their calorie intake. Someone who skips meals throughout the day may end up overeating at night; another might admit to stress eating; or another may be adding unnecessary nutrition supplements like protein shakes. Review Chapter 8 on everyday eating patterns for a preview of the various scenarios you will encounter and how to address them.

2. ***Keep a food journal without tracking calories.*** A magical thing happens when people start writing down their foods. Even without counting calories, they become aware of the extras–a cookie here, a piece of candy there; an afternoon habit; or some other recurring pattern. Even a short-term food log can help the patient identify which behaviors can be modified to help them reach their goals.

FAQ:
I'm not hungry for breakfast, but why am I so hungry at night?

A Common Eating Routine

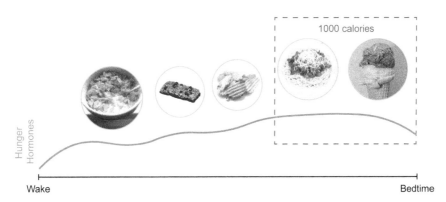

1000 calories

Hunger Hormones

Wake   Bedtime

Key Message
Skipped or unbalanced meals during the day can lead to increased hunger and overeating at night. Extra calories eaten at night are more likely to be stored as fat. Late night eating can prevent hunger in the morning.

FIGURE 14.3 A brief explanation about hunger hormones can help explain why skipping meals and/or unbalanced meals can lead to increased hunger at night. Learning about the existence of hunger hormones may help lessen the guilt about perceived "willpower."

Alternatively, for someone who describes themselves as a stress eater, suggest that they keep a "food and feeling" journal, in which they note their hunger level along with their emotions, especially when they are reaching for food outside of mealtimes. Frequent hunger may indicate a lack of balance in their meals or poor timing of eating. On the other hand, pausing to write before emotional eating can help the person address their feelings, gain perspective, become more mindful, and perhaps diffuse the severity of the situation.

3. ***Balance meals using the Plate Method.*** The Plate Method is an easy-to-understand approach to balanced meal planning. Using a standard nine-inch plate (often the salad plate), fill half the plate with non-starchy vegetables, one-quarter of the plate with lean protein, and the last quarter of the plate with carbohydrate (starch or fruit) (Figure 14.4).

This strategy has several benefits. First, it promotes a high intake of plant foods, ensuring adequate fiber, vitamins, minerals, and phytonutrients. Second, it encourages people to include a variety of food groups, which all provide different benefits–e.g., glucose for energy, protein for satiety and muscle maintenance, vegetables for fiber and micronutrients. Third, and pertinent to this section, it helps provide a full plate of food with maximal nutrition for minimal calories. The half plate of non-starchy vegetables is very low in calories, whereas the caloric protein and carbs are portion controlled.

FAQ:

FAQ:
How do I reduce calories, manage hunger, and boost my metabolism?

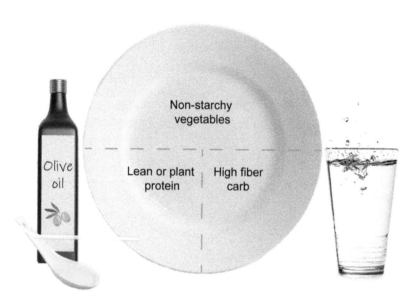

Fiber from vegetables
Keeps stomach full longer.
Prevents blood sugar spikes.

Fats/oils
Keeps stomach full longer.
Prevents blood sugar spikes.

Lean protein
Keeps stomach full longer.
Increases metabolism.
Prevents blood sugar spikes.

Water
Keeps stomach full.
Prevents salt cravings.

High fiber carbs
Stabilize blood sugar to
prevent hunger.

Timing
Space meals about 3 to 5 hours
apart. Include a snack if there is
a longer gap between meals.

Key Message
Protein, fat, fiber, and water help to feel full longer. The Plate Method provides proper balance and portions.

FIGURE 14.4   Explain the benefits of balanced meal planning beyond calories.

A typical Plate Method meal averages about 400 calories. Thus, if a person achieves this type of balance in breakfast, in lunch, and in dinner, total calorie intake is only 1,200 calories. If needed, a mindful snack can be included to manage hunger while still keeping calories below 1,500 calories. For those whose calorie needs are higher, additional healthy snacks can be added. Healthy snacks are typically around 200 calories or less. For example, a typical fruit serving is around 65 calories, or healthy fats like ¼ cup of almonds is about 170 calories.

3. *How much protein do I need?* The benefits of protein—let me count the ways: satiety, higher thermic effect, muscle development, and general body maintenance. A related question frequently asked is, "What can I eat to boost my metabolism?" to which protein would be a legitimate answer.

However, a common misconception among the general public is that adequate protein intake requires supplementation. The amount of grocery shelf space dedicated to protein bars, shakes, and other protein supplements reflects the extent of this misconception. While supplementation may be beneficial among elite athletes, the big business of protein supplements is incongruous to the portion of US adults who are athletically training. Less than one-quarter of US adults even meet the minimum physical activity guidelines (Elgaddal et al. 2022), let alone require a higher protein intake. For those who engage in general exercise, many are misled about protein through the media, and sometimes by personal trainers who are not adequately trained in nutrition therapy. Too many times, personal trainers give sports nutrition advice to their weight loss clients, such as consuming protein after exercise for recovery. While this advice may be appropriate for high-level athletes, those who see a trainer for an hour, three times a week, may unnecessarily be increasing their calorie intake.

Diet culture, with or without exercise, promotes high protein diets. Often, those attempting the ketogenic diet mistake the high-fat approach for a high protein diet. And while the higher thermic effect of protein does increase metabolism, weight loss is less likely if a calorie deficit is not concurrently achieved.

For general health, the recommended dietary allowance for protein is 0.8 g/kg/day (National Academies of Sciences, Engineering, and Medicine 2006)—adjusted for weight or fat-free mass if needed. For weight management, protein is well recognized as a satiety-inducing nutrient (Veldhorst et al. 2008). Consumption of up to 1.4 g/kg/day has been shown to be safe for those without renal impairment, especially in the form of plant protein (Ko et al. 2020; Knight et al. 2003). A typical Plate Method approach that includes an equivalent of three ounces of protein per plate typically provides more than the minimum requirement for most people. For example, a 160-lb moderately active woman would require 58 g of protein per day. Three Plate Method meals per day would provide approximately 90 g protein (or 1.25 g/kg for this example) and 90 g carbs in 1,200 calories, with a macronutrient profile of 30% protein, 30% carbohydrate, 40% fat, hitting many of the high notes of many popular diets. Again, through balanced, mindful choices, the numbers often just fall into place—without counting, without supplements, and without food restrictions.

4. *How do I manage my cravings for sugar?* Cravings for sweets or refined carbs are an undeniably common experience. Some even suspect that they are addicted to sugar. Their suspicion is not unfounded, as scientists have been studying this question for decades. Indeed, studies report several similarities in the behavioral, psychological, and neurobiological responses to sugar and drugs (DiNicolantonio et al. 2018). On the other hand,

some argue against the reproducibility of the neurobiological findings, or whether sugar induces withdrawal symptoms, a criteria for the diagnosis of addiction (Greenberg and St Peter 2021; DiNicolantonio et al. 2018). As was seen with the disease designation for obesity, a classification for sugar addiction would impact policy, research funding, treatment, and insurance coverage for treatment. In the meantime, while scientists continue to discover and debate, the outpatient dietitian is positioned at the front lines to support people who struggle with sugar. In these cases, each patient experience will individually determine how the dietitian treats their concern.

With or without addiction, the drive to sweets or carbs can be multifactorial. Physiological hunger, insulin resistance, psychological factors including coping skills or eating disorders, and environmental cues can each individually—or in concert—increase cravings for sweets. Through careful assessment and listening, the dietitian is likely to pick up on some factors that may be modifiable.

Highlighting the factors that are pertinent to the individual often brings the patient some relief. Many blame themselves for their sugar cravings. They use terms like "weakness" or "lack of willpower." However, if their everyday eating pattern may be exacerbating their desire for sweets, a discussion about the physiology of hunger helps to alleviate their self-blame. Similarly, for patients with insulin resistance, a description of the cyclical effect of blood sugar on cravings adds more clarity to their experiences. If emotional eating is a factor, brainstorming strategies for alternative coping strategies may empower them to be mindful and proactive. If they exhibit signs of psychological distress or eating disorder, a referral to a mental health professional may be required.

Whatever the cause of the patient's cravings, the nutrition counseling room is no space for debate. Hearing, understanding, and compassion are the heart of effective patient care.

5. *What snacks can I have?* At first glance, this seems like a very straightforward question. Certainly, it is handy to have a list of healthy snack ideas ready. Dietitian favorites might include fruit, Greek yogurt, whole grain crackers, air-popped popcorn, vegetables with hummus, or nuts. For those with a sweet tooth, a mindfully eaten dark chocolate square, a frozen fruit bar, or berries with whipped cream may hit the spot.

However, the concept of snacking can have different connotations for different people. While healthy snacks can help manage hunger and prevent overeating at meals, some people think snacks should be avoided. Some feel guilty about having a snack, and even try to avoid snacking, even if they are hungry. This can lead to increased hunger by mealtime, increasing the risk of overeating.

On the other hand, others feel that if the snack is healthy, they can indulge regardless of their hunger or calorie needs. For example, an evening snack in front of the TV is common practice, even if their dinner was sufficiently satisfying. For some, the evening snack is used to relax or de-stress at the end of the day but may exceed calorie needs. For example, a healthy snack of cut vegetables with two ounces of hummus is an additional 150 calories. In the absence of hunger, these calories may be unnecessary.

Therefore, in answer to this question, differentiating between well-timed snacks, habitual snacking, or emotional eating will be part of the discussion. For those who recognize that their snacking is more likely habitual or emotional, mindful eating strategies may be helpful.

"Mindfulness is awareness that arises through paying attention, on purpose, in the present moment, non-judgmentally…in the service of self-understanding and wisdom."

Jon Kabat-Zinn (Mindful 2017)

Some mindful eating strategies include:

1. Stop and think: Are you truly hungry? If so, a healthy snack would be appropriate.
2. If you are not truly hungry, what else are you feeling right now (e.g., boredom, anxiety, anger, etc.)?
3. If you want a snack due to boredom or emotion, is there a different way to handle the situation? For example, are there hobbies you enjoy to combat boredom, such as reading, listening to music, or knitting. For stress or anxiety, meditation has been shown to reduce emotional eating (Dalen et al. 2010). Going for a walk has also been shown to reduce cravings (Ledochowski 2015).

    Mindfulness strategies may help defuse the situation and either (a) the craving will subside or (b) the person may be more mindful about the portion of their snack. Mindful eating may not eradicate unnecessary snacking, but it may mean the difference between eating a whole sleeve of graham crackers versus a few squares. These small changes can add up significantly over time.

    For those with emotional eating tendencies, brainstorming strategies with them ahead of time can prepare them to take action when the moment presents itself.

6. ***What is the best exercise for weight loss?*** For general health, *The Physical Activity Guidelines for Americans, 2nd Edition* from the U.S. Department of Health and Human Services (2018) recommends at least 150 minutes per week of moderate aerobic activity, plus at least two days per week of muscle strengthening activity. However, the 2018 National Health Interview Survey conducted by the CDC's National Center for Health Statistics found that only about 24% of U.S. adults meet the recommended guidelines for both aerobic and strengthening activities.

    If your patient is not meeting the minimum recommendations, then the initial goal may be to incrementally increase their activity from their current level, with an eventual goal of reaching the minimum guidelines. As with nutrition counseling, empowering the patient to set goals that are acceptable, practical, and feasible for them supports their autonomy, a key factor in behavior change.

    However, the physical activity guidelines further specify that more aerobic activity is required for weight loss, recommending at least 300 minutes per week. These guidelines align with findings from the National Weight Control Registry, in which over 90% of participants exercise an average of one hour per day (NWCR n.d.). The National Weight Control Registry is a prospective study tracking over 10,000 individuals who have maintained a weight loss of at least 30 lbs for one year or longer. The registry was developed to identify the characteristics and behaviors of those who have achieved long-term weight loss (NWCR n.d.).

    Needless to say, these guidelines can feel daunting. However, the guidelines emphasize that these volumes can be achieved with bouts of any duration. For example, a 10-minute walk three times per day is as effective as 30 minutes all at once. Providing examples such as this can help make these goals seem more attainable.

60 MINUTES OF PHYSICAL ACTIVITY: SAMPLE DAY 1

Before work: Park further from the entrance -5 minutes

Lunch: Walk with a coworker for 10 minutes before or after eating.

Afternoon break: 10-minute walk

After work: Walk back to car -5 minutes

After dinner: 30-minute walk

For many, the concept of physical activity elicits images of gyms, classes, or high-intensity exercises like running. Clarifying the meaning of physical activity will be a key strategy in increasing a person's self-efficacy in this area. Listing examples like taking the stairs, parking at the back of the lot, or yardwork will show them that with mindful intention, the minutes can accumulate throughout the day (Figure 14.5).

60 MINUTES OF PHYSICAL ACTIVITY: SAMPLE DAY 2

Morning: Cutting the grass with a push mower -40 minutes

Walk after dinner: 20 minutes

Therefore, in answer to their question about the best exercise, the answers will be (1) the activities they can do and (2) the activities they enjoy. Also, all movement is good movement, as long as it is safe.

Of note, among NWCR participants, the most frequently reported form of activity was walking.

FAQ:

How can I get 60 minutes of physical activity in a day?

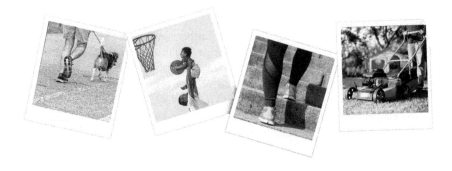

Key Message

Every minute counts.

FIGURE 14.5   Explaining that physical activity is not limited to formal exercise may help physical activity feel more attainable.

7. *Is there a menu I can follow?* Menus, Plate Method examples, and recipe ideas are beneficial for demonstrating the variety and flexibility that balanced meal planning can offer. Pictures are helpful in conveying that healthy, reduced-calorie meals can still be appetizing, flavorful, and filling. Including the calorie, protein, and carb counts illustrate how they can meet their needs while still keeping their intake within appropriate amounts.

Similarly, you can demonstrate a sample day with some of the foods they mentioned during their dietary recall. This strategy reassures people that they can still enjoy many of their favorite recipes. This approach is especially useful for those consuming traditional ethnic cuisines for which you may not have ready-to-go meal plans.

After reading hundreds of food records and creating dozens of sample meal plans, I have found that when people are mindful about their food choices and portions, the numbers tend to fall into place for calories, carbs, protein, sodium, or otherwise. While people often ask for specific meal plans, the issue is often less about meal ideas, and more often about behaviors. Identifying and addressing those behaviors are more likely to induce long-term lifestyle change rather than following a menu.

WHAT PATIENTS NEED TO KNOW?

1. *Basic metabolism.* With so many extreme diets and misconceptions about nutrition, a review of basic metabolism empowers people to filter through the hype. From which foods are carbs to the importance of glucose to the need for calories, this basic knowledge may help reframe how a person looks at food. As opposed to categorizing foods as "good" and "bad," learning the function of different foods may help them to achieve balanced nutrition in addition to weight loss.

Diet culture leads people to think that calories or carbs are bad. They read labels looking for the lowest numbers, and they avoid whole food groups. Earlier in this book, I described the tendency to "squeeze calories," where some restrict portions or meal sizes throughout the day, essentially under-fueling the most active part of their day. It is no wonder that one of the top complaints when dieting is that "I'm just so hungry."

While patients do not need to learn the biochemistry of metabolism, some basic concepts may reassure them that they can, indeed, eat food. That a yogurt cup does not have to be their whole meal. That an afternoon snack may be warranted. And yes, it is okay to eat a potato.

As will be covered in the chapter on health literacy, using everyday language, appropriate analogies, and simple visuals can help translate complicated topics into easy-to-understand, practical information. Some of the key concepts that will benefit many people include:

1. *Macronutrients.* Some popular diets have people counting macronutrients. Food tracking apps often calculate a percent of total calories from fat, protein, and carbs, provoking another common question, "What percentage should my macros be?"

   Start with the basics. Discuss that fat, protein, and carbs are the three main nutrients in our foods, and the key sources of calories in our diet. A brief description of the *benefits* of each of these nutrients will begin to dismantle some of the misconceptions your patient may have. As carbs currently carry more negative connotations in regard to weight, be sure to show examples of healthy carbohydrates and describe the nutrients they have to offer, including fiber, vitamins, minerals, phytonutrients, and glucose. Emphasize that all three macronutrients provide different benefits, so it is beneficial to include all of them.

During the nutrition assessment, the patient may have reported frequent hunger or some fatigue. If their dietary recall suggests that they are restricting carbohydrates, emphasize the role of glucose in energy production and brain function. If they are highly active, discuss the importance of glycogen replenishment for exercise performance.

2. *Glucose and insulin.* Explain the role of insulin in glucose metabolism and fat production. As blood glucose and insulin levels can impact hunger, cravings, and subsequent fat storage, describe how macronutrients and different types of foods affect these levels. Compare the glycemic and insulinemic responses to refined carbs versus high fiber carbs versus protein and fat. Emphasize how a combination of high fiber carbs, protein, and fat can help slow gastric emptying, helping them to feel full longer and mitigate spikes in blood sugar and insulin levels (Mourot et al. 1988; Gentilcore et al. 2006; Ma et al. 2009; Yu et al. 2014). Describe The Plate Method to illustrate how to properly achieve this balance of nutrients. Show several examples of Plate Method meals to reinforce the benefits of a varied diet.

For people with insulin resistance, such as with PCOS, prediabetes, or type 2 diabetes, emphasize the effect of physical activity in lowering insulin resistance (Richter and Hargreaves 2013) (see Figure 10.4). In regard to food choices, describe the effect of saturated fat on insulin resistance (Riccardi et al. 2004; Luukkonen et al. 2018), reinforcing the benefits of choosing lean proteins more often (see Figure 10.6)

3. *Timing of meals.* Discuss that gastric emptying and the rise and fall of blood sugar after a well-balanced meal typically occur over about four hours (Hellmig et al. 2006; Lu et al. 2022). Therefore, spacing balanced meals about four hours apart would be optimal in managing hunger, blood sugar, and insulin levels.

Discuss that physiological hunger signals typically align with blood glucose levels. As blood sugar rises and peaks after a meal, satiety signals increase. However, when blood sugar levels are lower about three or four hours later, cues to hunger will increase. The lower the blood sugar, the stronger the hunger signals, such as stomach grumbling, irritability, and increased cravings. Discuss the benefits of intuitive eating, which encourages people to recognize and eat according to their hunger and satiety cues (Cadena-Schlam et al. 2014).

While intuitive eating is a key strategy for weight management, research indicates that some people with obesity may have a blunted response to satiety cues (Barkeling et al. 2007). However, other studies suggest that "hunger training"—or eating in accordance to blood glucose levels—can restore responsiveness in some people (de Bruin et al. 2019). As hunger training requires blood sugar monitoring, this intervention may not be widely applicable at this time. However, providing the above information about basic metabolism, nutrients, meal timing, and balanced meal planning may encourage people to establish a more structured pattern of eating. Through increased mindfulness, they may develop an improved relationship with food, in which intuitive eating may be possible (Warren et al. 2017).

2. *Strategies for successful, long-term weight loss.* While various dietary patterns and interventions have shown benefits for initial weight loss, long-term maintenance continues to prove challenging. As mentioned above, many people have a history of weight cycling in which they repeatedly lose weight, regain, and repeat. Unsustainable or poor dietary practices, body composition changes, logistical barriers, underdeveloped meal

planning skills, low self-efficacy, lack of support, and emotional factors are just some causes that prevent long-term weight loss. However, that is not to say that weight loss maintenance is not possible.

EVIDENCED-BASED STRATEGIES FOR SUCCESSFUL WEIGHT LOSS

Reduced calorie intake: 1,200–1,500 kcal/day for women; 1,500–1,800 kcal/day for men

Physical activity: 200–300 minutes of aerobic physical activity per week plus at least 2 days of muscle strengthening exercises

Self-Monitoring: food, weight, and physical activity

Goal setting

Action planning and incremental changes

Mindful eating

Intensive lifestyle change program: group or individual

The National Weight Control Registry includes thousands of people who have maintained an average of 66-lb weight loss for over 5 years. The findings from this research highlight some behaviors that were common among them, such as:

Diet modification. Participants report reduced overall intake, minimal sugar and refined carbs, increased vegetables and fruit, drinking more water, elimination of sugary beverages and fast food, reduction in stress eating. Many participated in programs such as WW, diabetes or health education classes, or online support groups.

Increased physical activity. The most reported physical activity was walking. Average duration and frequency was 60 minutes most days of the week, which aligns with the *Physical Activity Guidelines for Americans* for weight loss.

Breakfast. While including—or skipping—breakfast can be a source of debate in regard to weight loss strategies, 75% of NWCR were breakfast eaters. Several studies also indicate metabolic benefit to including breakfast and detriment in skipping it (Alkhulaifi and Darkoh 2022).

  Many people report that they do not feel hungry in the morning. If the nutrition assessment reveals that they consume later dinners and/or evening snacks, that may be contributing to morning anorexia, and/or elevated fasting blood sugar. Adjusting their eating schedule to reduce late evening eating may restore their morning appetite.

Regular weighing. While tracking weight may not be appropriate, acceptable, or motivating for everybody, 75% of NWCR participants weigh themselves at least once a week. This strategy should be personalized to the individual.

Limited screen time. Most NWCR participants reported less than 10 hours of TV per week. This finding may be a surrogate measure of sedentary time. Limited exposure to food triggers, such as fast food commercials, may also explain this benefit. Also, as many people report a habit of snacking in front of the TV, reducing TV time may help to reduce snacking as well.

While the above actions may contribute to weight loss, concurrently applying strategies for long-term behavior change will be critical for maintenance, such as:

Goal setting. As discussed in the first part of this book, short-term action planning allows individuals to practice certain behaviors, increase their self-efficacy in performing these behaviors, and observe the outcome. Positive outcomes can reinforce the benefits and motivation to perform these behaviors. This practice is effective for both initial weight loss and long-term maintenance (Samdal et al. 2017).

Setting long-term goals allows the patient to explore their personal values and intrinsic motivation to maintain healthy behaviors. Some examples from NWCR participants included caring for children or grandchildren, disease prevention, health, and longevity. Sometimes, a health scare—often coupled with family experiences (e.g., a prediabetes diagnosis in someone whose parent suffered from diabetes)— triggers a long-term goal of health.

I once asked a patient who achieved significant weight loss and A1C reduction what motivated him to maintain his behavior changes. He answered, "Sometimes I get frustrated when I don't see my weight change, but then I remind myself that I'm making these changes for my health. So I keep up it up and eventually I start to lose weight again."

For the nutrition counselor, supporting the person's autonomy in goal setting continues to prove effective for long-term behavior change (Samdal et al. 2017).

Self-monitoring. Food and physical activity tracking often proves beneficial in making—and maintaining—change (Samdal et al. 2017). This is a common strategy employed in lifestyle change programs. While some people find it to be a burden, many who have kept a food log admit to its efficacy.

I first noted the significant effect of food tracking when I was a lifestyle coach for the Diabetes Prevention Program. At that time, the curriculum delayed food tracking until the fifth week. As I was tracking weekly weight data, I noticed a significant increase in the rate of weight loss after food journaling began. Participants noted increased awareness, more mindfulness in regard to snacking, and generally more accountability in their food choices.

On the other hand, on my first day as a dietetic intern, one of the first patients I observed stated, "I stopped tracking because the way I eat now is more of a habit." With that, I was sold. For patients starting out, I explain that food tracking is a proven strategy for long-term change. However, for those who exhibit resistance to the task, I reassure them that short-term tracking may be sufficient. Once new habits form, food tracking may be needed only during times when they need to get back on track.

Mindful eating has shown positive effects in managing emotional eating and eating in response to external cues and may prevent weight gain (Warren et al. 2017). As patients commonly report these factors as triggers for regression, mindfulness strategies may be effective for long-term maintenance in combination with other strategies.

Graded tasks (or progressively more challenging short-term goals), ***problem solving*** (described earlier in this book), ***regularly reviewing long-term goals***, and establishing ***social support*** are also associated with long-term behavior change (Samdal et al. 2017). Professional support and/or group support is generally found to be beneficial as well.

Whether you are facilitating a group program or counseling an individual, the more behavior change techniques each individual employs, the more likely long-term change can occur (Samdal et al. 2017).

3. ***Strategies for handling the weight loss plateau.*** The dreaded plateau. Almost everybody attempting weight loss comes to a point where they see a pause in their progress. Time and again, when patients recall past efforts at weight loss, they say they "hit a plateau," became upset, and just went back to old habits.

The plateau is an expected phase in weight loss. Some theories suggest a reduction in basal metabolic rate in response to weight loss and lower calorie intake (Sarwan and Rehman 2022). The "set point" theory suggests that metabolic changes occur to achieve homeostasis or weight regain (Trexler et al. 2014), perhaps ancient mechanisms designed for energy conservation and survival.

The plateau is a critical time during a weight loss journey. While physiological changes may be occurring, the psychological impact of the plateau may be a more detrimental issue. Individually and together, weight, body image, food, and eating behaviors are emotionally charging for many people. Without progress, the cost of the effort may seem to outweigh the benefit. If the patient is feeling particularly restricted in how they eat, or the time required for physical activity is too precious to spare, or dietary adjustments feel socially isolating, continuing the effort may not feel worthwhile.

Therefore, supporting the patient through this time should be built into the plan. Too often, a patient declines or discontinues follow up as they feel they received enough information. As part of the initial visit, explain the inevitability of the plateau and design a follow-up plan to address it. By preparing the patient ahead of time, they may react more mindfully and proactively when the plateau occurs. With ongoing support in action planning, problem solving, and reviewing their long-term goals, they may be able to maintain their motivation to continue healthy behaviors.

After facilitating several lifestyle change groups, I have observed many people break the plateau. While some may require additional nutrition changes, or a change to their physical activity routine, many people reported that when they just continued with what they were doing, the plateau broke itself. Again, through mindfulness, people may better manage the emotional aspect of the weight loss plateau. Therefore, an important message will be that while the plateau is inevitable, how people *react* to the plateau may ultimately determine its impact.

The increase in obesity over the past several decades coincides with the increase in metabolic disorders and chronic disease. Further, the well-documented metabolic actions of visceral fat as a contributor to insulin resistance and inflammation cannot be ignored. Therefore, obesity is a public health issue that requires continued research for effective treatment and prevention.

In individual nutrition counseling, compassion and respect for autonomy will be the foundation of care.

Thus, when asked about the best approach for weight loss, the answer will lie in their personalized PLANS.

PLANS should incorporate their:

P – Preferences (e.g., food choices, physical activity)
L – Labs, symptoms, and medical history
A – Attitude, feelings, and personal goals
N – Nutrition-related behaviors
S – Strategies for long-term change.

CLINICAL PRACTICE GUIDELINES, PROFESSIONAL AND PATIENT RESOURCES, AND MEAL PLANNING WEBSITES

Obesity in adults: a clinical practice guideline (Wharton et al. 2020)

2013 AHA/ACC/TOS Guideline for the Management of Overweight and Obesity in Adults (Jensen et al. 2014)

National Weight Control Registry – www.nwcr.ws/

National Diabetes Prevention Program – https://www.cdc.gov/diabetes/prevention/index.html

Food and physical activity tracking app – Cronometer.com

Calorie counting book and app – calorieking.com

Recipe Nutrition Calculator by Verywellfit – www.verywellfit.com/recipe-nutrition-analyzer-4157076

Educational slides and meal planning handouts are included with this book, available online at https://resourcecentre.routledge.com/books/9781032352459

REFERENCES

Alkhulaifi F, Darkoh C. Meal Timing, Meal Frequency and Metabolic Syndrome. *Nutrients*. 2022 Apr;14(9):1719. doi: 10.3390/nu14091719.

American Medical Association. *PolicyFinder: Obesity*; 1995–2023 [cited 23 June 2023]. Available from: https://policysearch.ama-assn.org/policyfinder/detail/obesity?uri=%2FAMADoc%2FHOD.xml-0-3858.xml.

Antonopoulos AS, Tousoulis D. The Molecular Mechanisms of Obesity Paradox. *Cardiovasc Res*. 2017 Jul;113(9):1074–1086. doi: 10.1093/cvr/cvx106.

Association for Size Diversity and Health. Health at Every Size(r) principles [Internet]; 2020 [cited 23 June 2023]. Available from https://asdah.org/health-at-every-size-haes-approach/.

Barkeling B, King NA, Näslund E, Blundell JE. Characterization of Obese Individuals Who Claim to Detect No Relationship between Their Eating Pattern and Sensations of Hunger or Fullness. *Int J Obes (Lond)*. 2007 Mar;31(3):435–9. doi: 10.1038/sj.ijo.0803449.

Cadena-Schlam L, López-Guimerà G. Intuitive Eating: An Emerging Approach to Eating Behavior. *Nutr Hosp*. 2014 Oct;31(3):995–1002. doi: 10.3305/nh.2015.31.3.7980.

Centers for Disease Control and Prevention. *Genes and Obesity* [Internet]; 2013 [cited 24 June 2023]. Available from: https://www.cdc.gov/genomics/resources/diseases/obesity/obesedit.htm.

Centers for Disease Control and Prevention. *Obesity, Race/Ethnicity, and COVID-19* [Internet]; 2022 [cited 24 June 2023]. Available from: https://www.cdc.gov/obesity/data/obesity-and-covid-19.html.

Dalen J, Smith BW, Shelley BM, Sloan AL, Leahigh L, Begay D. Pilot Study: Mindful Eating and Living (MEAL): Weight, Eating Behavior, and Psychological Outcomes Associated with a Mindfulness-Based Intervention for People with Obesity. *Complement Ther Med*. 2010 Dec;18(6):260–264. doi: 10.1016/j.ctim.2010.09.008.

de Bruin WE, Ward AL, Taylor RW, Jospe MR. 'Am I Really Hungry?' A Qualitative Exploration of Patients' Experience, Adherence and Behaviour Change During Hunger Training: A Pilot Study. *BMJ Open*. 2019 Dec;9(12):e032248. doi: 10.1136/bmjopen-2019-032248.

DiNicolantonio JJ, O'Keefe JH, Wilson WL. Sugar Addiction: Is It Real? A Narrative Review. *Br J Sports Med*. 2018 Jul;52(14):910–913. doi: 10.1136/bjsports-2017-097971.

Elgaddal N, Kramarow EA, Reuben C. Physical activity among adults aged 18 and over: United States, 2020. NCHS Data Brief, no 443. Hyattsville, MD: National Center for Health Statistics. 2022. https://dx.doi.org/10.15620/cdc:120213. Accessed 11/18/2023.

Evert AB, Dennison M, Gardner CD, Garvey WT, Lau KHK, MacLeod J, Mitri J, Pereira RF, Rawlings K, Robinson S, Saslow L, Uelmen S, Urbanski PB, Yancy WS Jr. Nutrition Therapy for Adults with Diabetes or Prediabetes: A Consensus Report. *Diabetes Care*. 2019 May;42(5):731–754. doi: 10.2337/dci19-0014.

Frazier C, Mehdi N. Forgetting Fatness: The Violent Co-Optation of the Body Positivity Movement. *Debates Aesthet*. 2021;16(1):13–28. Available from: https://debatesinaesthetics.org/debates-in-aesthetics-vol-16-no-1/#FRAZIERMEHDI.

Gentilcore D, Chaikomin R, Jones KL, Russo A, Feinle-Bisset C, Wishart JM, Rayner CK, Horowitz M. Effects of Fat on Gastric Emptying of and the Glycemic, Insulin, and Incretin Responses to a Carbohydrate Meal in Type 2 Diabetes. *J Clin Endocrinol Metab*. 2006 Jun;91(6):2062–2067. doi: 10.1210/jc.2005-2644.

Gillen MM. Associations Between Positive Body Image and Indicators of Men's and Women's Mental and Physical Health. *Body Image*. 2015 Mar;13:67–74. doi: 10.1016/j.bodyim.2015.01.002.

Greenberg D, St Peter JV. Sugars and Sweet Taste: Addictive or Rewarding? *Int J Environ Res Public Health*. 2021 Sep;18(18):9791. doi: 10.3390/ijerph18189791.

Gruberg L, Weissman NJ, Waksman R, Fuchs S, Deible R, Pinnow EE, Ahmed LM, Kent KM, Pichard AD, Suddath WO, Satler LF, Lindsay J Jr. The Impact of Obesity on the Short-Term and Long-Term Outcomes after Percutaneous Coronary Intervention: The Obesity Paradox? *J Am Coll Cardiol*. 2002 Feb;39(4):578–584. doi: 10.1016/s0735-1097(01)01802-2.

Hager ER, Quigg AM, Black MM, Coleman SM, Heeren T, Rose-Jacobs R, Cook JT, Ettinger de Cuba SA, Casey PH, Chilton M, Cutts DB, Meyers AF, Frank DA. Development and Validity of a 2-Item Screen to Identify Families at Risk for Food Insecurity. *Pediatrics*. 2010 Jul;126(1):e26–e32. doi: 10.1542/peds.2009-3146.

Hansen J. Explode and Die! A Fat Woman's Perspective on Prenatal Care and the Fat Panic Epidemic. *Narrat Inq Bioeth*. 2014;4(2):99–101. doi: 10.1353/nib.2014.0050. Accessed 2/14/2023.

Hellmig S, Von Schöning F, Gadow C, Katsoulis S, Hedderich J, Fölsch UR, Stüber E. Gastric Emptying Time of Fluids and Solids in Healthy Subjects Determined by 13C Breath Tests: Influence of Age, Sex and Body Mass Index. *J Gastroenterol Hepatol*. 2006 Dec;21(12):1832–1838. doi: 10.1111/j.1440-1746.2006.04449.x.

Hilbert A, Braehler E, Haeuser W, Zenger M. Weight Bias Internalization, Core Self-Evaluation, and Health in Overweight and Obese Persons. *Obesity*. 2014 Jan;22(1):79–85. doi: 10.1002/oby.20561.

Ingram DD, Mussolino ME. Weight Loss from Maximum Body Weight and Mortality: The Third National Health and Nutrition Examination Survey Linked Mortality File. *Int J Obes (Lond)*. 2010 Jun;34(6):1044–1050. doi: 10.1038/ijo.2010.41.

Jabbour J, Rihawi Y, Khamis AM, Ghamlouche L, Tabban B, Safadi G, Hammad N, Hadla R, Zeidan M, Andari D, Azar RN, Nasser N, Chakhtoura M. Long Term Weight Loss Diets and Obesity Indices: Results of a Network Meta-Analysis. *Front Nutr*. 2022 Apr;9:821096. doi: 10.3389/fnut.2022.821096.

Jensen MD, Ryan DH, Apovian CM, Ard JD, Comuzzie AG, Donato KA, Hu FB, Hubbard VS, Jakicic JM, Kushner RF, Loria CM, Millen BE, Nonas CA, Pi-Sunyer FX, Stevens J, Stevens VJ, Wadden TA, Wolfe BM, Yanovski SZ, Jordan HS, Kendall KA, Lux LJ, Mentor-Marcel R, Morgan LC, Trisolini MG, Wnek J, Anderson JL, Halperin JL, Albert NM, Bozkurt B, Brindis RG, Curtis LH, DeMets D, Hochman JS, Kovacs RJ, Ohman EM, Pressler SJ, Sellke FW, Shen WK, Smith SC Jr, Tomaselli GF, American College of Cardiology/American Heart Association Task Force on Practice Guidelines, Obesity Society. 2013 AHA/ACC/TOS Guideline for the Management of Overweight and Obesity in Adults: A Report of the American College of Cardiology/American Heart Association Task Force on Practice Guidelines and the Obesity Society. *Circulation*. 2014 Jun;129(25 Suppl 2):S102–S138. doi: 10.1161/01.cir.0000437739.71477.ee.

Johnston BC, Kanters S, Bandayrel K, Wu P, Naji F, Siemieniuk RA, Ball GD, Busse JW, Thorlund K, Guyatt G, Jansen JP, Mills EJ. Comparison of Weight Loss among Named Diet Programs in Overweight and Obese Adults: A Meta-Analysis. *JAMA*. 2014 Sep;312(9):923–933. doi: 10.1001/jama.2014.10397.

Kilpeläinen TO, Qi L, Brage S, Sharp SJ, Sonestedt E, Demerath E, Ahmad T, Mora S, Kaakinen M, Sandholt CH, Holzapfel C, Autenrieth CS, Hyppönen E, Cauchi S, He M, Kutalik Z, Kumari M, Stančáková A, Meidtner K, Balkau B, Tan JT, Mangino M, Timpson NJ, Song Y, Zillikens MC, Jablonski KA, Garcia ME, Johansson S, Bragg-Gresham JL, Wu Y, van Vliet-Ostaptchouk JV, Onland-Moret NC, Zimmermann E, Rivera NV, Tanaka T, Stringham HM, Silbernagel G, Kanoni S, Feitosa MF, Snitker S, Ruiz JR, Metter J, Larrad MT, Atalay M, Hakanen M, Amin N, Cavalcanti-Proença C, Grøntved A,

Hallmans G, Jansson JO, Kuusisto J, Kähönen M, Lutsey PL, Nolan JJ, Palla L, Pedersen O, Pérusse L, Renström F, Scott RA, Shungin D, Sovio U, Tammelin TH, Rönnemaa T, Lakka TA, Uusitupa M, Rios MS, Ferrucci L, Bouchard C, Meirhaeghe A, Fu M, Walker M, Borecki IB, Dedoussis GV, Fritsche A, Ohlsson C, Boehnke M, Bandinelli S, van Duijn CM, Ebrahim S, Lawlor DA, Gudnason V, Harris TB, Sørensen TI, Mohlke KL, Hofman A, Uitterlinden AG, Tuomilehto J, Lehtimäki T, Raitakari O, Isomaa B, Njølstad PR, Florez JC, Liu S, Ness A, Spector TD, Tai ES, Froguel P, Boeing H, Laakso M, Marmot M, Bergmann S, Power C, Khaw KT, Chasman D, Ridker P, Hansen T, Monda KL, Illig T, Järvelin MR, Wareham NJ, Hu FB, Groop LC, Orho-Melander M, Ekelund U, Franks PW, Loos RJ. Physical Activity Attenuates the Influence of FTO Variants on Obesity Risk: A Meta-Analysis of 218,166 Adults and 19,268 Children. *PLoS Med.* 2011 Nov;8(11):e1001116. doi: 10.1371/journal.pmed.1001116.

Knight EL, Stampfer MJ, Hankinson SE, Spiegelman D, Curhan GC. The Impact of Protein Intake on Renal Function Decline in Women with Normal Renal Function or Mild Renal Insufficiency. *Ann Intern Med.* 2003 Mar;138(6):460–467. doi: 10.7326/0003-4819-138-6-200303180-00009.

Ko GJ, Rhee CM, Kalantar-Zadeh K, Joshi S. The Effects of High-Protein Diets on Kidney Health and Longevity. *J Am Soc Nephrol.* 2020 Aug;31(8):1667–1679. doi: 10.1681/ASN.2020010028.

Kyle TK, Dhurandhar EJ, Allison DB. Regarding Obesity as a Disease: Evolving Policies and Their Implications. *Endocrinol Metab Clin North Am.* 2016 Sep;45(3):511–520. doi: 10.1016/j.ecl.2016.04.004.

Ledochowski L, Ruedl G, Taylor AH, Kopp M. Acute Effects of Brisk Walking on Sugary Snack Cravings in Overweight People, Affect and Responses to a Manipulated Stress Situation and to a Sugary Snack Cue: A Crossover Study. *PLoS One.* 2015 Mar ;10(3):e0119278. doi: 10.1371/journal.pone.0119278.

Lu X, Fan Z, Liu A, Liu R, Lou X, Hu J. Extended Inter-Meal Interval Negatively Impacted the Glycemic and Insulinemic Responses after Both Lunch and Dinner in Healthy Subjects. *Nutrients.* 2022 Sep;14(17):3617. doi: 10.3390/nu14173617.

Luukkonen PK, Sädevirta S, Zhou Y, Kayser B, Ali A, Ahonen L, Lallukka S, Pelloux V, Gaggini M, Jian C, Hakkarainen A, Lundbom N, Gylling H, Salonen A, Orešič M, Hyötyläinen T, Orho-Melander M, Rissanen A, Gastaldelli A, Clément K, Hodson L, Yki-Järvinen H. Saturated Fat Is More Metabolically Harmful for the Human Liver Than Unsaturated Fat or Simple Sugars. *Diabetes Care.* 2018 Aug;41(8):1732–1739. doi: 10.2337/dc18-0071.

Ma J, Stevens JE, Cukier K, Maddox AF, Wishart JM, Jones KL, Clifton PM, Horowitz M, Rayner CK. Effects of a Protein Preload on Gastric Emptying, Glycemia, and Gut Hormones after a Carbohydrate Meal in Diet-Controlled Type 2 Diabetes. *Diabetes Care.* 2009 Sep;32(9):1600–1602. doi: 10.2337/dc09-0723.

Matheson EM, King DE, Everett CJ. Healthy Lifestyle Habits and Mortality in Overweight and Obese Individuals. *J Am Board Fam Med.* 2012 Jan-Feb;25(1):9–15. doi: 10.3122/jabfm.2012.01.110164.

Mindful staff. *Jon Kabat-Zinn: Defining Mindfulness. Mindful: Healthy Mind, Healthy Life.* [Internet]. Chicago, IL: Mindful Communications & Such, PBC; 2017 [cited 2023 June 23]. Available from: https://www.mindful.org/jon-kabat-zinn-defining-mindfulness/

Mourot J, Thouvenot P, Couet C, Antoine JM, Krobicka A, Debry G. Relationship between the Rate of Gastric Emptying and Glucose and Insulin Responses to Starchy Foods in Young Healthy Adults. *Am J Clin Nutr.* 1988 Oct;48(4):1035–1040. doi: 10.1093/ajcn/48.4.1035.

National Academies of Sciences, Engineering, and Medicine. 2006. Dietary Reference Intakes: The Essential Guide to Nutrient Requirements. Washington, DC: The National Academies Press. https://doi.org/10.17226/11537.

National Institutes of Health. Clinical Guidelines on the Identification, Evaluation, and Treatment of Overweight and Obesity in Adults--The Evidence Report. *Obes Res.* 1998 Sep;6(Suppl 2):51S–209S.

National Weight Control Registry. NWCR Facts [Internet]. Providence, RI: n.d. Available from: http://www.nwcr.ws/Research/default.htm. Accessed 11/18/2023.

Nield L, Moore HJ, Hooper L, Cruickshank JK, Vyas A, Whittaker V, Summerbell CD. Dietary Advice for Treatment of Type 2 Diabetes Mellitus in Adults. *Cochrane Database Syst Rev.* 2007 Jul;2007(3):CD004097. doi: 10.1002/14651858.CD004097.pub4.

Ospina MS. 11 Influencers Talk Body Pos versus Fat Acceptance. *Bustle* [Internet]. 2016 [cited 2023 June 23]. Available from: https://www.bustle.com/articles/170978-11-influencers-discuss-the-differences-between-body-positivity-fat-acceptance

Pan L, Sherry B, Njai R, Blanck HM. Food Insecurity is Associated with Obesity among US Adults in 12 States. *J Acad Nutr Diet.* 2012 Sep;112(9):1403–1409. doi: 10.1016/j.jand.2012.06.011.

Phelan SM, Burgess DJ, Yeazel MW, Hellerstedt WL, Griffin JM, van Ryn M. Impact of Weight Bias and Stigma on Quality of Care and Outcomes for Patients with Obesity. *Obes Rev.* 2015 Apr;16(4):319–326. doi: 10.1111/obr.12266.

Rabast U, Vornberger KH, Ehl M. Loss of Weight, Sodium and Water in Obese Persons Consuming a High- or Low-Carbohydrate Diet. *Ann Nutr Metab.* 1981;25(6):341–349. doi: 10.1159/000176515.

Riccardi G, Giacco R, Rivellese AA. Dietary Fat, Insulin Sensitivity and the Metabolic Syndrome. *Clin Nutr.* 2004 Aug;23(4):447–456. doi: 10.1016/j.clnu.2004.02.006.

Richter EA, Hargreaves M. Exercise, GLUT4, and Skeletal Muscle Glucose Uptake. *Physiol Rev.* 2013 Jul;93(3):993–1017. doi: 10.1152/physrev.00038.2012.

Sacks FM, Bray GA, Carey VJ, Smith SR, Ryan DH, Anton SD, McManus K, Champagne CM, Bishop LM, Laranjo N, Leboff MS, Rood JC, de Jonge L, Greenway FL, Loria CM, Obarzanek E, Williamson DA. Comparison of Weight-Loss Diets with Different Compositions of Fat, Protein, and Carbohydrates. *N Engl J Med.* 2009 Feb;360(9):859–873. doi: 10.1056/NEJMoa0804748.

Samdal GB, Eide GE, Barth T, Williams G, Meland E. Effective Behaviour Change Techniques for Physical Activity and Healthy Eating in Overweight and Obese Adults; Systematic Review and Meta-Regression Analyses. *Int J Behav Nutr Phys Act.* 2017 Mar;14(1):42. doi: 10.1186/s12966-017-0494-y.

Sarwan G, Rehman A. "Management of Weight Loss Plateau." 2022. In: *StatPearls* [Internet]. Treasure Island, FL: StatPearls Publishing; 2022

Stierman B, Afful J, Carroll MD, Chen TC, Davy O, Fink S, Fryar CD, Gu Q, Hales CM, Hughes JP, Ostchega Y, Storandt RJ, Akinbami LJ. National Health and Nutrition Examination Survey 2017-March 2020 Prepandemic Data Files Development of Files and Prevalence Estimates for Selected Health Outcomes. *National Health Statistics Report* [Internet]. 2021 [cited 6/24/2023]; NHSR No. 158. Available from: https://stacks.cdc.gov/view/cdc/106273.

Trexler ET, Smith-Ryan AE, Norton LE. Metabolic Adaptation to Weight Loss: Implications for the Athlete. *J Int Soc Sports Nutr.* 2014 Feb;11(1):7. doi: 10.1186/1550-2783-11-7.

U.S. Department of Health and Human Services. Physical Activity Guidelines for Americans, 2nd edition. 2018. Available from: https://health.gov/paguidelines/second-edition/pdf/Physical_Activity_Guidelines_2nd_edition.pdf. Accessed 11/18/2023.

U.S. Food & Drug Administration. *Weight Loss Drugs* [Internet]. Silver Spring, MD; 2015 [cited 2023 June 24]. Available from: https://www.fda.gov/drugs/information-drug-class/weight-loss-drugs

U.S. Food & Drug Administration. *FDA Approves New Drug Treatment for Chronic Weight Management, First Since 2014* [Internet]. Silver Spring, MD; 2021 [cited 2023 June 24]. Available from: https://www.fda.gov/news-events/press-announcements/fda-approves-new-drug-treatment-chronic-weight-management-first-2014

U.S. Food & Drug Administration. *Tainted Weight Loss Products* [Internet]. Silver Spring, MD; 2023 [cited 2023 June 24]. Available from: https://www.fda.gov/drugs/medication-health-fraud/tainted-weight-loss-products

Veldhorst M, Smeets A, Soenen S, Hochstenbach-Waelen A, Hursel R, Diepvens K, Lejeune M, Luscombe-Marsh N, Westerterp-Plantenga M. Protein-Induced Satiety: Effects and Mechanisms of Different Proteins. *Physiol Behav.* 2008;94(2):300–307. doi: 10.1016/j.physbeh.2008.01.003.

Warren JM, Smith N, Ashwell M. A Structured Literature Review on the Role of Mindfulness, Mindful Eating and Intuitive Eating in Changing Eating Behaviours: Effectiveness and Associated Potential Mechanisms. *Nutr Res Rev.* 2017 Dec;30(2):272–283. doi: 10.1017/S0954422417000154.

Wharton S, Lau DCW, Vallis M, Sharma AM, Biertho L, Campbell-Scherer D, Adamo K, Alberga A, Bell R, Boulé N, Boyling E, Brown J, Calam B, Clarke C, Crowshoe L, Divalentino D, Forhan M, Freedhoff Y, Gagner M, Glazer S, Grand C, Green M, Hahn M, Hawa R, Henderson R, Hong D, Hung P, Janssen I, Jacklin K, Johnson-Stoklossa C, Kemp A, Kirk S, Kuk J, Langlois MF, Lear S, McInnes A, Macklin D, Naji L, Manjoo P, Morin MP, Nerenberg K, Patton I, Pedersen S, Pereira L, Piccinini-Vallis H, Poddar

M, Poirier P, Prud'homme D, Salas XR, Rueda-Clausen C, Russell-Mayhew S, Shiau J, Sherifali D, Sievenpiper J, Sockalingam S, Taylor V, Toth E, Twells L, Tytus R, Walji S, Walker L, Wicklum S. Obesity in Adults: A Clinical Practice Guideline. *CMAJ.* 2020 Aug;192(31):E875–E891. doi: 10.1503/cmaj.191707.

Wijayatunga NN, Bailey D, Klobodu SS, Dawson JA, Knight K, Dhurandhar EJ. A Short, Attribution Theory-Based Video Intervention Does Not Reduce Weight Bias in a Nationally Representative Sample of Registered Dietitians: A Randomized Trial. *Int J Obes (Lond).* 2021 Apr;45(4):787–794. doi: 10.1038/s41366-021-00740-6.

Wu YK, Berry DC. Impact of Weight Stigma on Physiological and Psychological Health Outcomes for Overweight and Obese Adults: A Systematic Review. *J Adv Nurs.* 2018 May;74(5):1030–1042. doi: 10.1111/jan.13511.

Yu K, Ke MY, Li WH, Zhang SQ, Fang XC. The Impact of Soluble Dietary Fibre on Gastric Emptying, Postprandial Blood Glucose and Insulin in Patients with Type 2 Diabetes. *Asia Pac J Clin Nutr.* 2014;23(2):210–218. doi: 10.6133/apjcn.2014.23.2.01.

Part IV

Putting It All Together

15 Health Literacy

Soon after earning my dietetics degree, I was fully ingrained with nutrition information. So much so, that I believed much of it was common knowledge. After two years of grad school—and to be honest, a lifetime of interest in food—I figured everybody already knew how to read labels, count calories, or identify which foods belonged to which food groups. In my early efforts to be respectful to the patient, and to avoid being condescending, I practiced on this assumption by glossing over some nutrition "basics," thinking they already had this knowledge. But soon, I realized that not everybody was as interested in nutrition as I was. In fact, a lack of nutrition knowledge may be a contributor to the development of disease. My misconceptions caused me to mismanage my time, as I would find out too late in the session that I needed to provide more information. In general, I found that even with my most educated patients, nutrition knowledge and meal planning skills are not a given. Even with other health professionals, nutrition is not everybody's area of expertise.

Since then, I have learned that people appreciate more information, not less. Even for those who have been reading labels and counting calories, a quick review never hurts and rarely offends. And for other health professionals, they are more often thankful for a comprehensive review rather than dismissive of it. As discussed in Part One of this book, implicit biases are often wrong and prohibit patient-entered care. As such, the Health Literate Care Model suggests to approach all patients with the assumption that they are at risk of not understanding their health conditions or how to deal with them (Koh et al. 2013).

Statistically speaking, the odds that your patient needs more information are high. The National Center for Education Statistics reports that 36% of U.S. adults have a basic or below basic level of health literacy, 53% have an intermediate level, and only 11% of adults were rated as proficient (Kutner et al. 2006).

WHAT IS HEALTH LITERACY?

The Healthy People 2030 initiative defines *health literacy* as follows:

> *Personal health literacy* is the degree to which individuals have the ability to find, understand, and use information and services to inform health-related decisions and actions for themselves and others.
>
> *Organizational health literacy* is the degree to which organizations equitably enable individuals to find, understand, and use information and services to inform health-related decisions and actions for themselves and others.

This two-part definition recognizes that acting on information is as important as understanding it; that health literacy is not the sole responsibility of the individual; and that health organizations and practitioners are responsible for providing easy-to-understand information and services to support people in taking action (Santana et al. 2021). The definition incorporates the concepts of shared decision-making, empowerment, and action planning, as espoused throughout this book.

Thus, in daily practice, the challenge for the healthcare provider is in translating complex health information into plain language, employing communication skills that appeal to various learning styles and literacy levels, and verifying that the patient not only understands the information, but is also ready and able to make meaningful change.

DOI: 10.1201/9781003326038-19

KNOW YOUR AUDIENCE

Learning styles and barriers vary by age, cultural background, level of education, and other factors. For example, advances in technology provide an opportunity to incorporate various modes of teaching. Videos, computer presentations, Internet resources, and interactive video games may appeal to visual, hands-on, and auditory learners. However, younger adults may be more comfortable with technology-based learning and resources compared to older adults (Romanelli et al. 2009).

Age has been found to be inversely related to health literacy (Cutilli 2007). In addition to the digital divide, age-related physiological changes such as hearing, vision, and cognition are also a challenge (CDC 2009). A vast majority of older adults also have difficulty using print materials, forms, charts and graphs, and numerical calculations (Kutner et al. 2006). For patients with lower health literacy, providing a system that includes specific directions with easy-to-follow steps, clear graphics, daily instructions, and charts to fill out has been shown to help people achieve successful self-care (DeWalt et al. 2004). Examples of self-care charts may be blood glucose, blood pressure, or medication logs.

Other factors that can affect the education experience include socioeconomic barriers, language, culture, and physical or cognitive impairments (Romanelli et al. 2009; Beagley 2011), as well as readiness and motivation to learn (Knowles 1970).

In addition to understanding health literacy, educators must recognize when the curriculum itself presents barriers. In efforts to provide a comprehensive education, the information may be too much or too complex (Kandula et al. 2011), or may not provide actionable recommendations (Hill-Briggs and Smith 2008). If the information is too general, it may not speak to the individual's personal concerns and motivations. If the information does not resonate, it may not be memorable.

TAILOR THE EDUCATION

In nutrition counseling, breaking the ice at the start of the session can help determine what key pieces of information the patient needs most (see Chapter 2 for "Breaking the Ice"). By establishing an open, comfortable environment, not only will the patient express what they want to know, but the educator can also glean what information they need to know. Thus, to avoid information overload, tailor the session to the patient's immediate needs. For example, in diabetes education, self-care topics may include healthy eating, physical activity, testing blood sugar, and taking medication, among other daily concerns. However, effectively addressing all of these topics in one 60-minute session would not be possible. If the assessment reveals that they are not taking their insulin properly, tailoring the session to explain how the medication works would be a priority. After all, without enough insulin, even those following the healthiest diet would have high glucose levels. Other topics can be addressed in follow up sessions as needed.

CONSIDER LEARNING AND TEACHING STYLES

When I first imagined the purpose of this book, I recalled my early days in practice when I had not yet curated my go-to educational resources. The clinic I worked for had files of printed handouts for various nutrition topics, collected from various sources throughout the years. There was more than could be easily sifted through for a newbie, especially for spur-of-the-moment, unanticipated questions during patient encounters. For example, for a common question like, "How much protein do I need?" the answer does not stop with a number based on 0.8 g/kg/day. A list of foods and their protein content, examples of how protein adds up in each meal and throughout the day, and a discussion about the benefits of lean protein and plant proteins are important to discuss as well.

Without ready-to-go educational materials, the counselor is limited to verbal explanations, with hopes that the patient will remember the information they heard after the session is over. However, studies have shown that health education participants forget about half the information two weeks after the session (Kandula et al. 2011).

Remembering the information will be dependent on the patient's ability to understand the information in the first place. Therefore, the patient's learning style, as well as the educator's teaching style, must be considered. For some, a verbal explanation may be sufficient; for others, reading materials may be more effective; others require hands-on experience, demonstrations, pictures or video, or writing and taking notes (Beagley 2011). For many, multiple modes of learning are preferred and sometimes required. For the educator, providing a variety of teaching modalities can help accommodate various learning styles and provide a more inclusive environment (Romanelli et al. 2009).

USE VARIOUS TEACHING MODALITIES

Teaching modalities may vary among in-person, one-on-one sessions, group classes, and virtual care. However, in all cases, a variety of communications can be employed, including:

Discussion and verbal explanation. When speaking with the patient, apply the *plain language* guidelines described by the Plain Language Action and Information Network (2011). Just as in writing, use common, everyday words (e.g., high blood pressure instead of hypertension) and define terminology that they need to know (e.g., blood glucose is the same as blood sugar). Avoid presenting unnecessary details that the patient may not remember or use. For example, telling a patient that olive oil contains polyphenols may not resonate with them. But telling them that using olive oil may help prevent a heart attack might. Similarly, specifying that "soluble fiber" helps to lower cholesterol may not easily translate into actionable steps. However, explaining that high fiber foods such as oatmeal, brown rice, beans, and lentils can help lower cholesterol may influence their food choices.

On the other hand, if you assess that the patient applies unsafe or unnecessary nutrition practices, then providing more clarification may be appropriate. For example, if someone is taking a B-complex vitamin supplement without a true deficiency, you might mention that proteins and whole grains will sufficiently provide what they need. You might add that B vitamins are water soluble, explaining that extra intake is simply lost in the urine.

However, some information may be more important to discuss than others. As your time is limited, be sure to prioritize the information that they want and need most. For example, while a patient may be wasting money on vitamin supplements, there may be bigger fish to fry. If that patient is seeing you for hypertension and you find that they dine out frequently, a discussion about sodium, dining out strategies, and/or quick and easy meal prep may take priority over the efficacy of vitamin supplements. Jumping from topic to topic may reduce recall. Instead, focus on the topic that needs immediate attention. Additional topics can be covered in later sessions as needed.

Whichever topics you and your patient decide to discuss, keep your explanations concise and purposeful. Smaller chunks of information may be easier for them to remember later. Therefore, focus on key pieces of information that they need to know, want to know, and will be able to use.

As you present information, stop frequently to assess understanding. Avoid asking questions with binary "yes or no" answers such as "Do you have any questions?" If they simply answer no, you would be unable to assess if they truly comprehend the information, or were just too shy to ask. Instead, ask how the information applies to them. For example, if discussing physical activity guidelines, ask, "What type of activities are you able to do?" Or if describing the Plate Method, ask, "How might you adjust your meals to be similar to this plate?" These types of questions allow the patient to further process the information and imagine how they can apply it in their daily lives. They will begin to generate ideas that may be later incorporated into an action plan. They may recall similar actions that they have successfully taken in the past, which may revive their self-efficacy in performing those behaviors again.

Relate the information to the patient as often as possible. For example, when describing how food affects blood sugar to a patient with diabetes, compare their blood sugar log to their dietary recall to demonstrate your point. Or when describing how FODMAPs attract water into the bowel to a patient with IBS-D, connect this information to their symptoms. Or if advising calorie reduction for weight loss, refer to their dietary recall or food log to identify sources of excess calories. Often, while the relationship between their behaviors and their symptoms is clear to you, the connection is not always clear to them. By helping them put the puzzle pieces together, they achieve clarity about what actions they can take to improve their condition. What once seemed confusing may start to feel manageable. A sense of empowerment may foster hope.

Storytelling. Sharing stories is an age-old strategy for sharing knowledge and influencing behavior (Brooks et al. 2022). From nursery rhymes and fairy tales to movies and media, stories engage the listener through entertainment, relatable content, memorable imagery, and emotional connection. In healthcare, stories can help a patient visualize healthy behaviors applied in real life. For example, one of my first patients told me that whenever her blood sugar is high, she starts vacuuming the house. Afterward, her blood sugar is back to normal. I have never forgotten that story. The **imagery** is vivid. Her motivation to lower her blood sugar is **relatable**. The action is **practical** and, for many, **achievable**. I retell that story whenever I discuss physical activity in diabetes education. I follow the story with a joke, saying that we will all have cleaner houses after the class. The more engaged the listener can be with the story, the more likely they may remember it.

Sharing other patients' stories provides an element of role modeling, which may further influence behavior change (Shunk 1987 as cited by Glanz et al. 2008). Their stories are testimony of proof that a behavior is effective. Hearing that others in similar situations can perform a behavior may increase the listener's self-efficacy that they, too, can take action (Bandura 2004 as cited by Glanz et al. 2008). Group education formats are especially conducive to sharing stories and modeling, along with the benefit of peer support.

When first entering the field, you may not yet have many stories to share. However, over time, the things you learn from your patients will allow you to pass that knowledge on to others. That is even more reason to "start with a blank page" and allow the patient to explain their point of view, their feelings, and their actions. The key to becoming a good storyteller is to be a good listener.

You may feel compelled to share your own success stories. However, take caution with this strategy. As a provider, the patient may not find you relatable. As you are already a figure of authority, detailing your behaviors may make you appear superior or arrogant, or insensitive to their limitations and barriers. For example, a healthy-appearing dietitian proclaiming that they exercise first thing in the morning to get it out of the way may not resonate with someone who has to be at dialysis by 7 o'clock in the morning. Unless you have the same condition, your success stories may cause a disconnect between you and the patient, resulting in the opposite effect of what you intended.

That is not to say that you cannot find common ground with the patient. Perhaps you have had similar struggles. Or you have a loved one with health concerns. See Chapter 3 for more information about cultivating empathy and communicating compassion, which can help to build a relationship of trust with the patient.

If your experiences are not directly relevant, focus on theirs. Listen to their stories. Acknowledging their fears, frustrations, confusion, and anger will help them feel heard. The more you hear, the more you will learn, and the more you can help. Again, listening more than speaking will go a long way.

Visual aids. Simple graphics in handouts or presentation slides can help illustrate your verbal explanations. For many, hearing the information and seeing examples may help enhance understanding, recall, and skills. With so many images available on the Internet, designing engaging materials is attainable for most professionals, and the possibilities are inexpensive and limitless. For example, your clinic may not have the budget for a variety of anatomical or food models, but you can easily copy and paste pictures and illustrations into a presentation slide or a handout (be sure to use images according to their copyright license—see Table 15.1). You may not be able to include physical activity in your session, but you can show pictures of people similar to your patient population walking, using exercise equipment, or taking the stairs. Like storytelling, seeing images of people similar to themselves engaging in health behaviors may increase their confidence in trying it themselves.

A note about image licenses and copyright. A common mistake that educators make when designing presentations and handouts is taking images from the Internet without regard to their copyright restrictions. This practice often goes unnoticed for small, one-time presentations. However, if your intention is to design a work that you will distribute regularly in your practice, or present to a large audience, take caution not to infringe on a creator's copyright. Doing so may subject you or your employer to legal action.

Many educators have limited, if any, budget for creating materials. In these cases, royalty-free artwork with no cost is the most desirable image. See Table 15.1 for a description of various image licenses, how to use them, as well as various resources for high-quality images.

TABLE 15.1

Image Licenses, Terms of Use, and Available Resources

Free, Royalty-Free* Images

Creative Commons Licenses

Images are free to use but with specific guidelines

CC By	Images can be used, adapted, and distributed in any format as long as attribution is given to the creator
CC By – SA	Images can be used, adapted, and distributed as long as attribution is given to the creator. The modified material must be licensed in the same way
CC-By-NC	Images can be used, adapted, and distributed in any format FOR NON-COMMERCIAL PURPOSES ONLY. Attribution must be given to the creator
CC-By-NC-SA	Images can be used, adapted, and distributed in any format FOR NON-COMMERCIAL PURPOSES ONLY. Attribution must be given to the creator. The modified material must be licensed in the same way
CC-By-ND	The image can be copied and distributed in any format but WITHOUT modification. Attribution must be given to the creator

(Continued)

TABLE 15.1 (*Continued*)

Image Licenses, Terms of Use, and Available Resources

Free, Royalty-Free* Images

CC-By-ND-NC	The image can be copied and distributed in any format but WITHOUT modification FOR NON-COMMERCIAL USE ONLY. Attribution must be given to the creator
CC0 (aka CC zero) or public domain	Users can copy, modify, and distribute in any format with no conditions. No attribution required. Either the copyright expired, or the creator waived their right. At the time of this writing, all U.S. works created before 1926 are in the public domain

The information above was adapted from "About CC Licenses," Creative Commons, under the CC by 4.0 license, available from: https://creativecommons.org/about/cclicenses/

Google Images and other online image searches allow filtering by creative commons licenses.

Bing.com allows further filtering by "public domain"

Some websites provide a collection of public domain or otherwise free-to-use images such as **pixabay.com** (some restrictions may apply)

Royalty-Free Stock Images for Purchase

Companies like **Shutterstock.com** or **istock.com** provide high-quality, royalty-free photos and illustrations for individual purchase or by subscription. Once purchased, no attribution is required, but licensing restrictions will apply

Platemethodpics.com is a stock photography website specializing in plate method pictures. Photos are affordable and royalty-free. No attribution is required. Some licensing restrictions apply.

The Fair Use Doctrine (U.S. Copyright Office, 2023)

Fair use is a legal doctrine that promotes freedom of expression by permitting the unlicensed use of copyright-protected works in certain circumstances. For example, an image used for non-profit educational purposes may be permitted, depending on how much of the work is used, how it affects the copyright holder, and other considerations. Fair use is determined on a case-by-case basis. In the case of stock photography, if the copyright holder's livelihood is dependent on the sale of his artwork, unpermitted use is likely not protected by this doctrine. For more information, visit the U.S. Copyright Office Fair Use Index at https://www.copyright.gov/fair-use/

When in doubt, either (1) follow the licensing restrictions, (2) request permission from the copyright holder, or (3) find another image.

*Royalty-free does not mean free of charge. It means that you can use the content as often as you want, with some limitations, without paying the creator each time. However, an initial fee to purchase the rights to the image may apply. Images with a Creative Commons license are free of charge. Be sure to read the license details to see if your usage falls within the scope of the license

Showing pictures of food and appetizing meals is especially important in nutrition counseling. For many people, the concept of healthy meals evokes images of only grilled chicken and salad. People often feel restricted in what they can eat. Pulling up recipe websites is a great way to demonstrate how much variety people can have. Health organizations like the American Heart Association, American Diabetes Association, or the National Kidney Foundation often have recipes with appetizing photos on their websites. You can also find examples for a variety of cuisines such as Southern, Asian, Middle Eastern, Mexican, Indian, and others. Quick and easy, budget-friendly, and snack ideas are also highly available. Again, with the Internet, the possibilities are endless, even if the budget is not.

Patients may ask about specific food products or restaurants. With the Internet, you can pull up nutrition information and nutrition facts labels for foods that they ask about. The Internet is especially useful for foods that are unfamiliar to you. For example, a patient recently told me that she drank three bottles of Birds Nest a day. I had never heard of the beverage before. The patient explained that it was a beverage made with the saliva of swallows. The saliva was historically used in Chinese medicine. As I was unfamiliar with the product, I was able to quickly pull up the nutrition label on the Internet. Upon seeing that it had 15 g of added sugar, I explained that each bottle contained about three teaspoons of sugar. Both the patient and her Mandarin interpreter were astonished at this information. Again, in nutrition counseling, the educator's role is to provide information, while the patient determines how they value that information. More about cultural competency in nutrition counseling is discussed in Chapter 16.

Today's technology provides ample opportunity to respond to your patient's specific questions and to personalize the education. The more tailored the education, the more memorable and applicable it will be for them. In face-to-face sessions, a laptop or tablet can be set up between the educator and patient to view images, slides, videos, or online resources. You can use your own smartphone to demonstrate apps like food databases or trackers. In virtual care, sharing the screen also allows for a multimedia experience. As telehealth has its limitations in regard to hands-on demonstrations, optimizing visual presentations is especially important. However, you can provide a hands-on experience for your patients by having them use products and objects that are in their home. For example, they can practice reading labels from packages in their kitchen, or measure food onto a plate for a demonstration of portion control. More about virtual counseling is discussed later in this book.

Presentation slides are a practical and affordable vehicle for presenting pictures and images, whether to an individual or in a group setting. Like verbal explanations, present the information in small chunks, as if telling a story from a picture book. Organize the information in a step-by-step, progressive fashion. As with written materials, the design should be easy to understand for a broad range of literacy levels. Use more graphics and less text, as you will be verbally explaining the information. Too many words on the screen may distract the reader from hearing what you are saying, which can undermine your efforts to tailor the information to the patient. However, be prepared to provide supplemental handouts that reinforce the presentation with written detail, as those who learn by reading can reference them later. Also, patients will frequently ask, "Can I have a copy of your slides?" Be sure the slides can stand alone as education materials or provide supplemental handouts that reinforce the presentation with more information. The education materials provided with this book are examples of coordinated written and digital materials.

Food, scales, measuring cups, measuring spoons, plates, cups, and glasses can help patients visualize real world portion sizes. Patients can arrange food models on a plate to practice balanced meal planning. Non-perishable foods like dried macaroni or nuts can be used to practice weighing food and reading labels. Comparing food to items like a deck of cards, a computer mouse, or a baseball can also help patients learn how to estimate portions.

Other visual aids used in health education include food models, anatomical models, and packages of food. For educators with arts and crafts skills, creating models can be an economical option. For example, one of my coworkers attached sugar cubes to a red, foam ball to describe hemoglobin A1C. Another crafted a stomach and esophagus out of felt to help explain GERD. A commonly used DIY model is a drained soda pop bottle filled with the amount of sugar contained in that beverage. A little creativity can go a long way.

Handouts, brochures, and other printed materials. Most health educators will find themselves designing their own materials at one time or another. As nutrition trends change frequently, patient questions will change, and you will need to adjust your education accordingly. While the Internet provides a wealth of educational materials, sometimes it is difficult to find information specific to your population. Or your organization discourages outside materials. Or you simply cannot find adequate resources. A common project for dietetic interns is to create educational materials. Therefore, understanding the basic concepts of graphic design and health communications is a useful skill.

Good design can convey key messages at a glance. The material should entice the learner to take a closer look for more detail. If a reader must search for the purpose of the handout, they are less likely to engage with it. While visual materials should be attractive and engaging, the layout should guide the eye to key messages. Pictures should be used with intention, not just for decoration. Images might be placed to direct the reader to important information. Or to convey relatability. Or to model behavior. Or to build skills or self-efficacy (Figure 15.1).

Some common errors in creating education materials is designing without regard to readability; or simply for aesthetics, without regard to messaging; or simply for providing information, without regard to learning style. Again, the materials should appeal to a broad audience. While text and graphics are effective for readers and visual learners, interactive elements can engage those who learn by doing, writing, or reflecting. For example, in addition to showing a sample meal plan, include a section for the learner to plan their own sample meals. A shopping list form organized by food groups can help a learner stock up on healthy staples. Goal setting and action planning pages can guide a patient in reflecting on their intrinsic motivation, their intentions, and their abilities.

The *CDC Clear Communication Guide* is a useful resource for developing effective health education materials (Centers for Disease Control and Prevention Office of the Associate Director of Communication 2019). The guide describes the research and development process, layout and design principles, plain language guidelines, numeracy considerations, behavior change strategies, and effective messaging. They even provide a scoring sheet to guide you in assessing your educational piece. This guide is available online.

Demonstrations and hands-on activities. While technology has allowed more flexibility in creating and using visual aids, hands-on experience is especially effective for increasing skills, knowledge, self-efficacy, and ultimately behavior change.

Both cooking demonstrations and hands-on classes have been shown to improve diet quality and self-efficacy in behavior change (Alpaugh et al. 2020; Hasan et al. 2019). Grocery store tours and gardening are other avenues of hands-on learning (Nikolaus et al. 2016; Palar et al. 2019). While demonstrations and hands-on activities have shown benefits, the latter has shown a greater effect (Hasan et al. 2019).

Due to the time and cost required for hands-on activities, they are typically more practical for group settings. Group education, in turn, has additional benefits in behavior change, where participants learn not only from the activity, but from each other. Such settings allow for peer modeling and social support, both of which can enhance self-efficacy (Bandura 2004 as cited by Glanz et al. 2008).

Group classes versus individual counseling. Nutrition interventions have been found effective in both group and individual settings (Bolognese et al. 2020; Canuto et al. 2021; Hwee et al. 2014; Gajewska et al. 2019). Therefore, the education format will depend on patient preference, patient cost, and available resources for the provider.

Group education can be cost-effective for both the provider and the patient. For the provider, less time is required to treat more people. Cost savings typically result in reduced participation fees for the participants. If applicable, insurance coverage is often better for group interventions versus individual nutrition counseling.

Oftentimes, group classes allow for more frequent interaction with the participants. Classes are typically designed to provide several sessions, often at weekly intervals. Through this format, more information can be delivered and in smaller chunks. The frequency allows for more immediate evaluation and troubleshooting of action plans and behavioral experiments. Again, the format is also conducive to hands-on learning, demonstrations, and educational trips like grocery store tours.

Attention-Grabbing Header:
What does the reader want to know?

Use plain language.
Use everyday words and shorter sentences. A rule of thumb is to write at the fourth or fifth grade level. Keep explanations brief. Use subheads to help the reader find the information they want most.

Use pictures with purpose.
Graphics are more than decoration. Images should convey information that answers the reader's question. Simple illustrations and pictures can explain complex topics, model behaviors, or both.

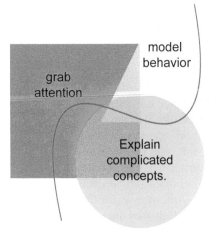

Use images to show the reader what, why, and how this information applies to them.

Key messages should stand out on the page. Prioritize the information. Vary font sizes, use subheads, or box information to guide the eye.

Define terms they should know. At times, you will have to define health terminology. They will see these terms in their chart or on the Internet. Empower them with knowledge. They are reading this to learn something new.

Include a call-to-action.
If the reader only reads one thing, what do you want it to be? What should the reader do with this information?

For more information about designing health communications, visit https://npin.cdc.gov/pages/health-communication-language-and-literacy.

FIGURE 15.1 Health communications should engage the reader with eye-catching visuals, messages that resonate, and information that is easy to understand and actionable.

Care must be taken to keep the number of participants manageable and beneficial. Too few can feel awkward, undermine perceptions of social norms, reduce motivation, and lead to attrition. Also, the benefits of peer modeling and social support are compromised. Too many participants, on the other hand, prohibit personalized attention and active participation in discussion. Some participants may feel intimidated to speak or ask questions in a large group setting. For the facilitator, time utilization during class or in administrative time may be compromised.

The impact of class size may vary between in-person and virtual programs. In my experience, an in-person class with 15 participants is comfortable for both the patients and the facilitator. In contrast, 15 participants in a virtual setting feels more impersonal. The flow of communication differs in a virtual setting, where some people are more inclined to observe passively. Audio and visual limitations impair dynamic discussion and feedback through body language. The ability to build camaraderie and foster social support is limited.

Individual counseling, on the other hand, allows for more precise personalization. Education can be tailored specifically to the patient's needs. A more intimate exchange of information may take place in which the provider may identify if additional support is needed. For example, the patient may report symptoms that require further evaluation from their doctor. Or they may report emotional issues that require mental health care coordination.

Unfortunately, the cost of individual counseling may inhibit the number or frequency of visits. Therefore, follow-up, feedback, and ongoing support may be limited. A month could pass until the next visit, over which time the patient's motivation may wane. With the passage of time, if the person feels they did not make progress, they may not return for fear of judgment, feelings of failure, or a sense that the visit is not worthwhile. On many occasions, patients have said to me, "I almost didn't come today because I haven't changed anything since last time."

Ironically, the best reason to return for support is to revisit goals, troubleshoot barriers, and nurture motivation. Therefore, setting expectations at the initial visit may help forge a reason for them to return.

Retention and return visits. The likelihood that someone will return for ongoing support is impacted by a variety of factors, including: their interest and attitude toward coming to the first visit, their personal goals, their experience during the first visit, their expectations of what future visits can provide, and logistical barriers such as time constraints, transportation, or costs (Delahanty 2010). As discussed earlier in this book, establishing rapport and building trust are critical for patient satisfaction, retention, and ultimately treatment outcomes.

PRACTICE TIP: STRATEGIES TO PREVENT ATTRITION (DELAHANTY 2010)

1. Assess and address expectations throughout the intervention or during each visit.
2. Identify anticipated challenges, reassure ongoing support, and demonstrate confidence in the patient's ability to succeed.
3. Accommodate the patient's schedule and time constraints and immediately reschedule missed appointments.
4. Behavior change strategies such as goal setting, action planning, problem solving, positive feedback, planning ahead for barriers, and addressing self-efficacy can also encourage ongoing participation.
5. Define and frame measures of success to mitigate feelings of failure or frustration. For example, one of the tools used in the Diabetes Prevention Program is a weight loss graph that charts weekly weight loss along a 5% trend line (see Figure 15.2). This visual helps patients confirm that they are making progress with incremental changes in their weight.

Weekly Weight Chart

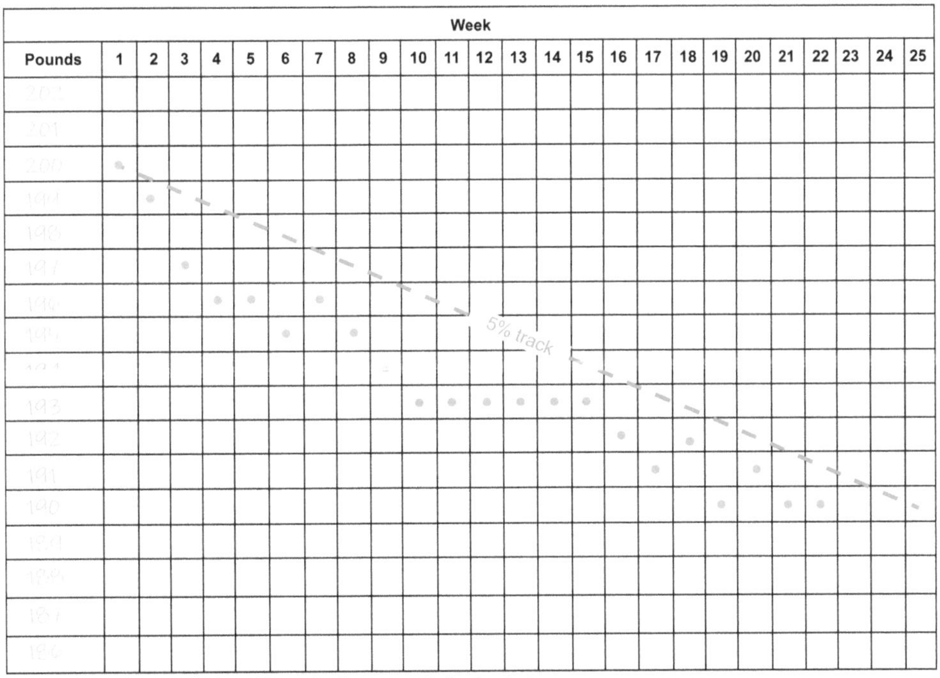

Adapted from the National Diabetes Prevention Program curriculum handouts.

FIGURE 15.2 Define and frame measures of success. In the above weight tracking grid, the plotted points illustrate that incremental changes, occasional increases, and some plateaus can still be on track.

From building trust to delivering education to motivating change, nutrition counseling is a multifaceted process that requires several skills. The outpatient dietitian is simultaneously a nutrition expert, educator, and counselor. At times, the dietitian must also write and design effective health communications. Some of these skills are developed in school. Some are developed through additional training. Some are innate to the provider. All will continue to improve with experience. But just as the patient's progress will be reinforced by your feedback, their feedback, in turn, will reinforce yours. How will you know you have delivered an effective education? Your patients will tell you.

REFERENCES

Alpaugh M, Pope L, Trubek A, Skelly J, Harvey J. Cooking as a Health Behavior: Examining the Role of Cooking Classes in a Weight Loss Intervention. *Nutrients*. 2020 Nov;12(12):3669. doi: 10.3390/nu12123669.

Bandura A. Health Promotion by Social Cognitive Means. *Health Educ Behav*. 2004 Apr;31(2):143–164. doi: 10.1177/1090198104263660.

Beagley L. Educating Patients: Understanding Barriers, Learning Styles, and Teaching Techniques. *J Perianesth Nurs*. 2011 Oct;26(5):331–337. doi: 10.1016/j.jopan.2011.06.002.

Bolognese MA, Franco CB, Ferrari A, Bennemann RM, Lopes SMA, Bertolini SMMG, Júnior NN, Branco BHM. Group Nutrition Counseling or Individualized Prescription for Women With Obesity? A Clinical Trial. *Front Public Health*. 2020 Apr;8:127. doi: 10.3389/fpubh.2020.00127.

Brooks SP, Zimmermann GL, Lang M, Scott SD, Thomson D, Wilkes G, Hartling L. A Framework to Guide Storytelling as a Knowledge Translation Intervention for Health-Promoting Behaviour Change. *Implement Sci Commun*. 2022 Mar;3(1):35. doi: 10.1186/s43058-022-00282-6.

Canuto R, Garcez A, de Souza RV, Kac G, Olinto MTA. Nutritional Intervention Strategies for the Management of Overweight and Obesity in Primary Health Care: A Systematic Review with Meta-analysis. *Obes Rev.* 2021 Mar;22(3):e13143. doi: 10.1111/obr.13143.

Centers for Disease Control and Prevention. *Improving Health Literacy for Older Adults: Expert Panel Report 2009.* Atlanta, GA: U.S. Department of Health and Human Services; 2009.

Centers for Disease Control and Prevention Office of the Associate Director of Communication. *CDC Clear Communication Index: A Tool for Developing and Assessing CDC Public Communication Products - User Guide* [Internet]. 2019 [cited 28 June 2023]. Available from: https://www.cdc.gov/ccindex/pdf/clear-communication-user-guide.pdf

Cutilli CC. Health Literacy in Geriatric Patients: An Integrative Review of the Literature. *Orthop Nurs.* 2007 Jan-Feb;26(1):43–48. doi: 10.1097/00006416-200701000-00014.

Delahanty LM. An Expanded Role for Dietitians in Maximising Retention in Nutrition and Lifestyle Intervention Trials: Implications for Clinical Practice. *J Hum Nutr Diet.* 2010 Aug;23(4):336–343. doi: 10.1111/j.1365-277X.2009.01037.x.

DeWalt DA, Pignone M, Malone R, Rawls C, Kosnar MC, George G, Bryant B, Rothman RL, Angel B. Development and Pilot Testing of a Disease Management Program for Low Literacy Patients with Heart Failure. *Patient Educ Couns.* 2004 Oct;55(1):78–86. doi: 10.1016/j.pec.2003.06.002.

Gajewska D, Kucharska A, Kozak M, Wunderlich S, Niegowska J. Effectiveness of Individual Nutrition Education Compared to Group Education, in Improving Anthropometric and Biochemical Indices among Hypertensive Adults with Excessive Body Weight: A Randomized Controlled Trial. *Nutrients.* 2019 Dec;11(12):2921. doi: 10.3390/nu11122921.

Hasan B, Thompson WG, Almasri J, Wang Z, Lakis S, Prokop LJ, Hensrud DD, Frie KS, Wirtz MJ, Murad AL, Ewoldt JS, Murad MH. The Effect of Culinary Interventions (Cooking Classes) on Dietary Intake and Behavioral Change: A Systematic Review and Evidence Map. *BMC Nutr.* 2019 May;5:29. doi: 10.1186/s40795-019-0293-8.

Hill-Briggs F, Smith AS. Evaluation of Diabetes and Cardiovascular Disease Print Patient Education Materials for Use with Low-Health Literate Populations. *Diabetes Care.* 2008 Apr;31(4):667–671. doi: 10.2337/dc07-1365.

Hwee J, Cauch-Dudek K, Victor JC, Ng R, Shah BR. Diabetes Education Through Group Classes Leads to Better Care and Outcomes Than Individual Counselling in Adults: A Population-Based Cohort Study. *Can J Public Health.* 2014 May;105(3):e192–e197. doi: 10.17269/cjph.105.4309.

Kandula NR, Malli T, Zei CP, Larsen E, Baker DW. Literacy and Retention of Information after a Multimedia Diabetes Education Program and Teach-Back. *J Health Commun.* 2011;16(Suppl 3):89–102. doi: 10.1080/10810730.2011.604382.

Knowles M. *Andragogy: An Emerging Technology for Adult Learning. The Modern Practice of Adult Education.* New York: Association Press; 1970. pp 37–55.

Koh HK, Brach C, Harris LM, Parchman ML. A Proposed 'Health Literate Care Model' Would Constitute a Systems Approach to Improving Patients' Engagement in Care. *Health Aff (Millwood).* 2013 Feb;32(2):357–367. doi: 10.1377/hlthaff.2012.1205.

Kutner M, Greenberg E, Jin Y, Paulsen C. *The Health Literacy of America's Adults: Results from the 2003 National Assessment of Adult Literacy* [Internet]. Washington, DC: Institute of Education Sciences, National Center for Education Statistics, U.S. Department of Education; 2006 [cited 2023 June 28]. Available from: https://nces.ed.gov/pubsearch/pubsinfo.asp?pubid=2006483

Nikolaus CJ, Muzaffar H, Nickols-Richardson SM. Grocery Store (or Supermarket) Tours as an Effective Nutrition Education Medium: A Systematic Review. *J Nutr Educ Behav.* 2016 Sep;48(8):544-554.e1. doi: 10.1016/j.jneb.2016.05.016.

Palar K, Lemus Hufstedler E, Hernandez K, Chang A, Ferguson L, Lozano R, Weiser SD. Nutrition and Health Improvements after Participation in an Urban Home Garden Program. *J Nutr Educ Behav.* 2019 Oct;51(9):1037–1046. doi: 10.1016/j.jneb.2019.06.028.

Plain Language Action and Information Network. *Federal Plain Language Guidelines* [Internet]. 2011 [Revised 2011 May, cited 28 June 2023]. Available from: https://www.plainlanguage.gov/guidelines/.

Romanelli F, Bird E, Ryan M. Learning Styles: A Review of Theory, Application, and Best Practices. *Am J Pharm Educ.* 2009 Feb;73(1):9. doi: 10.5688/aj730109.

Santana S, Brach C, Harris L, Ochiai E, Blakey C, Bevington F, Kleinman D, Pronk N. Updating Health Literacy for Healthy People 2030: Defining Its Importance for a New Decade in Public Health. *J Public Health Manag Pract*. 2021 Nov-Dec;27(Suppl 6):S258–S264. doi: 10.1097/PHH. 0000000000001324.

Shunk DH. Peer Models and Children's Behavioral Change. *Rev Educ Res*. 1987;52(2):149–174.

U.S. Copyright Office. *U.S. Copyright Office Fair Use Index* [Internet]. Washington, DC; 2023 February [cited 27 June 2023]. Available from: https://www.copyright.gov/fair-use/.

16 Cultural Competence

When I present to dietetics students, one question that always comes up is, "How do you counsel people from different cultural backgrounds?"

For me, this question elicits so many emotions, memories, and perspectives that the answer is surely not a quick one. As a first generation, Filipina-American raised in a Detroit suburb with a master's degree in nutrition, I have a complicated relationship with food, culture, and nutrition. Early in my career, I struggled with conflict between my nutrition knowledge and the foods of my upbringing. While I found comfort in many traditional Filipino dishes, I regarded them with caution for their high sodium seasonings, refined carbohydrates, and high fat content.

In my family's home, a rice cooker was always full on the counter. I recall my last trip to the Philippines when my cousin said to me, "We eat rice for breakfast, for lunch, for dinner, and for snacks!" Filipinos often combined white rice with noodle dishes, fried pork, or processed meat like canned corned beef and Spam. For breakfast, we seasoned the rice with soy sauce and fried it in oil. While I trimmed the fat from my meat, my mom would say, "That's the best part!" Fish was often fried, crispy, and salty, as were the egg rolls filled with pork. I often teased my mom that she used vegetables as a decoration.

To be fair, Filipino food was not the only thing I ate growing up. Like other Americans, I was a frequent consumer of McDonald's, Burger King, Pizza Hut, and other fast-food chains. Various sugary cereals topped our refrigerator. My main beverage at home was soda. In high school, I pulled a Hawaiian Punch and Hostess Apple Pie out of the vending machine on a daily basis. For lunch, I dipped chicken nuggets in nacho cheese sauce.

Many dietitians may similarly struggle with conflict between their nutrition knowledge and their social background. Due to their expertise in nutrition, they may eat differently from their own family members, their next-door neighbor, and their friends, thus experience a similar type of cultural divide. A dietitian's own eating pattern and values might seem foreign to many of their patients, even if they share similar cultural or ethnic backgrounds. Navigating these interactions, either personally or professionally, requires a similar approach of respect, understanding, and self-awareness.

Therefore, one step toward cultural competence in nutrition counseling is recognizing that eating behaviors vary from person to person, not just from culture to culture. Thus, patient-centered care will still be the primary approach for each interaction.

WHAT IS CULTURAL COMPETENCE?

Cultural competence is "the ability to collaborate effectively with individuals from different cultures" (Nair and Adetayo 2019). The word **culture** refers to "the integrated pattern of human behavior that includes thoughts, communications, actions, customs, beliefs, values, and institutions of a racial, ethnic, religious, or social group" (Cross et al. 1989).

Due to the diversity of the American population, most dietitians in the United States can expect to encounter patients of different ethnicities, races, and religious backgrounds. Becoming familiar with various ethnic cuisines is only part of the challenge. Understanding the values, beliefs, and behavioral practices around food and health is another. Perceptions of health, body image, and physical activity can vary among different ethnic populations (Mathew Joseph et al. 2018) and can therefore affect their health behaviors. Religious practices can affect which foods are allowed, when they can be

DOI: 10.1201/9781003326038-20

consumed, and in what combinations. Some practices can be a concern for certain conditions, such as fasting for patients with diabetes who are at risk for hypoglycemia. A wealth of literature is available online to learn about foods, social practices, values, and beliefs.

For those serving specific populations, dietitians can develop an expertise in their culture as their interactions will be more immersive. However, for those who serve a more diverse population, developing an expertise for every culture they encounter would be more challenging.

However, rest assured that your patients likely do not expect you to be an expert in their culture. They, themselves, are culturally competent enough to know that different ethnicities eat different foods. For example, I do not expect every reader of this book to know lechon or puto, which are staple dishes at any Filipino celebration. What I would expect, however, is that if you do not know, you simply ask, "Can you describe that for me?"

Ask questions. There is nothing offensive about asking to learn more. In fact, in my personal experience, the only people who have been offended when I did not know something are other Filipinos. They say, "Why don't you know that? That is part of your culture!" Otherwise, most people are willing to describe their food for you. As you conduct a dietary recall, patients will often provide details without prompting. When discussing foods specific to their culture, many recognize that the dietitian may not be familiar with them and are willing to describe them. Or they may ask if you know it, at which point you can ask for more information. For example, when conducting a 24-hour recall with a patient from Sri Lanka, he stated that for breakfast he consumed "milk rice" and asked if I had heard of it. I admitted that I had not but asked if he could describe it, and he obliged, saying it was "rice made with coconut milk." Food preparations may vary from culture to culture, but the food groups and ingredients are typically recognizable.

Perhaps you may be wondering how to handle a situation where the food they describe has questionable ingredients. As in the example above, coconut milk is high in saturated fat, but is a staple ingredient in his culture. Again, patient-centered care will determine which nutrition issues to address. In this case, if metabolic disorders are present, such as hyperlipidemia or insulin resistance, then a deeper investigation into frequency, portions, and other sources of saturated fat in the diet would be warranted, followed by an objective explanation about the concerns about saturated fat. On the other hand, if the patient exhibits mindfulness, portion control, and an otherwise varied diet, and there are no metabolic concerns, then specifically targeting coconut milk may not be necessary. The same could be said about somebody who mentions pizza in their 24-hour recall. In most cases, overall eating pattern and lifestyle are determinants of health, not individual foods or nutrients.

Therefore, do not be afraid to ask questions. As in any social interaction, people appreciate when you take an interest in them and want to learn more about them. In healthcare, your patients will appreciate the personalized care.

Beware of implicit bias. While each culture may have age-old traditions, each person within a culture may uphold these traditions to varying degrees. To assume that everybody within a specific ethnic group follows tradition would be an implicit bias. Age, life experience, socioeconomic status, political belief, and other factors can all affect one's cultural practice (Epner and Baile 2012). Furthermore, culture can refer to a variety of social groups and belief systems that transcend ethnicity and race. As such, individuals may belong to multiple social groups and engage in a variety of cultural practices.

I recall a time when I invited my cousin and his family over for dinner. I had not seen my cousin since I was a child visiting the Philippines. As adults, we were both living in California and I was new to the area. It would be the first time we spoke in a decade. I had decided to serve pork chops. While I was not cooking a Filipino dish specifically, pork is a main protein in Filipino culture. Imagine my surprise when my cousin arrived and said, "Oh, I'm sorry Joyce, we do not eat pork. We're Seventh Day Adventists now." I realize I had made two assumptions because he was Filipino. One, that he ate pork. And two, that he was Catholic like me, the predominant religion in the Philippines. Needless to say, I learned a lot about implicit bias that day. As I said in Chapter 3, I have found that when I make assumptions, I am often wrong.

Therefore, implicit bias is likely a larger concern in cross-cultural counseling rather than cultural expertise. Review Chapter 3 for information about mindfully identifying and addressing implicit bias.

Consider various "food cultures." In the field of health and nutrition, the term "culture" can be applied to various lifestyles. For example, "fitness culture" includes a variety of nutrition practices that can be further broken down by type of training—i.e., endurance trainers may practice carb loading strategies while bodybuilders may focus more on protein. "Diet culture," on the other hand, may be committed to reduced-calorie, low carb, or fasting strategies. For those following vegan or vegetarian diets, their values around nutrition may be based on animal rights, on health, on the environment, or on all three. People can be as passionate about their food culture as they are about any other cultural aspect of their lives. As such, those values and beliefs must be similarly understood and respected.

Create an inclusive healthcare environment. Cultural competence and healthcare disparity must be addressed at the organizational level. Some interventions include (1) training in diversity, equity and inclusion (DEI) for providers and staff, (2) achieving a diverse workforce, especially one that reflects the patient population, (3) interpreter services for non-English speaking patients, (4) and education materials that are culturally and linguistically appropriate (Nair and Adetayo 2019; Anderson et al. 2003).

In turn, each individual provider should seek opportunities to learn and grow. Participate in professional development training, or request training if your organization has not offered it to you. Search online for educational materials in different languages and for more information about your patient populations. If your organization does not have interpreter services, work with them to find a service provider.

Ideally, those studying to become healthcare professionals will have DEI training as part of their education curriculum. However, learning does not stop at graduation. Competence will develop over time as you gain more experience interacting with different people.

Seek knowledge. Ten years after I started working in nutrition, the COVID-19 pandemic hit. By this time, I had personally logged hundreds of food records documenting my food choices which included whole grains, plenty of vegetables, and lean proteins. I was fully indoctrinated into the world of nutrition with pious devotion. Sheltering in place, I started binge-watching food documentaries on various streaming services. I also started listening to as many food podcasts as I could find. From award winning chefs, locally renowned cooks, entrepreneurial immigrants, and food historians, I learned about the histories of various cuisines. I realized that many foods were born of necessity. For example, the comforting dishes of the South were crafted by enslaved Africans with the foods they brought to America, the rations provided by the slave owners, and the plants they were allowed to grow and keep. Around the world, foods were created with what was locally available—the corn of North America, the rice of Asia, the plantains of the Caribbean, all cultivated to feed the people of those lands. Foods designed for portability like breads stuffed with meat were often created to support working people. Curing meat was critical for preserving food to survive migration or cold weather or to prevent food waste. Even food processing technologies were invented to deliver food to people in urban areas who did not have the means to farm their own food.

I learned about the artisanal skills required for the creation of foods like cheese, soy sauce, breads, pasta, and even beer, wine, spirits, and chocolate. I gained an appreciation for the toil and effort required to grow, harvest, and prepare various types of ingredients. I marvel at the various cooking methods invented over the years, from barbecue pits to clay ovens to bamboo steamers. I wonder at discoveries like fermentation and oil pressing. I better understand the tenacity and passion of food sellers in market stalls, food trucks, and restaurants around the world, as well as the customers who rely on those foods to feed themselves and their families.

Respect the food. While I champion the research behind the Mediterranean Diet, I have come to appreciate the healthful qualities of cuisines around the world. Corn, beans, squash, root vegetables, and other native plant foods are traditional staples for the indigenous groups of the Americas. Asian diets are high in fish and seafood, as are those in other seaside regions. Indian spices like turmeric, cinnamon, and cumin are frequently researched for their antioxidant and anti-inflammatory properties. Legumes like beans and lentils are used around the world. Quinoa, teff, barley, buckwheat, farro, and spelt are grains originating from outside of the United States. Vegetables and fruits are ubiquitous to all cultures.

In contrast, the American diet is often characterized by ultra-processed foods, fast food, and excess. The industrial age allowed for the wide distribution of food, but advances in science and technology outpaced our understanding about its overall impact on health. The spread of the Western diet and lifestyle around the world is associated with the spread of obesity and chronic diseases (Kopp 2019). American food and beverage empires like McDonald's and Coca-Cola notoriously market their goods globally such that families worldwide are regularly consuming their products.

Learn by eating. As my perspective on food evolved, my interaction with it changed as well. Instead of screening foods for their health value, I started to seek them out for their cultural significance. I take advantage of the diversity of restaurants in my area or on my travels. I choose foods on the menus that are representative of that cuisine. When I meet people from various backgrounds, whether coworkers or patients or neighbors or Uber drivers, I ask them which restaurants they recommend for authentic, traditional meals. The more foods I try, the more acquainted I become with the vocabulary of various cuisines. I notice the similarities among different cultures, like the naan, roti, and chapati of India, the pita of the Mediterranean and Middle East, the tortilla of Mexico and Central America, and the injera of Ethiopia. I have learned how foods migrated around the world, largely through the slave trade and colonialism. The cuisine of my own Filipino heritage demonstrates the global influence of food, such as the Spanish-inspired adobo, menudo, afritada, and leche flan, or pancit and lumpia, adaptations of Chinese noodles and egg rolls.

However, there is no better example of the confluence of international cuisine than the United States. A country built on immigration, cultures from around the world coexist and combine to create a culinary landscape as varied as its population. Metro Detroit, where I grew up, boasts some of the most authentic Southern, Mexican, Polish, Middle Eastern, and Greek restaurants in the Midwest. Fusions of Asian and Mexican cuisine are a common concept. Chinatowns and Italian villages are prominent in large cities around the country. Even American ketchup has its roots in Chinese fish sauce.

While many ethnic restaurants put an American spin on their food, they offer opportunities to become introduced to their signature flavors, ingredients, and cooking styles. From my experience, if you want good Filipino food, go where the Filipinos go—and apply that tip to any type of cuisine.

Expand your view. The more I learned about the history of food, the more I realized how skewed my view about nutrition had been. The lens of nutrition counseling is more like a kaleidoscope than a microscope, where several angles can be viewed together and adjusted. When I teased my mom about using vegetables for decoration, I missed the fact that she stood at the counter finely slicing fresh vegetables every day. The pork in her sinigang, a Filipino soup, was actually outweighed by large chunks of cabbage, carrot, green beans, and eggplant. The fish she fried was bought fresh and hand dipped in breadcrumbs, not laden with additives and preservatives and frozen in a box. And the lumpia, only made for special occasions, were hand-rolled one by one, a process that can take several days. Today, my mother's rice cooker is always filled with brown rice. She uses the loin cuts for her pork dishes. Her daily staple is a smoothie made with milk, oatmeal, frozen fruit, and peanut butter. And she beams with pride whenever she shows me her lab values.

For individuals, food is simultaneously a source of nourishment, cultural identification, and emotional comfort. Socially, it brings together families and friends. Economically, it sustains farmers, food producers, small business owners, the employees of large companies, and the communities in which they live. Medically, it can be therapeutic.

SHARE. While these themes are wide and varied, nutrition counseling has a singular starting point: the patient. Therefore, the SHARE process is equally useful in counseling people of various cultural backgrounds. When you give them the time and space to speak freely, they will tell you their concerns, beliefs, and eating practices. During the dietary recall, people will tell you what they eat, what they do not, and why. They are willing to provide details of the types of foods they include in their meals. In my experience, people are rarely—if ever—offended when asked for more clarification. In fact, more often than not, they are appreciative of a personalized experience that incorporates their preferences, culture, and traditions. As with many people, the concern may not be what they eat, but how much, how often, when, and why.

I recently saw a patient who was newly diagnosed with diabetes. He was Mexican American, and he was accompanied by his mother, who was visiting from Mexico. At the time of our visit, he had already made many changes. He ate more vegetables, cut out soda, and reduced corn tortillas to two or three per meal. During our discussion, I showed pictures of foods to limit—namely, ultra-processed foods, high fat meats, and fast food. When he saw the picture, he and his mom exchanged a look. Then he looked back at me and said, "That is how I used to eat!" By starting with the patient—and not their ethnicity—we were able to uncover the specific nutritional changes that were important for him. And it had nothing to do with Mexican food.

Similarly, patients can use pictures to educate the dietitian. On so many occasions, people have turned to their smartphones to look up pictures of food they were unable to describe. By sharing information, both the patient and the dietitian can grow and learn.

ONLINE RESOURCES FOR TRANSLATED
MATERIALS OR MEAL PLANNING

The USDA's Food and Nutrition Services provides MyPlate tip sheets and graphics in 21 different languages at https://www.myplate.gov/resources/myplate-multiple-languages.

The Institute for Family Health provides images of "Healthy Plates around the World" at https://institute.org/health-care/services/diabetes-care/healthyplates/. Plate examples include Latin American, American, Soul Food, and West African meals.

Learning About Diabetes, Inc., provides Plate Method handouts and other diabetes care information translated in several languages at https://learningaboutdiabetes.org/.

Oldways provides information and recipe ideas for a variety of traditional diets including Mediterranean, African, Asian, Latin American, and Vegetarian/Vegan diets at https://oldwayspt.org/traditional-diets.

Empathize. While cultural values vary, nobody wants to be sick. Many have seen the devastating effects that diabetes, heart disease, and other nutrition-related conditions have had on family or friends. They may be scared. They may not feel well. They are often confused about what they can or cannot eat. But they are often ready to change. In fact, by the time they see a dietitian, many people have already made changes. Large portions, snacks, sweets, and sugary beverages are often the first to go. Increasing vegetables is also intuitive for many. Unfortunately, some nutrition misconceptions manage to cross language barriers. For example, from all walks of life, people with diabetes report that they "avoid carbs," whether it is rice or tortilla or bread or potatoes. When faced with disease, many are willing to make changes—even if they are not yet sure what changes they need to make.

Regardless of where your patient is from, the role of the dietitian is to educate them on how food affects their health, and how to achieve balance with foods that they enjoy. Every culture has protein, fruit, vegetables, and grains. In all cases, patient-centered care will guide the education. Recommendations should be personalized to the preferences and needs of the patient. As with any patient, assess their eating behaviors and their education needs. Then through shared decision-making, the patient will be empowered to make changes that align with their values and beliefs.

In nutrition counseling, both the provider and the patient educate and learn. Listen. Ask questions. Continue to seek more information and experiences. Embrace your own cultural heritage. And eat food. Lots of it.

So in answer to the question, "How do you counsel people from different backgrounds?"

With respect. Not just for the patient. But also for the food.

REFERENCES

Anderson LM, Scrimshaw SC, Fullilove MT, Fielding JE, Normand J, Task Force on Community Preventive Services. Culturally Competent Healthcare Systems. A Systematic Review. *Am J Prev Med.* 2003 Apr;24(3 Suppl):68–79. doi: 10.1016/s0749-3797(02)00657-8.

Cross TL,et al., Towards a Culturally Competent System of Care: A Monograph on Effective Services for Minority Children Who Are Severely Emotionally Disturbed [Internet]. Washington, DC: Georgetown Univ. Child Development Center; 1989 [cited 2023 June 29]. Available from: https://eric.ed.gov/?id=ED330171.

Epner DE, Baile WF. Patient-Centered Care: The Key to Cultural Competence. *Ann Oncol.* 2012 Apr;23(Suppl 3):33–42. doi: 10.1093/annonc/mds086.

Kopp W. How Western Diet and Lifestyle Drive the Pandemic of Obesity and Civilization Diseases. *Diabetes Metab Syndr Obes.* 2019 Oct;12:2221–2236. doi: 10.2147/DMSO.S216791.

Mathew Joseph N, Ramaswamy P, Wang J. Cultural Factors Associated with Physical Activity among U.S. Adults: An Integrative Review. *Appl Nurs Res.* 2018 Aug;42:98–110. doi: 10.1016/j.apnr.2018.06.006.

Nair L, Adetayo OA. Cultural Competence and Ethnic Diversity in Healthcare. *Plast Reconstr Surg Glob Open.* 2019 May;7(5):e2219. doi: 10.1097/GOX.0000000000002219.

17 SHARE Your Screen – and Other Virtual Care Tips

The first time the little green video icon lit up in the electronic medical record, my heart rate kicked up a notch. After years of providing diabetes education to both individuals and groups, delivering virtual health care was making my palms sweat.

Like many educators, I relied on a variety of props, visual aids, drawings, and handouts to explain diabetes and how to manage it. Many of us employ a multi-media approach to drive home key messages. In turn, we look for physical clues from the patient that indicate if they are engaged and comprehending. We watch for the moment they lean in, when the light bulb goes off, and they respond, "nobody has ever explained it that way before."

Over the years, I had developed an arsenal of tools and strategies to tackle the variety of questions that come up in diabetes education. I had mastered the art of whiteboard illustrations, explaining digestion, absorption, insulin release, and glucose uptake in a way a fifth grader could understand. Then COVID-19 hit, and I had to find a different way. Ambulatory clinics were shut down. In-person care was limited to necessary and urgent procedures only. We were told to work from home, but just figuring out how to log into the healthcare system from my bedroom raised my cortisol level. How was I going to empower patients through a video camera?

Like many dietitians across the country, I was faced with learning new technology rapidly. Then the technology changed. And then it changed again. Within three weeks, we went from using tablets to meeting websites to the updated EMR. HIPAA[1] compliance had us scrambling for approvals. We installed phone apps for telephone visits. Simultaneously, we had to convince our patients to switch to video visits and educate them on how to log in. The learning curve was steep for us all.

As we were figuring out the technology, we also had to rethink our education strategies. Without that whiteboard, how could we help patients visualize complicated health information? How do you create a safe, comfortable learning environment in a two-dimensional setting?

At that time, I was sure that the quality of care would suffer. I was not the only one. Earlier in the pandemic, surveys indicated that many providers felt the same way (Chu et al. 2022). Indeed, there was an acclimation period. We had to learn what was possible and not possible through a video visit. As an educator, I found myself starting from scratch. Like my early days, I was verbally explaining complicated concepts without visual aids, hands-on activities, or other tools to enhance learning and recall. We had to find ways to efficiently distribute class books and handouts through the patient portal. Including interpreter services was challenging as they were also still figuring out how to effectively join the video visits. Even today, there are times when my patient is on the video, the interpreter is present by phone conference, and I hope that the images I show are strong enough to convey the message.[1]

Compared to providers, patients reported a higher acceptance rate of virtual care early in the pandemic, with most saying that they would not have sought care if the video visit was not available (Chu et al. 2022). Consistent with these findings, the number of virtual visits including return visits quickly increased. In my practice, the number of scheduled video and phone visits increased

---

[1] The Health Insurance Portability and Accountability Act of 1996 insures that people have rights over their own health information including privacy and security (U.S. Office for Civil Rights 2022).

DOI: 10.1201/9781003326038-21

to back-to-back patients with fewer no shows. During the pandemic, many people were working remotely or sheltering at home, making it easier for them to keep their appointments. Not only did patients log in to the first visit, but they were willing to schedule more frequent follow-ups. With the increased patient load, providers had to increase efficiency during the visit. As time online moves at a snail's pace, patients exhibited less tolerance for late starts.

In the post-pandemic era, providers are much more comfortable with the virtual environment. We have learned from trial, error, and as always, from listening to our patients. Clinics are now open for in-person care. However, as long as their insurance covers it, patients are still requesting virtual visits, indicating an overall positive experience. Schedules continue to be full. Online class sizes continue to increase. Video visits have allowed us to expand our reach as patients log in from around the state. The time spent teaching and troubleshooting the technology is lessening as the world becomes more comfortable with videoconferencing. With increased modes of access, the new challenge is in accommodating increased referrals and appointment requests. In my department, the demand has justified the hiring of more educators, and a hybrid format allows for a larger team despite office space limitations.

While there will continue to be limitations in virtual care, both patients and providers have found benefits. Many patients find it more convenient as they do not have to leave home, and in some cases, they even log in from work (Donelan et al. 2019). They may save money as they do not have to take time off work or spend money on transportation, gas, or parking. As providers have become more comfortable with the format, they too are now more likely to recommend virtual care (Chu et al. 2022). For patients, increased follow-up may improve outcomes. For providers, fuller schedules translate to increased revenue.

LESSONS LEARNED

Today, as the dust is beginning to settle, I continue to tidy up my approach to video visits. I reflect on what has worked, what has not, and what I can improve. I continue to explore online tools to consider new things to try and to keep up with new and changing technology.

Patient-centered care. For educators, the types of tools available will continue to grow and change over time. However, the foundations of patient-centered care will endure. Empathy, compassion, empowerment, and shared decision-making will continue to enhance patient satisfaction and, subsequently, outcomes. Access and equitable care must always be a priority. Education must be inclusive and easy to understand. While all of this goes without saying, the virtual environment does pose different challenges in these areas.

As discussed earlier in this book, ***implicit bias*** can affect what and how much information an educator provides as well as how they provide it. In addition to the biases related to race, gender, age, weight, and other characteristics prone to prejudice, technology introduces additional assumptions. For example, while a digital divide is often cited between younger and older adults, assuming that your older patients are unable to engage in technology risks withholding tools that can enhance care. For example, for patients with diabetes, continuous glucose monitors can improve self-management of the disease, and online data sharing allows for remote monitoring. Throughout the pandemic, training on those devices sometimes occurred online. Today, as more patients are logging in from further away, virtual visits can address distance barriers. Therefore, online device training and data sharing may still be a better option for some people. While in-person, hands-on training has inherent advantages, keeping the options open allows for increased access. As in all treatment decisions, determining whether online care is appropriate must be determined on an individual basis and in collaboration with the patient.

Similarly, just because a patient is younger, it should not be assumed that they are comfortable with technology. Other factors can also affect a patient's ability to participate in virtual care.

Experience with technology can vary depending on financial, environmental, cognitive, or emotional barriers. For example, a young adult living with roommates may not have enough privacy at home to engage in an open discussion with their healthcare provider online. Or if they do not have a private space at work, they may be relegated to log in from their cars, which may not be conducive to learning. While patients often opt for video visits even with such barriers, the option for an in-person visit should always be available.

Situational factors can also trigger bias. For example, early in the pandemic, if somebody did not log on at their scheduled time, I assumed that they either forgot about the visit or were choosing not to participate, and thus were not engaged in their self-care. More often than not, upon calling the patient by phone, I found that they were having technology issues—either technical or skill related. Thus, making assumptions about their interest in the visit initially jeopardized my approach to their care.

When logging in from home, some patients may be lying in bed or eating at the kitchen table. While we often look to body language for signs of engagement and understanding, we still cannot make assumptions. How people act in the comfort of their own home may differ from their behaviors in a clinic or classroom. For decades, people have fully engaged with information on their TVs, computers, laptops, and phones from their dining table or their beds. Therefore, unless the patient explicitly declines the information, the educator must provide the education with the same commitment as they would for someone logging in from an office space or present in the clinic.

Videoconferencing may also increase the risk of reinforcing common stereotypes (Dhawan et al. 2021). A woman whose children are in the room, a higher weight person logging in from their couch, or a person of color logging in from their car may all trigger implicit biases. As discussed earlier in this book, providers must be mindfully aware of their thoughts and behaviors to identify and address any tendency toward bias.

In virtual care, *empathy* must extend to the patient's struggles with technology. For many patients, medical appointments alone can increase anxiety, let alone their concerns about their health. Add to that an unfamiliarity with new technology and/or a tedious online check-in process, and it is no wonder that patients are sometimes agitated upon arrival. Providers need to only remember the early days of virtual care to recall their own struggles with the technology to cultivate empathy.

Initially, I was concerned that communicating through a screen would pose a barrier to building rapport or conveying *compassion*. Maintaining eye contact can be tricky over video. A quiet space is not guaranteed. The comfort of proximity is lost. However, I quickly found that applying the concepts of patient-centered care does not change online. Assuming there are no distractions in the background, both patient and provider focus on their screens, creating the semblance of a shared space. Similar to in-person visits, when the clinician "starts with a blank page" and allows the patient to freeflow their questions and concerns, the clinician is pulled into their world. By cultivating a sincere interest in the patient and asking clarifying questions, the provider can enter their world even further to find how, specifically, they can help during that visit. As the patient detects your interest and feels heard, they become more receptive to you as a provider. You build trust. Patient satisfaction increases. They are more likely to return. In other words, listening goes a long way.

Time management. Listening, however, takes time. Therefore, time management is more critical than ever. As with every advance in technology, when more can be done in less time, patience wanes. Even though a patient did not have to travel to the clinic, the time it takes to complete online questionnaires can be agitating for them. Also, compared to a 10-minute delay in the clinic waiting area, 5 minutes waiting online can feel excessive. As discussed earlier, the convenience of virtual care has increased patient load, resulting in back-to-back scheduling with fewer no shows.

Not only must the provider allow time to interact with each patient, but there must also be time for care coordination and documentation. For the provider, developing new efficiencies is necessary to keep on schedule.

Learning needs and follow-up. Fortunately, the convenience of virtual visits has also increased the willingness of patients to follow up sooner and more frequently. Therefore, instead of trying to cover as much as possible in their allotted hour, the dietitian or health educator can home in on a topic of priority with a plan to cover additional topics in subsequent visits. Instead of waiting one month for a follow-up visit, the patient may be able to return online in two weeks, sometimes sooner if scheduling allows. In regard to insurance coverage, allowable hours can be spread out in shorter, more frequent visits. Not only does this allow for a more efficient session, it also may be more conducive to learning. As discussed in the health literacy chapter, smaller chunks of information are easier to recall, and may be easier to apply. For example, if a patient visits for weight management, an educator may feel compelled to comprehensively cover nutrition, meal planning, physical activity, and lifestyle change strategies. With the convenience of virtual care, patients may be able to establish some weekly sessions to cover each topic, spreading out their insurance hours accordingly. Not only may the information volume be easier to remember, but like in a lifestyle change program, it may be more actionable as well.

Access and health disparity. While virtual care expanded access for some people, others found an increased disparity. For example, during the pandemic, while more people could enroll in group classes, those who could not join by video went without. Not everybody has an Internet connection, a smartphone, or a tablet. Those with vision impairment either could not log on or, if they did, they could not see the information presented on the screen. For those with hearing impairment, unless closed captioning was enabled or a sign language interpreter was present, they could not listen to the presentation. While the technology continues to be updated to address some of these barriers, a digital divide remains. Some programs have not yet resumed in-person classes as the majority of people prefer the online format. Thus, those with sensory impairments, or lack of Internet or technology, or lack of knowledge or self-efficacy in using the technology are still unable to participate. While clinics are now open for in-person visits, the cost is higher for those who have to travel, take time off work, coordinate childcare, or enlist the help of a support person or caregiver.

Insurance coverage may include phone visits as part of their telehealth benefit, which may help reach those who are unable to participate by video. While audio formats have some inherent limitations, they can serve as a way to increase follow-up without burdening the patient with frequent trips to the clinic. For comprehensive education, visual or hands-on learners may be at a disadvantage. However, an education plan may be developed that could include both formats. Or if an in-person session is not possible, perhaps education materials could be sent to the patient ahead of time, and the educator could refer to the materials during the phone visit.

For patients with visual impairment, the Commission for the Blind may be able to provide adaptive equipment for learning and self-care. For example, readers, magnifiers, self-monitoring equipment like talking blood sugar meters, or medication dosing devices are available to support independence (Camporeale 2001). A multidisciplinary team that includes the doctor, nurse, dietitian, social worker, and occupational therapist can help patients learn how to obtain and use the equipment. For nutrition counseling, tactile stickers can be used for patients to identify measuring cups. Talking food scales are also available. In-person visits or home care from the occupational therapist would be necessary for initial training, but once the patient is acclimated to these tools, ongoing support and education can be provided by phone.

For patients with hearing impairments, sign language interpreters and closed captioning can be used in video visits. For phone visits, adaptive technologies and services are available to either magnify sound or translate speech to text. If the patient is not already aware of these options, a referral to the social worker and occupational therapist is necessary. For the nutrition educator, confirming that the patient's needs are met ahead of the education is important to ensure an effective learning experience.

Despite advances in technology, equitable health care continues to be a challenge, often due to lack of training for the care provider. For the health educator, identifying and accommodating all learning needs is critical. On one hand, lack of experience may be due to a lack of encounters with various disabilities. On the other hand, the lack of encounters is likely due to the lack of accessibility. As for all marginalized groups, when faced with bias or an atmosphere of exclusion, many opt out of seeking care. Ongoing promotion, advocacy, and training will be the responsibility of all levels of healthcare in order to increase access for all.

BEST PRACTICES, CHALLENGES, AND OPPORTUNITIES

Virtual group programs. Below are some tips for transforming the two-dimensional video class into a personalized experience that answers your patients' questions, helps them to build new skills, and shows them how to apply the information in their everyday lives.

1. **As in traditional group classes, start out with an introduction to the program.** Remind them about the duration and end time and when they can expect a break. Let them know if there will be handouts or other class materials and how they will receive them—whether through patient portal, email, an online file-sharing service, or mail.
2. **Briefly introduce yourself.** To establish your credibility, include your title and related certifications, as well as your experience with the program. If you have personal experience with the topic, including that information can enhance your credibility and relatability.
3. **Present an outline of the session** so participants will know which topics will be covered. This often reassures them that their questions are on the agenda. If their topic of interest is not listed, they can prepare to ask about it.
4. **Provide a quick tour of the videoconference features** to familiarize them with the basic tools they can use to participate—including the microphone, video, chat function, and gesture signs.

    If the group is large and/or if there is excessive background noise, instruct them to stay muted if they are not speaking. However, encourage them to unmute whenever they have a question or comment. As discussion can enhance learning and allows the group to learn from each other, encourage participation. For those who are uncomfortable speaking to the group, show them how to ask questions using the chat or comment fields.

    Become familiar with how to mute participants or stop their video in case the necessity arises.
5. **Introductions**. If time permits and the class size is appropriate, invite each participant to introduce themselves. If the class is large, invite a few volunteers. Share your screen with a slide of guiding questions:
    1. What is your name?
    2. What would you like to learn?
    3. What is a fun fact about you?
    4. Also include guiding questions that are specific to the class topic. For example, if the class is for patients with kidney disease, you might ask what stage of kidney disease they are in, and whether or not they are on dialysis. Or if they have diabetes, you might ask them to say how long ago they were diagnosed.

By sharing their stories, questions, and some personal information, participants will be reassured that they are not alone. Many people have the same questions, fears. and challenges. Breaking the ice can help establish rapport among participants and with you.

6. **Just as in traditional classes, provide multiple modes of learning** to accommodate different learning styles—e.g., visual, reading, listening, doing, and demonstrations. As discussed in the health literacy chapter, many people learn best when multiple modes are used.

Well-designed *presentation slides* can help illustrate the information you are presenting and are helpful for visual learners. Design your slides with minimal text and large simple graphics. The text and graphics should convey the main message of the slide while you present the details verbally.

Be sure to provide *supplemental materials* that include the same images with more written details for those who learn by reading.

Use *plain language* when you speak and in your education materials.

Images of people should reflect the diversity of your audience to promote inclusivity as well as role modeling. However, take caution not to promote stereotypes in imagery.

Throughout the session, include opportunities for *participation.* Many videoconference platforms allow for *in-session polling* that tabulates the results in real time. For example, you might assess knowledge with a multiple-choice question such as, "Which food is a carbohydrate? (1) carrots, (2) nuts, or (3) yogurt." Or simply include a slide with a question to spur *discussion*. For example, you might ask the group, "What types of physical activity do you enjoy?"

For *hands-on learning*, you can ask participants to use objects in their own home. For example, to teach label reading, ask the participants to get a packaged food from their kitchen. Ask for volunteers to read the serving sizes and relevant nutrition information.

Demonstrations are useful for introducing new tools. For example, share your screen to show them how to use online food trackers, calorie databases, recipe websites, or nutrition calculators. Demonstrations are often eye-opening experiences that leave indelible impressions. For example, some restaurants have nutrition calculators on their websites. Upon building an order—for example, a burrito—the nutrition calculator totals the calories, protein, sodium, and other nutrients with each topping, side, and beverage added. The results often spur lively discussion. Even without a calculator, most restaurants have their nutrition information available online in the form of PDFs. Displaying the file and highlighting popular menu items can be enlightening.

Demonstrations can also be an engaging and entertaining way to get a point across. For example, ask them how many teaspoons they think are in one cup of orange juice, then measure teaspoons of sugar into a glass as you count out loud. Many people will be surprised to hear you count seven teaspoons, and the image of the sugar in the glass will likely be memorable.

Videos can also be a good teaching tool for your visual and auditory learners. You may be able to find short, animated videos online to help illustrate complicated concepts. For example, Monash University has a brief video that demonstrates how FODMAPs affect the GI tract. Videos are also useful for demonstrating physical activity such as walking videos or seated exercises. Be mindful to show activities that are appropriate for your population. Showing videos with people who reflect your audience is helpful for role modeling.

If the time and topic allow, including a three-minute *physical activity* can be useful for building skills and self-efficacy. Including activity also reinforces the importance of minimizing sedentary time and shows ways to get a few minutes of movement throughout the day. Keep the activity simple, short, and safe, such as gentle stretches, marching in place, arm exercises, calf raises and chair squats.

7. **Take breaks if needed.** Depending on the topic and the number of sessions in the program, a session might range from 60 minutes to 2 hours—sometimes longer. If longer than an hour, be sure to incorporate breaks.
8. **At the end of the session, discuss goal setting and action planning.** Provide guidance in developing an action plan, and allow time for the participants to share their plan with the group. Encourage them to write their plan down, which increases their chances of meeting their goal.
9. **As in all classes, invite questions** throughout the session and at the end.

The increasing size of online classes is testament to the reach and satisfaction that virtual care provides. No longer limited by classroom sizes, more people can log in at a time. Thus, more information is distributed to more people. However, whether in person or online, the larger the class, the less personal the experience. Time constraints may prohibit the opportunity for everybody to introduce themselves. Those who are uncomfortable in large group settings are less likely to ask questions or participate in discussion. Also, with more people present, some who want to ask questions may not get the opportunity. Many participants prefer to keep their cameras off and listen passively, making it difficult for the educator to assess their engagement or understanding. In turn, a reduction in feedback from the participants may cause educators to be lax in their own engagement, energy, and effort.

Access to the class materials can be challenging as well. While they can be distributed per patient preference—i.e., digitally versus mail—many programs default to electronic distribution. As such, patients must take the extra step to open emails or log in to file-sharing websites. Many people do not like to read materials on screen and therefore would need to print the materials—an option they either may not have or choose not to do. Those who do not have computers or tablets would be relegated to downloading and reading files on their phone, which would be unappealing to many. Those who were not fully engaged in the class may not seek out the materials afterwards.

Despite some limitations, the demand and cost efficiency of virtual care are apparent. As a result, many programs have been slow to return to in-person classes. Therefore, programs and educators must implement continuous quality improvement to ensure that they are meeting the needs of their population. Staffing must be developed and trained to deliver quality education. Smaller, more frequent class offerings may be needed to enhance personal interactions and improve the individual experience. Individual visits may be needed as an alternative option or for follow-up.

Individual sessions. For individual visits, time is more limited. Just like in-person visits, it's important to identify early which topics should be prioritized. Making the patient comfortable and establishing trust from the beginning will help them open up, reveal their biggest concerns, and let you know what information they need most.

Opening up to a stranger is awkward enough. Opening up through a video camera is even harder. Before drilling the patient with personal questions, build trust by introducing yourself and your experience. Give a brief explanation of what types of information you provide as a nutrition counselor. Perhaps share a little of what you already know about the patient, demonstrating that this experience will be personalized to them.

Once you have introduced yourself, the **SHARE** approach outlined in the first part of this book can similarly guide your virtual session.

S - Start with a blank page.
H - Hear and understand.
A - Assess their learning needs.
R - Review the information they need most.
E - Empower them to develop a plan that is right for them.

Start with a blank page. Once you have established your credibility, ask the patient what they would like to learn during that session. Allowing them to set the agenda results in a more efficient session, and the information you provide will better resonate with them. As discussed in Chapter 2, once you break the ice, the patient will reveal what they need most.

Hear and understand. Allow the patient to speak freely with minimal interruption. Ask clarifying questions that encourage them to share their experience with their condition, such as symptoms, meal planning challenges, or emotional barriers to self-management.

Assess and review. As their story unfolds, assess their learning needs. Listen for what they know, what they want to know, and what they need to know. Then review the information that will be most helpful for that session. An hour is not enough time to provide a comprehensive education, but by addressing their main concerns, the session will be more resonating, relevant, and actionable for the patient. A more positive experience for the patient increases the likelihood that they will schedule another session with you for additional information. In each session, various teaching modes can be applied, similar to those described above for group classes.

The more involved you can make the patient in the learning process—from discussion to engaging visuals to some hands-on demonstrations—the more likely they will retain the information, build skills, increase self-efficacy, and return for more.

Empower. Nutrition counseling and health education have evolved to be more of an exchange of information rather than a didactic experience. After the patient explains their experiences with their disease, the educator provides information about the disease itself. With more information, the patient is empowered to make informed decisions about which self-care actions align with their values and preferences (Funnell and Anderson 2004). The exchange is collaborative between the patient and educator. In addition to providing information, the educator also guides them through the goal setting and action planning process while allowing them to determine what next steps are right for them.

As with in-person care, developing a relationship of trust with the patient will improve their likelihood of following up. Follow-up not only may improve outcomes for the patient, but is also beneficial for your practice. However, not all encounters will be positive. Even if the educator applied the concepts of motivational interviewing, empowerment, and shared decision-making to the best of their abilities, there will always be some patients who are not engaged. The ease of virtual care may increase the number of patients who schedule the appointment simply because their doctor advised them to do so. In the past, if a person was not interested in nutrition counseling, they may have been less likely to schedule the appointment due to time or travel requirements. As those barriers are minimized, many will log in to please their doctor. However, the SHARE approach can still be applied in these cases. Through a patient-centered approach, some may even be converted during the visit. It is not uncommon for a patient to respond, "I wasn't going to come today, but I'm glad I did!" While not all will be responsive, providing a personalized education may still leave an impression. While they may not agree to follow up, they may remember you later when they become ready for change.

As more people become comfortable with the technology, telehealth has increased the patient load for many providers. As mentioned earlier, back-to-back patients require the provider to more efficiently focus on the visit. Increased follow-up visits, however, further fill up the schedule. Whether in-person or by video, patients are encountering longer wait times for appointments.

Providers, in turn, are feeling more overwhelmed with increased patient loads. Healthcare burnout is an increasing concern. This need may allow for increased staffing, but ramping up takes time. While organizations must prioritize the well-being of their staff, individuals must be engaged in their own self-care and mental health. Mindfulness strategies that enhance a provider's sense of professional purpose can help mitigate the stress. For many, seeking the support of a mental health professional would be beneficial.

As with all advances in technology, there is a learning curve. Organizations are learning how to develop virtual programs. Providers are learning how to deliver effective care online. Together, they must ensure that resources, professional development, and support are available to ensure a quality experience for everyone.

Telehealth had been working its way into the healthcare system even before the COVID-19 crisis. Online lifestyle change programs have long employed webinars, email coaching, and motivational text messages. However, insurance coverage and privacy policies dictated careful implementation in the clinic setting. While the pandemic required lightning-speed adoption, virtual health care is now here to stay. As educators, we will continue to develop new strategies for delivering information in creative and meaningful ways. But if there is one guiding principle that will stand the test of time, it's this one: Listen. Your patients will tell you what they need.

REFERENCES

Camporeale J. Teaching an Insulin-Dependent Blind Patient about Self-Care. *Home Healthc Nurse.* 2001 Apr;19(4):247–50. doi: 10.1097/00004045-200104000-00016.

Chu C, Nayyar D, Bhattacharyya O, Martin D, Agarwal P, Mukerji G. Patient and Provider Experiences with Virtual Care in a Large, Ambulatory Care Hospital in Ontario, Canada During the COVID-19 Pandemic: Observational Study. *J Med Internet Res.* 2022 Oct;24(10):e38604. doi: 10.2196/38604.

Dhawan N, Carnes M, Byars-Winston A, Duma N. Videoconferencing Etiquette: Promoting Gender Equity during Virtual Meetings. *J Womens Health (Larchmt).* 2021 Apr;30(4):460–465. doi: 10.1089/jwh.2020.8881.

Donelan K, Barreto EA, Sossong S, Michael C, Estrada JJ, Cohen AB, Wozniak J, Schwamm LH. Patient and Clinician Experiences with Telehealth for Patient Follow-up Care. *Am J Manag Care.* 2019 Jan;25(1):40–44.

Funnell MM, Anderson RM. Empowerment and Self-Management of Diabetes. *Clin Diabetes.* 2004;22(3):123–127.

U.S. Department of Health & Human Services Office for Civil Rights. *Privacy, Security, and Electronic Health Records* [Internet]. Washington, DC: U.S. Department of Health and Human Services; 2022 [cited 30 June 2023]. Available from: https://www.hhs.gov/sites/default/files/ocr/privacy/hipaa/understanding/consumers/privacy-security-electronic-records.pdf.

18 Making PLANS and Taking Action

I originally became a dietitian to help people enjoy food. Whether they had food allergies, weight loss goals, or metabolic conditions, I wanted to share my experience in learning how to cook, substitute ingredients, and overall live healthfully. The more I learned about how food affects the body, the more motivated I became to eat more vegetables, choose leaner proteins, limit processed foods, and all those other phrases that dietitians say daily. I thought that surely if I shared this knowledge with other people, they too would be able to make lifestyle changes. After all, who would want saturated fat if it drives up their cholesterol levels? Or sodium if it increases blood pressure? Or sugary soda if it causes insulin and blood sugar to spike?

I quickly learned, however, that knowledge alone was not a motivator. For me, I had several underlying reasons to care about what I ate and what I served my family. My children's food allergies were an easy motivator to avoid certain ingredients. My husband's food intolerances were another. For myself, my father's diabetes, coronary artery disease, kidney failure, and early death certainly impacted me, along with my own struggles with body image. For me, as for others, knowledge merely informed me of what I had to do. *Wanting* to do it came from a deeper place. I do it for the love I have for my family. For my desire to stay strong. For my hopes to live long and enjoy as much as I can.

One particular memory comes to mind that embodies my long-term vision for myself. My husband and I were hiking in Red Rock Canyon in Las Vegas. We had climbed up onto a large rock to enjoy the view. While we were up there, an older man also climbed up and joined us. We chatted for a while, and he told us that he belonged to a hiking club. He and his wife were retired and hiked several times a week. He detailed some of the other places they had visited. He talked about his kids and his grandkids, and the trips they have taken together. Needless to say, he appeared fit and healthy, and most of all, happy.

When I think of my own future, I remember this man. I also remember the dietitian who taught my first nutrition class in college, who said, "What kind of old person do you want to be?" For me, these words resonated. After watching my father slowly deteriorate until his death, I know how debilitating disease can be. I remember the difficulty he had walking on our outings. I remember when he became homebound. I remember the dialysis, the signs of malnutrition, and the last day. Consequently, my motivation to live healthfully comes not from knowledge, but from personal experience.

Personal experience will be a factor for each individual you encounter–experiences that have affected them in the past as well as those they want for the future. The source of motivation will be different for each individual. For patients who feel the immediate effects that diet has on their health—whether in GI symptoms or allergic reactions or other symptoms—those experiences may drive them to make changes. For others like myself, memories of family members who struggled with disease may motivate them. A desire to live for kids or grandkids is another commonly reported motivation. However, motivation is neither a given nor an obligation. There will be some who are not willing to change anything, regardless of their symptoms or risks.

DOI: 10.1201/9781003326038-22

Nutrition counselors use motivational interviewing in hopes of drawing out their patient's intrinsic drive to manage their health. We hope to provide education in a way that is understandable enough to be actionable. We aim to clear the path for them to move forward toward their goals.

What we cannot do, however, is set those goals for them. With nutrition counseling, identifying behaviors to change is the easy part for the dietitian. If a patient is experiencing symptoms or has abnormal lab values, you will often find something in their diet or lifestyle that needs addressing. Even those following a generally healthy diet may not be aware of specific guidelines for their individual condition. Not all tenets of healthy eating apply to all conditions. For example, a patient with IBS may not be aware of FODMAPS, which can be high in some legumes, which are often recommended as an excellent source of fiber and plant protein. Or a patient with gastroparesis may not realize that a high fiber, vegetable salad can actually worsen their symptoms. Or for someone with defective lipoprotein lipase activity, even healthy fats may be problematic and elevate triglyceride levels. And of course, there are nutrition misconceptions, where people think they are eating healthfully but may in fact be putting themselves at risk. For example, a person with reactive hypoglycemia may have been told to "avoid carbohydrates," only to be frequently reaching for glucose tablets to get their blood sugar back up.

Wherever your patient lies on the readiness scale, the SHARE approach ensures that you understand their viewpoint, and that you have provided information that is relevant to them. Once they are empowered with information, the final step in the session would be to make a plan, even if the plan is not to change anything at all.

MAKING PLANS

PLANS should incorporate the following:

  P – Patient preferences.
  L – Labs, symptoms, and medical history.
  A – Attitude, feelings, and personal goals.
  N – Nutrition-related behaviors.
  S – Strategies for long-term change.

Patient preferences. During your nutrition assessment, you will learn what foods they enjoy, whether or not they like to cook, what lifestyle change strategies they have tried in the past, and what types of physical activity they do. For meal planning, most people can identify a variety of lean proteins, vegetables, starches, and fruits that they enjoy. Use those foods when describing sample meals. For example, if a patient mentioned pork in their dietary recall, include pork loin chops or tenderloin in a sample dinner. Or pull up a recipe website and search for pork recipes. If they dine out frequently, pull up the websites of their favorite restaurants and explore the menu for healthier choices. If they rely on frozen or prepared meals, search products online to demonstrate how to read nutrition labels for good choices.

Labs, symptoms, and medical history. Review relevant lab results with them. Describe what the labs measure and define the lab goals. Provide an overview of the specific nutrition guidelines for their diagnosis. During your education, explain how certain foods in their diet are affecting their lab values or symptoms. For example, if someone has hyperkalemia but they frequently consume sports drinks, search for the nutrition label online to demonstrate its potassium content.

Attitude, feelings, and goals. Throughout your interaction with a patient, they may indicate through their words, body language, or behavior how they feel about making change. Some will appear very engaged and eager. Others may appear ambivalent. Some may arrive angry about their diagnosis or past experiences with other health care providers. In each of these cases, be sure to acknowledge their experiences and communicate compassion. Acknowledging their feelings can go a long way in how they react to you and your education. When it comes to making a plan, their feelings will determine how much change they are ready and willing to make. For the counselor, resist the temptation to push an additional goal or a more aggressive change. Allowing the patient their autonomy will reinforce that they are ultimately responsible for their own self-care. While you may fear that they are not planning enough change, rest assured that if they decide to engage in one change, they are likely to make additional changes as well, even if they did not mention it in your visit. Time and again, I have seen patients leave with a physical activity goal, then return with an improved diet as well. However, the opposite is also true. Some who appear highly motivated and eager to change sometimes return with little to report or do not return at all.

Beware of implicit bias. You can never truly know what is on someone's mind when they speak to you, or what will happen after they leave. What you can ensure, however, is that you answer the questions they have, provide information they need, and are available for ongoing support if they want.

Nutrition-related behaviors. During the nutrition assessment, you may have picked up on recurring nutrition-related behaviors that are prohibiting them from achieving their goals. As discussed in Part 2 of this book, examples of everyday eating routines include night snacking, frequent dining out, fad dieting, and others. Highlight how these behaviors may relate to their nutrition concerns, and which factors may be reinforcing the behaviors. For example, the person who is starving by dinner and consequently overeats at night may not realize that skipping meals during the day exacerbates his hunger. With this knowledge, he may be reassured that there is an actionable solution such as including a balanced lunch, rather than simply struggling with restraint and willpower at night.

Strategies for long-term change. Goal setting, incremental changes, and self-monitoring are evidence-based strategies for long-term lifestyle change (Samdal et al. 2017). Long-term goal setting may help a patient envision their future and draw out their intrinsic motivation for change. Short-term, achievable goals for incremental change are more actionable and can help build self-efficacy in adopting new behaviors. Self-monitoring increases awareness and provides feedback that the changes they are making are effective. Depending on their condition, examples of self-monitoring include blood sugar logs, blood pressure records, food/symptom/feeling diaries, weight records, physical activity logs, or a medication log. In addition to behavior modification, establishing a network of support that includes family, friends, peers, community programs, online resources, and the appropriate professional support may also make long-term change more achievable.

TURNING PLANS INTO ACTION

In nutrition counseling, assisting the patient in making informed PLANS is the ultimate goal of the session. Through careful listening, clear communication, and objective guidance, patients leave with a greater awareness of their everyday eating routines, and how they can improve their health. By personalizing the education, they can identify actionable, incremental changes that are specific to them.

However, upon leaving the session, the patient is faced with putting their plan into action. For that, more information may be needed. Ideally, the patient will have learned the basics of balanced meal planning during the session and will be able to apply those concepts to their own food preferences. However, patients often request more ideas. For example, someone may have a goal of including a balanced breakfast. Breakfast, however, can be a challenging meal to plan. On many days, people are rushing out the door to get to school or work. Or people have difficulty thinking beyond oatmeal, cereal, or eggs and bacon. Providing balanced breakfast ideas helps to further translate general concepts into actionable steps. By seeing different ways that nutrition guidelines are applied, people may be able to generate more ideas of their own.

While there may be time to develop some sample meals and snacks, a counseling session typically does not include enough time to develop a full, personalized meal plan. For more ideas, recipe websites are one tool you can recommend. However, that does require the patient to take extra steps to remember the website, log on, and search for their specific interests. Recipe books are another tool but can be a cost to the patient. Oftentimes, patients can incorporate the foods and recipes they already enjoy into a healthy meal plan, but need guidance on how to properly balance their meals. Providing handouts for their specific questions can give them tangible references that they can easily look at later and can help them remember the key messages of the education. Handouts are also helpful for those who do not regularly use the Internet.

I have found that there are certain questions that patients frequently ask. Having ready-to-go materials for these FAQs allows you to quickly provide a thorough answer. This book includes supplemental materials that can be used to answer these questions, plus other tools for nutrition counseling and education. The materials are available online. They include printable handouts, as well as downloadable presentation slides that can be used in group or individual sessions, in person or online. Also included are counseling worksheets for goal setting, action planning, and food tracking.

Handouts for FAQs

1. What can I have for breakfast?
2. What can I have for snacks?
3. How much protein do I need?
4. How can I find time to cook?
5. How can I eat healthy on a budget?

Educational Slides

1. Prediabetes and Type 2 Diabetes
2. Nutrition and Heart Health
3. Protecting Your Kidneys
4. IBS and the Low FODMAP diet
5. Nutrition and Weight Management

Counseling Handouts

1. Goal setting and action planning worksheet
2. Tips for successful food and physical activity tracking

To access these handouts, https://resourcecentre.routledge.com/books/9781032352459

Over time, you will pick up on other frequently asked questions for your specialty. You may need to develop your own educational materials. Refer to the chapter on health literacy for tips on writing and designing health communications.

Patient education materials, recipes, and articles are also available online from various organizations such as the USDA Food and Nutrition Service, Academy of Nutrition and Dietetics, the American Heart Association, the American Diabetes Association, and other professional societies. Key organizations and resources for the conditions covered in this book are listed in their respective chapters in Part 3.

You will also learn a lot from your patients. They will tell you about various diets, programs, supplements, meal services, cookbooks, or websites that they have used. While some may not be valid, or may be unsafe, others may be useful to add to your toolkit. For example, many meal delivery kits use fresh, healthy ingredients. Similarly, many weight loss programs or apps promote portion control, healthy choices, and mindfulness. Patients often find healthful products with minimal additives that are quick and convenient. Or they may share tips for how they make time for meal planning, physical activity, or other healthy strategies.

Nutrition education and counseling is a bi-directional learning experience. The provider and patient share information and stories, and they learn from each other. With every patient, you will gain insight into both the struggles and successes that are possible with disease management. As your expertise grows, so will your toolkit.

Over time, nutrition guidelines will fluctuate. Popular diets will come and go. Your patients will continue to question what works, what does not, and what is right for them. They will come to you looking for answers. The crux of their questions will be, "What can I eat?"

While research will continue to uncover new information, the source for the answer will remain the same: the patients themselves. While nutrition guidelines specify how food affects health, the patient will tell you how their lives affect their food choices. Through mindful listening, clarifying questions, and careful review of their medical history, you will home in on recommendations that are specific to them. As an educator, you will consider their learning style. As a communicator, you will consider which messages will resonate most. And as a counselor, you will guide them through the behavior change process.

In other words, you will think like a dietitian.

REFERENCE

Samdal GB, Eide GE, Barth T, Williams G, Meland E. Effective Behaviour Change Techniques for Physical Activity and Healthy Eating in Overweight and Obese Adults; Systematic Review and Meta-Regression Analyses. *Int J Behav Nutr Phys Act.* 2017 Mar;14(1):42.

Index

Note: **Bold** page numbers refer to tables; *italic* page numbers refer to figures.

A1C 75, 77, 79–80, 83, 88, 90, 130–131
abdominal obesity 89
Academy of Nutrition and Dietetics 15, 58, 210
"a calorie is a calorie," concept of 158
action planning 36–41
active listening 4, 15, 17, 19–20
AHA *see* American Heart Association
allergy-friendly foods 15
American College of Cardiology 94, 108
American College of Gastroenterology 70, 137
American College of Gastroenterology Clinical
    Guidelines 149
American Diabetes Association 75, 184, 210
American Heart Association (AHA) 94, 103, 108,
    184, 210
anorexia nervosa (AN) 57, 58
autonomy 37, 39

barriers 45–46, 48
BC-ADM *see* Board Certified in Advanced Diabetes
    Management
binge eating disorder (BED) 57, 58
blood sugar 8, 29, 41, 47, 51, 57, 60, 72–75, 79–83, 88, 91,
    131, 168
BMI *see* body mass index
BN *see* bulimia nervosa
Board Certified in Advanced Diabetes Management
    (BC-ADM) 74
body mass index (BMI) 151
body positivity movement 151, 152
bulimia nervosa (BN) 58

carb counting 77, 79
carbohydrate metabolism 81–83
CDC *see* Centers for Disease Control and Prevention
CDC Clear Communication Guide 186
CDCES *see* Certified Diabetes Care and Education
    Specialist
CEDRD *see* Certified Eating Disorders Registered
    Dietitian credential
Celiac Disease 8, 139, 143
Centers for Disease Control and Prevention (CDC)
    155, 165
Certified Diabetes Care and Education Specialist
    (CDCES) 74
Certified Eating Disorders Registered Dietitian credential
    (CEDRD) 58
chasing hunger 56–57
chronic kidney disease (CKD) 114, 115, 122–135
    7-point subjective global assessment 125, **126–127**
    balanced diets for 125, 127, *129,* **133–134**
    comorbidities 125
    food additives 127, **128**

improving function 128–129
nutritional management for 131–132
potassium and phosphorus levels 125, **126,** 127–128,
    129, 132, 134
reduced appetite and malnutrition 125
related with diabetes and heart health 129–131, *130, 132*
role of kidneys 129–130
stages **124,** 124–125
CKD *see* chronic kidney disease
Commission on Dietetic Registration 138, 153
common eating patterns *see* eating patterns
communication skills 16, 179
community-supported agriculture (CSA) programs 111
compassion 15, 17–20, 23, 80, 81, 151, 153, 164, 182, 199,
    200, 209
cooking skills 61
corticosteroids 155
counter-stereotypic imaging 24
countertransference 20–21
COVID-19 pandemic 61, 194, 198, 206
CSA *see* community-supported agriculture programs
cultural competence 192–197
    cultural significance of food 195
    cultural values 197
    definition 192–193
    food cultures 194
    healthcare disparity 194
    history of food 195–196
    implicit bias 193–194
    SHARE process 196

DASH diet *see* Dietary Approaches to Stop
    Hypertension diet
dawn phenomenon 55
DGA *see* Dietary Guidelines for Americans
diabetes 69
    assessment 74–75
    basic carbohydrate metabolism 82–83, *83*
    carbohydrate metabolism with 82–83
    dietary pattern 75–80
    insulin resistance (*see* insulin resistance)
    managing without medication 80
    meal planning for 90–91
    Plate Method *77,* 77–78
    prediabetes and diabetes 81–82
    progressive nature of diabetes 83
Diabetes Prevention Program 45, 90, 170, 188
diabetic ketoacidosis 55
dialysis 124–125, 128
Dietary Approach to Stop Hypertension (DASH) diet 7,
    50, 75, 78, *79,* 94, 108–110, 115–116, *117*
Dietary Guidelines Advisory Committee 116
Dietary Guidelines for Americans (DGA) 77, 78, 116, 143

dietary recall 12–14, 48, 51, 54, 141, 167
diet culture 56, 163, 167, 194
digital divide 180, 199
dyslipidemia 95–99

eating disorders 50, 57–58, 141, 156–157
eating patterns 50–64
    "all or nothing" mentality 59
    eating out 60–61
    emotional eating 57–58
    factors affecting 46
    grazing 59–60
    habit cycling 61–63, *62*
    Intermittent Fasting (IF) 54–55
    Ketogenic Diet (KD) 54–55
    multifactorial pattern 63–64
    nighttime eating 50–51, **51–53**
    skipping meals 51, 54
    squeezing calories and chasing hunger 56–57
EBM *see* evidence-based medicine
EER *see* estimated energy requirements; everyday eating
    routine (EER)
eGFR *see* estimated glomeruler filtration rate
80/20 rule 33, *100*
electrolytes 115, 124
emotional eating 47–48, 50, 57–58, 60, 161, 164
emotional sensitivity 16
emotions 16, 25
empathy 15–20, 23, 56, 182, 197, 199, 200
empowerment 4, 35–41, 51, 90, 179, 182, 199, 205
estimated energy requirements (EER) 47–49, 159
estimated glomeruler filtration rate (eGFR) 129
everyday eating routine (EER) 48–49
evidence-based medicine (EBM) 35

FDA *see* Food and Drug Administration
Feeding America 157
fitness culture 194
FODMAP Friendly 138, 144
FODMAP(s) 203
    definition 142–143
    elimination approach 50
    high and low FODMAP foods 141, 143–147, *144*
    trial 11, 139
food allergies 7, 15, 17, 207
Food and Drug Administration (FDA) 103, 148, 155
Food Insecurity Screening Toolkit 157

gastric emptying 50, 168
gastrointestinal (GI) issues 7, 70, 80, 137, 139, 140, 148
GLP-1 agonists 155
gluconeogenesis 55
glucose 29, 35, 41, 50, 54, 72, 75, 78, 81, 82, 168
gluten 137, 143
gluten-free diet 47, 137
goal setting 36–41, 45, 170, 186, 188, 204, 205, 209, 210
Good and Cheap: Eat Well on $4/Day (Brown) 157, 158
grazing 59–60
grehlin 54

HBM *see* Health Belief Model
HDL 105

Health at Every Size® 151
health behavior 15–17, 38, 45, 48, 151, 152, 183, 192
    theory 16
Health Belief Model (HBM) 45–46
health communications 6, 185, *187,* 189, 210
health education 16, 169, 181, 185, 186, 205
health literacy 33, 34, 179–189, 205
    definition 179
    demonstrations and hands-on activities 186
    discussion and verbal explanation 181–182
    group classes *vs.* individual counseling 186, 188
    handouts, brochures and printed materials
        185–186, *187*
    image licenses and copyright 183, **183–184**
    learning and teaching styles 180–181
    learning styles and barriers 180
    retention and return visits 188–189
    storytelling 182
    tailoring session 180
    visual aids 183–185
Health Literate Care Model 179
healthy eating 6, 30, 32, 47, 48, 56, 75, 79, 88
healthy fat 7, 30, 45, 50, 56, 77, 78, 98, 100, 102
Healthy People 2030 initiative 179
heart disease prevention and management 69, 77,
    94–118
    bad and good fats 100–102
    causes of high LDL 105–106
    dyslipidemia 95–99
    eating pattern 100
    egg consumption 103–104
    hypertension (*see* hypertension)
    lipid values 105, 107
    lowering LDL levels 99–100, *101*
    omega-3 supplementation 103
    raising good cholesterol 105
    triglycerides 106, *107*
    ultra-processed and restaurant foods **103**
    ultra-processed foods 95–99
heart health 50, 107, 115, 122, 124, 129–131, *130, 132*
heart healthy diet 88, 94, 97, 98, 105, 118
hemodialysis 125
hunger hormones 51, 54, *160*
hydration 8
hypercholesterolemia 96
hyperglycemia 55
    risk factors for **76**
hyperglycemic rebounds 55
hyperkalemia 130–132
hyperlipidemia 8, 30
hyperphosphatemia 131
hypertension 108–118
    assessment 110
    categories **115**
    coffee 113
    dairy alternatives 112
    diet and lifestyle modification 109–110, 116, **117,** 118
    potassium, calcium, and magnesium in 116
    risk for complications *114,* 114–115
    sodium 115
hypoglycemia 55, 74, 91, 131
    risk factors for **76**

iaedp *see* International Association of Eating Disorders
Professionals
IBS *see* irritable bowel syndrome
IF *see* Intermittent Fasting
implicit bias 4, 21–24, 193–194, 199,
200, 209
individuation 24
insulin 55, 81–83, 168
insulin resistance 81–83, *86*, 130, 164, 168
causes 86
improving 90–91
physical activity 87–88, *88*
saturated fat 88–89, *89*
weight loss 90
insulin-to-carb ratio regimen 73, 77
insurance coverage 164, 186, 201, 206
Intermittent Fasting (IF) 47, 51, 54–55
International Association of Eating Disorders
Professionals (iaedp) 58
International Foundation for Gastrointestinal
Disorders 148
intuitive eating 168
irritable bowel syndrome (IBS) 70, 137–149
assessment 139–141
benefits of physical activity 148
classification 140–141
diagnostic criteria 140–141
dining out tips 148
eating disorders 141
exacerbating foods and lifestyle habits 141
fiber supplements 147
FODMAPs, definition 142–143
GI symptoms 139
gluten intolerance 143
low FODMAP diet 138, 141, 143–147
natural laxatives 148
packaged foods 148
pharmacological therapy 148–149
stress and anxiety 141
symptoms 140
vitamin and mineral supplements for 148

KD *see* Ketogenic Diet
*KDOQI Clinical Practice Guidelines for Nutrition in
CKD: 2020 Update* 124, 125
ketogenesis 55
Ketogenic Diet (KD) 47, 54–55, 60, 158

Latent Autoimmune Diabetes in Adults (LADA) 73
LDL-cholesterol 88, 99, 100, 101, 103
leptin 54
lifestyle
change 3, 6, 14, 25, 30, 33, 36, 45, 46
counseling 13, 30
factors 108
listening and acknowledging 24–25
long-term goal 38, 170, 171
low carb diets 47

Mature Onset Diabetes of the Young (MODY) 73
meal skipping 51, 54
medical nutrition therapy 3, 6, 7, 57, 73, 94, 109, 125, 154

Mediterranean Diet 30, 50, 75–76, 78, *79,* 94, 102,
106–108, 122, 124, 195
methylcellulose 147
Mifflin-St. Jeor calculator 48, 160
mindful listening 19–20
mindfulness 18–19, 23, 56, 80, 165
Mindfulness-Based Stress Reduction program 20
MODY *see* Mature Onset Diabetes of the Young
Monash Low FODMAP app 144, 148
Monash University 138, 147, 148, 149, 203
motivational interviewing 15, 37, 41, 208
motivations 45–46
MyPlate 77, 78, *78,* 143

National Center for Education Statistics 179
National Center for Health Statistics 165
National Diabetes Prevention Program 56
National Health and Nutrition Survey 116, 152
National Health Interview Survey (2018) 165
National Heart, Lung and Blood Institute 94
National Institute of Mental Health 58
National Kidney Foundation 184
National Weight Control Registry (NWCR) 165, 166, 169
NCGS *see* Non-Celiac Gluten Sensitivity
night cravings 50, 51, **52–53**
nighttime eating 50–51, **51–53**
Non-Celiac Gluten Sensitivity (NCGS) 143
NOVA Classification of foods 95
nutrient deficiencies 13, 15
nutrition assessments 3, 7–9, 29, 31, 33, 49, 51, 137, 139,
141, 157, 168, 169, 208, 209
nutrition care process 4, 7
nutrition counseling 4, 7, 9–10, 15–17, 21, 45, 46, 70,
205, 208
assumptions and consequences in **22**
nutrition science knowledge 16
NWCR *see* National Weight Control Registry

obesity 8, 29, 54, 58, 70, 151–153
omega-3 fats 102, 103
omega-3 supplementation 102
"Online FODMAP and IBS Training for Dietitians"
138, 149

packaged foods 47, 89, 96
Paleo Diet 47, 100
partial meal replacement (PMR) 29
patient-centered approach 21, 70
patient-centered care 15–17, 19, 28, 54, 193
patient-dietitian relationship 15–16
people with diabetes (PWD) 55, 77, 103
peritoneal dialysis 125
personal distress 18
person-centered care 4, 9, 199–200
perspective taking 18, 24
philosophy of patient empowerment 35
physical activity 7, 35, 37, 39, 74, 80, 84, 87–88, *88,* 97,
110, 148, 165–166, *166,* 203
The Physical Activity Guidelines for Americans 87
*The Physical Activity Guidelines for Americans, 2nd
Edition* 165
physiological causes 50

Plain Language Action and Information Network 181

PLANS 208–209

    attitude, feelings, and goals 208–209

    labs, symptoms, and medical history 208

    nutrition-related behaviors 209

    patient preferences 208

    strategies for long-term change 209

plant foods 29, 72, 78, 82, 94, 95, 97, 98, 107, 122, 127, 161

Plate Method 56, *77*, 77–81, 90, 91, 143, 161–163, 167, 168

PMR *see* partial meal replacement

post-bariatric hypoglycemia 11

post-kidney transplantation 124

postprandial hyperglycemia 91

post-transplant diabetes 73

prediabetes 72, 73, 80–82

probiotics 147–148

problem solving 36–41, 63

Project Implicit® 21–22

psyllium husk 147

PWD *see* people with diabetes (PWD)

RDNs *see* registered dietitian nutritionists

referrals to dietitian 69–71, **70**

refined carbohydrates 89, 90, 97, 168

refined sugars 81

registered dietitian nutritionists (RDNs) 12, 16, 21, 49, 54, 55, 137

saturated fat 88–89, *89*, 96, 97, 100, 101, 103, 105, *106*

SCOFF questionnaire 58, **58**

self-awareness 4, 21

self-care 3, 20, 25

Self-Determination Theory 37

self-efficacy 37, 39, 40, 46, 170, 203

self-management 16, 75

SGLT-2 inhibitors 55

Share, Hear, Assess, Review and Empower (SHARE) approach 4, 36, 37, 40, 196, 204, 208

shared decision-making 35

short-term goal 38

SNAP *see* USDA Supplemental Nutrition Assistance Program

stereotype replacement 24

steroid-induced diabetes 73

stress eaters/eating 57, 60

stress management 20, 57

stroke 115

sugar-free beverages 80

sugary beverages 80

telehealth 16, 185, 201, 205, 206

time management 7, 13

transference 20

Transtheoretical Model of Change 36

triglycerides 106, *107*

2017 Scope of Practice document 16

type 1 diabetes 29, 73

type 2 diabetes 72, 73, 75, 77, 81–84, 86, *87*, 90

typical American diet 89, 95, 106, 107, 115

ultra-processed foods 29, 47, 73, 79, 89, 95–99, 106, 122

United States Department of Agriculture Economic Research Service 61

University of Michigan 138

USDA Food and Nutrition Service 6, 210

USDA Supplemental Nutrition Assistance Program (SNAP) 157

U.S. Department of Health and Human Services 165

videoconferencing 199, 200, 202, 203

virtual health care 198–206

    access and health disparity 201–202

    compassion 200

    demonstrations 203

    empathy 200

    hands-on learning 203

    individual sessions 204

    in-session polling 203

    learning needs and follow-up 201

    person-centered care 199–200

    physical activity 203

    plain language and images of people 203

    presentation slides and supplemental materials 203

    SHARE approach 204–205

    size of online classes 204

    time management 200–201

    videos 203

    virtual group programs 202–206

weight counseling 70, 151–172

    balanced meals using Plate Method 161, *162,* 163

    basic metabolism 167

    behavior change techniques 170

    benefits of protein 163

    counting calories in 152–153, 158–161, *159*

    diet modification 169

    diets to lose weight 158

    eating disorders 156–157

    factors causing unintentional weight gain 154–155

    genetic disorders 155

    glucose and insulin 168

    handling weight loss plateau 171

    long-term weight loss 168–169

    macronutrients 167–168

    managing sugar cravings 163–164

    medications and nutrition 155

    menus and recipe ideas 167

    mindful eating 165, 170

    physical activity 165–166, *166,* 169

    self-monitoring 170

    setting long-term goals 170

    socioeconomic barriers 157–158

    timing of meals 168

    tracking weight 169

    weight loss medications 155

    weight loss strategies 156

weight loss 29–30, 90, 151

    medications 155

    strategies 156

weight management 70, 71, 90, 152

yo-yo dieting 55, 153

For Product Safety Concerns and Information please contact our EU
representative GPSR@taylorandfrancis.com
Taylor & Francis Verlag GmbH, Kaufingerstraße 24, 80331 München, Germany

www.ingramcontent.com/pod-product-compliance
Ingram Content Group UK Ltd.
Pitfield, Milton Keynes, MK11 3LW, UK
UKHW050931180425
457613UK00015B/358